ELECTRONIC HEALTH RECORDS

Challenges in Design and Implementation

ELECTRONIC HEALTH RECORDS
Challenges in Design and Implementation

Edited by
Dean F. Sittig, PhD

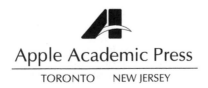

Apple Academic Press

TORONTO   NEW JERSEY

Apple Academic Press Inc. | Apple Academic Press Inc.
3333 Mistwell Crescent | 9 Spinnaker Way
Oakville, ON L6L 0A2 | Waretown, NJ 08758
Canada | USA

©2014 by Apple Academic Press, Inc.

First issued in paperback 2021

Exclusive worldwide distribution by CRC Press, a member of Taylor & Francis Group
No claim to original U.S. Government works

ISBN 13: 978-1-77463-311-3 (pbk)
ISBN 13: 978-1-926895-93-2 (hbk)

Library of Congress Control Number: 2013948330

Library and Archives Canada Cataloguing in Publication

Electronic health records: challenges in design and implementation/edited by
Dean F. Sittig, PhD.

Chapters in this book were previously published in various formats and in various places.
Includes bibliographical references and index.
ISBN 978-1-926895-93-2
1. Medical records--Data processing. 2. Medical records--Data processing--Safety measures. 3. Clinical medicine--Decision making--Data processing. 4. Health services administration--Data processing. I. Sittig, Dean F., author, writer of introduction, editor of compilation

R858.E44 2013   610.285   C2013-905900-8

Apple Academic Press also publishes its books in a variety of electronic formats. Some content that appears in print may not be available in electronic format. For information about Apple Academic Press products, visit our website at **www.appleacademicpress.com** and the CRC Press website at **www.crcpress.com**

ABOUT THE EDITOR

DEAN F. SITTIG, PhD

Dean F. Sittig, PhD, is a Professor at the School of Biomedical Informatics at The University of Texas Health Science Center at Houston and a member of the UT Houston-Memorial Hermann Center for Healthcare Quality and Safety. Dr. Sittig's research interests center on the design, development, implementation, and evaluation of all aspects of clinical information systems. In addition to Dr. Sittig's work on measuring the impact of clinical information systems on a large scale, he is working to improve our understanding of both the factors that lead to success, as well as the unintended consequences associated with computer-based clinical decision support and provider order entry systems.

CONTENTS

ACKNOWLEDGMENT AND HOW TO CITE

The chapters in this book were previously published in various places and in various formats. By bringing them together here in one place, we offer the reader a comprehensive perspective on recent investigations of electronic health records. Each chapter is added to and enriched by being placed within the context of the larger investigative landscape.

We wish to thank the authors who made their research available for this book, whether by granting their permission individually or by releasing their research as Open Source articles. When citing information contained within this book, please do the authors the courtesy of attributing them by name, referring back to their original articles, using the credits provided at the end of each chapter.

LIST OF CONTRIBUTORS

Patricia Abbott
Johns Hopkins University

Joan S. Ash
Department of Medical Informatics and Clinical Epidemiology, Oregon Health & Science University, Mail Code: BICC, 3181 SW Sam Jackson Park Road, Portland, OR 97239-3098, USA

David W. Bates
Department of Medicine, Brigham and Women's Hospital, Harvard Medical School, Boston, Massachusetts, USA, The Department of Health Policy and Management, Harvard School of Public Health, Boston, Massachusetts, USA

Elmer Victor Bernstam
School of Biomedical Informatics, The University of Texas Health Science Center at Houston (UTHealth), Houston, Texas, USA, Department of Internal Medicine, Medical School, The University of Texas Health Science Center at Houston (UTHealth), Houston, Texas, USA

David Brick
NYU Langone Medical Center

Arwen Bunce
Oregon Health & Science University, Portland, OR, USA

Emily M. Campbell
Department of Medical Informatics and Clinical Epidemiology, Oregon Health & Science University, Mail Code: BICC, 3181 SW Sam Jackson Park Road, Portland, OR 97239-3098, USA

James D. Carpenter
Providence Health & Services, Portland, OR, USA

Kathrin M. Cresswell
The School of Health in Social Science, The University of Edinburgh, Edinburgh, UK

Richard H. Dykstra
Department of Medical Informatics and Clinical Epidemiology, Oregon Health & Science University, Mail Code: BICC, 3181 SW Sam Jackson Park Road, Portland, OR 97239-3098, USA

Adol Esquivel
Department of Clinical Effectiveness and Performance Measurement, St. Luke's Episcopal Health System, Houston, TX

Donna Espadas
The Center of Inquiry to Improve Outpatient Safety Through Effective Electronic Communication and the Houston VA HSR&D Center of Excellence at the Michael E DeBakey Veterans Affairs Medical Center, VA Medical Center (152) 2002 Holcombe Blvd, Houston, TX 77030, USA

Joshua C. Feblowitz
Brigham & Women's Hospital, Boston, MA, USA, Partners HealthCare, Boston, MA, USA

Greg Fraser
Mid-valley Independent Physicians Association, Salem, Oregon, USA

Tejal Gandhi
Division of General Medicine, Department of Medicine, Partners Healthcare Systems and Harvard Medical School, Boston, Massachusetts

Michael C. Gibbons
Johns Hopkins University

Kenneth P. Guappone
Department of Medical Informatics and Clinical Epidemiology, Oregon Health & Science University, Mail Code: BICC, 3181 SW Sam Jackson Park Road, Portland, OR 97239-3098, USA, Providence Portland Medical Center, Portland, OR, USA

Michael G. Kahn
Department of Pediatrics, University of Colorado Denver, Aurora, Colorado, USA

Kanav Kahol
Public Health Foundation of India, New Delhi, India

Ramin Khorasani
Division of General Medicine, Department of Radiology, Partners Healthcare Systems and Harvard Medical School, Boston, Massachusetts

Anne Kittler
Partners HealthCare Information Systems, Clinical and Quality Analysis, Partners Healthcare Systems and Harvard Medical School, Boston, Massachusetts

Michael A. Krall
Kaiser Permanente Northwest, Portland, OR, USA

Gilad J. Kuperman
Division of General Medicine, Department of Medicine and Clinical Informatics Research and Development, Partners Healthcare Systems and Harvard Medical School, Boston, Massachusetts

Svetlana Z. Lowry
National Institute of Standards and Technology

Saverio M. Maviglia
Brigham and Women's Hospital, Boston, Massachusetts, USA, Harvard Medical School, Boston, Massachusetts, USA, Partners HealthCare, Boston, Massachusetts, USA

Allison B. McCoy
School of Biomedical Informatics, The University of Texas Health Science Center at Houston (UTHealth), Houston, Texas, USA

Carmit McMullen
Kaiser Permanente Center for Health Research, Portland, Oregon, USA

Blackford Middleton
Brigham & Women's Hospital, Boston, MA, USA, Partners HealthCare, Boston, MA, USA, Harvard Medical School, Boston, MA, USA

Daniel R. Murphy
Houston VA HSR&D Center of Excellence and The Center of Inquiry to Improve Outpatient Safety Through Effective Electronic Communication, both at the Michael E. DeBakey Veterans Affairs Medical Center and the Section of Health Services Research, Department of Medicine, Baylor College of Medicine, VA Medical Center (152), 2002 Holcombe Blvd, Houston 77030, TX, USA

W. Paul Nichol
Patient Care Services, Veterans Health Administration, VACO, Washington, DC, USA, Division of General Internal Medicine, University of Washington, Seattle, Washington, USA

Emily S. Patterson
Ohio State University

Laura A. Petersen
The Center of Inquiry to Improve Outpatient Safety Through Effective Electronic Communication and the Houston VA HSR&D Center of Excellence at the Michael E DeBakey Veterans Affairs Medical Center, VA Medical Center (152) 2002 Holcombe Blvd, Houston, TX 77030, USA, Section of Health Services Research, Department of Medicine, Baylor College of Medicine, Michael E DeBakey Veterans Affairs Medical Center (MEDVAMC), HSR&D Center of Excellence (152) 2002 Holcombe Boulevard, Houston, TX 77030 USA

Jerome A. Osheroff
Thomson Micromedex, Denver, Colorado, Department of Medicine, University of Pennsylvania, School of Medicine, Philadelphia, Pennsylvania

Justine E. Pang
Brigham & Women's Hospital, Boston, MA, USA, Partners HealthCare, Boston, MA, USA

Emily S. Patterson
Getting at Patient Safety (GAPS) Center, Veterans Affairs Medical Center (VAMC), Cincinnati, and
Clinical Medicine, University of Cincinnati, Cincinnati

Matthew T. Quinn
National Institute of Standards and Technology

Mala Ramaiah
National Institute of Standards and Technology

Brian Reis
The Center of Inquiry to Improve Outpatient Safety Through Effective Electronic Communication and
the Houston VA HSR&D Center of Excellence at the Michael E DeBakey Veterans Affairs Medical
Center, VA Medical Center (152) 2002 Holcombe Blvd, Houston, TX 77030, USA

Marta L. Render
VA GAPS Center, and Professor of Clinical Medicine, University of Cincinnati

Joshua Richardson
Weill Cornell Medical College, New York, NY, USA

Michelle L. Rogers
Getting at Patient Safety (GAPS) Center, Veterans Affairs Medical Center (VAMC), Cincinnati, and
Clinical Medicine, University of Cincinnati, Cincinnati

Mona K. Sawhney
The Center of Inquiry to Improve Outpatient Safety Through Effective Electronic Communication and
the Houston VA HSR&D Center of Excellence at the Michael E DeBakey Veterans Affairs Medical
Center, VA Medical Center (152) 2002 Holcombe Blvd, Houston, TX 77030, USA

M. Michael Shabot
Departments of Surgery and Enterprise Information Services, Cedars-Sinai Medical Center, Los An-
geles, California

Jason S. Shapiro
Department of Emergency Medicine, Mount Sinai School of Medicine, New York, New York, USA

Michael Shapiro
Oregon Health & Science University, Portland, OR, USA

Aziz Sheikh
eHealth Research Group, Centre for Population Health Sciences, The University of Edinburgh, Edinburgh, UK

Hardeep Singh
Houston VA Health Services Research and Development Center of Excellence and The Center of Inquiry to Improve Outpatient Safety Through Effective Electronic Communication, Michael E. DeBakey Veterans Affairs Medical Center and the Section of Health Services Research, Department of Medicine, Baylor College of Medicine, Houston

Dean F. Sittig
University of Texas School of Health Information Sciences and the UT-Memorial Hermann Center for Healthcare Quality and Safety, Houston

Cynthia Spurr
Partners HealthCare Information Systems, Clinical Informatics Research and Development, Partners Healthcare Systems and Harvard Medical School, Boston, Massachusetts

Jack Starmer
Vanderbilt University Medical Center, Nashville, Tennessee, USA

Milenko Tanasijevic
Division of General Medicine, Department of Pathology, Partners Healthcare Systems and Harvard Medical School, Boston, Massachusetts

Jonathan M. Teich
Elsevier Health Sciences, Philadelphia, Pennsylvania, Department of Medicine, Harvard University, Boston, Massachusetts

Meena S. Vij
Diagnostic & Therapeutic Care Line Executive and Chief of Radiology, Michael E. DeBakey VA Medical Center, and Associate Professor of Radiology at Baylor College of Medicine

Lynn Volk
Partners HealthCare Information Systems, Clinical and Quality Analysis, Partners Healthcare Systems and Harvard Medical School, Boston, Massachusetts

Samuel Wang
Clinical Informatics Research and Development, Partners Healthcare Systems and Harvard Medical School, Boston, Massachusetts

Lindsey Wilson
The Center of Inquiry to Improve Outpatient Safety Through Effective Electronic Communication and the Houston VA HSR&D Center of Excellence at the Michael E DeBakey Veterans Affairs Medical Center, VA Medical Center (152) 2002 Holcombe Blvd, Houston, TX 77030, USA

Adam Wright
Brigham and Women's Hospital, Harvard Medical School, Boston, Massachusetts, USA

Jiajie Zhang
School of Health Information Sciences, University of Texas, Houston, Texas

INTRODUCTION

Establishing a safe and effective electronic health record (EHR)-enabled health care delivery system is one of the most important and complex challenges facing clinicians and the healthcare organizations they work for today. Since the passage of the Health Information Technology for Economic and Clinical Health (HITECH) Act, a portion of the American Recovery and Reinvestment Act of 2009, the proportion of clinicians using EHRs on a routine basis has increased from less than 20% to over 60%. Concomitantly, the number of certified EHR vendors in the United States has increased from 60 to more than 1700. When coupled together, this influx of healthcare organizations and clinicians that are new to the uses of health information technology, along with a myriad of new EHR vendors, stands to create significant new and often unanticipated challenges. The goal of this book is to provide an overview of the challenges in EHR design and implementation along with an introduction to the "best practices" that have been identified over the past several years. The book is divided into and introduction and eight subsections. Each subsection focuses on a key implementation issue or a specific component of an EHR.

The first section provides an overview of the issues at hand. In the first chapter, Sittig and Singh looks at some of the concerns surrounding EHR use and proposes eight rights of safe EHR use. These rights are grounded in Carayon's Systems Engineering Initiative for Patient Safety, a human factors engineering model that addresses work-system design for patient safety.

In Chapter 2, Cresswell and colleagues argue that the implementation of health information technology interventions is at the forefront of most policy agendas internationally. However, such undertakings are often far from straightforward as they require complex strategic planning accompanying the systemic organizational changes associated with such programs. Building on experiences of designing and evaluating the implementation of large-scale health information technology interventions in the USA and the UK, the authors highlight key lessons learned in the hope of inform-ing the ongoing international efforts of policymakers, health directorates, healthcare management, and senior clinicians.

Part II, titled "Identifying and Preventing EHR Safety Concerns," ex-amines the many organizations in the midst of implementing Electronic Health Records (EHRs). Research and experience gained over the past 20 years has shown that implementing EHRs is difficult, time-consuming, and expensive. In addition, recent reports indicate that many organizations continue to experience various types of unintended adverse consequences. The goal of this section is to illustrate how an organization can identify specific EHR-related safety concerns as well as begin their understanding of what they should do to remedy these situations before tragedy strikes.

In Chapter 3, Sittig and Singh find that despite the promise of health in-formation technology (HIT), recent literature has revealed possible safety hazards associated with its use. The Office of the National Coordinator for HIT recently sponsored an Institute of Medicine committee to synthesize evidence and experience from the field on how HIT affects patient safety. To lay the groundwork for defining, measuring, and analyzing HIT-related safety hazards, they propose that HIT-related error occurs any time HIT is unavailable for use, malfunctions during use, is used incorrectly by some-one, or when HIT interacts with another system component incorrectly, re-sulting in data being lost or incorrectly entered, displayed, or transmitted. These errors, or the decisions that result from them, significantly increase the risk of adverse events and patient harm. They describe how a socio-technical approach can be used to understand the complex origins of HIT errors, which may have roots in rapidly evolving technological, profes-sional, organizational, and policy initiatives.

The next chapter details how although electronic health records (EHRs) have a significant potential to improve patient safety, EHR-related safety concerns have begun to emerge. Sittig and Singh analyzed 369 responses to a survey sent to the memberships of the American Society for Health-care Risk Management and the American Health Lawyers Association and supplemented by their previous work in EHR-related patient safety, the authors identified the following common EHR-related safety concerns: 1) Incorrect patient identification; 2) Extended EHR unavailability (either planned or unplanned); 3) Failure to heed a computer-generated warning or alert; 4) System-to-system interface errors; 5) Failure to identify, find, or use the most recent patient data; 6) Misunderstandings about time; 7) Incorrect item selected from a list of items; 8) Open or incomplete orders. In this paper, the authors present a "red flag"-based approach that can be used by risk managers to identify potential EHR safety concerns in their institutions. An organization that routinely conducts EHR-related surveillance activities, such as the ones proposed here, can significantly reduce risks associated with EHR implementation and use.

Chapter 5, by McCoy et al., seeks to quantify the percentage of records with matching identifiers as an indicator for duplicate or potentially duplicate patient records in electronic health records in five different healthcare organizations, describe the patient safety issues that may arise, and present solutions for managing duplicate records or records with matching identifiers. For each institution, they retrieved de-identified counts of records with an exact match of patient first and last names and dates of birth and determined the number of patient records existing for the top 250 most frequently occurring first and last name pairs. They also identified methods for managing duplicate records or records with matching identifiers, reporting the adoption rate of each across institutions. They found that the occurrence of matching first and last name in two or more individuals ranged from 16.49% to 40.66% of records; inclusion of date of birth reduced the rates to range from 0.16% to 15.47%. The number of records existing for the most frequently occurring name at each site ranged from 41 to 2552. Institutions varied widely in the methods they implemented for preventing, detecting and removing duplicate records, and mitigating resulting errors. The percentage of records having matching patient identifiers is high in several organizations, indicating that the rate of duplicate records or records may also be high. Further efforts are necessary to improve management of duplicate records or records with matching identifiers and minimize the risk for patient harm.

Part III is titled "EHR Users and Usability"; the rapid increase in the rate of EHR adoption following the HITECH Act of 2009 has highlighted many shortcomings of existing EHR technology. Many of these shortcomings revolve around the concept of EHR usability as exemplified by the need for users to engage in data entry, communication, and review. A major confounder in the usability debate revolves around the multiple

users of the EHR; each with a distinct and often conflicting set of requirements. A major challenge is to identify the myriad EHR users and the
key tasks they need to accomplish, for example, clinicians need to record
their thoughts and actions regarding patients past medical history, current
presenting complaints, and future plans including ordering diagnostic tests
and therapy. The EHR is also used as a front-end to the billing process that
requires documentation using a distinct set of billing codes that record
exactly what the clinician did (i.e., physiologic systems examined, procedures performed, tests and therapies ordered) during the encounter. The
same data are also used by the organization's administration to measure
and monitor the quality of care provided across the organization. Attempts
to improve EHR usability must take a comprehensive view of this problem
considering the viewpoints of all potential users.

In Chapter 6, Sittig and Singh argue that despite the potential benefits
of electronic health records, clinicians have experienced several challenges in their adoption and use. To encourage debate on strategies to overcome these challenges, they developed a set of 10 "rights" of clinicians
that represent important features, functions and user privileges of electronic health records that clinicians need to provide safe, high·quality care.
Each right is accompanied by a corresponding responsibility of clinicians,
without which the ultimate goal of improving quality of health care might
not be achieved.

Lowry and colleagues examine the practice of EHR in pediatric medicine in Chapter 7. Adoption of electronic health record (EHR) systems in
hospitals and physician practices is accelerating. Usability of EHRs has
been identified as an important factor impacting patient safety, and recommendations for improvement have been provided. Pediatric patients
have unique characteristics that translate into unique EHR usability challenges. It is not surprising, then, that the adoption of EHRs by pediatric
care providers has lagged behind adoption for adult care providers. In this
document, we highlight important user interactions that are especially salient for pediatric care and hence to the EHR user-centered design process. These interactions and associated usability recommendations were
identified by consensus during a series of teleconferences with experts
representing the disciplines of human factors engineering, usability, informatics, and pediatrics in ambulatory care and pediatric intensive care.

In addition, extensive peer review was provided by experts in pediatric informatics, emergency medicine, neonatology, pediatrics, human factors engineering, usability engineering, and software development and implementation. This report details recommendations to enhance EHR usability when supporting pediatric patient care and also identifies promising areas for EHR innovation. Finally, the authors illustrate unique pediatric considerations in the context of representative clinical scenarios that may be helpful for formative user-centered design approaches and summative usability evaluations.

Chapter 8 examines a different challenge of adopting EHR practices, this time in developing countries. Sittig, Kahol, and Singh examine the potential for health information technology (IT) to enhance quality of care is limited by unanticipated problems following adoption of new systems and technologies. Proactive assessment of system vulnerabilities can help improve existing systems and ease implementation of new innovations. The authors applied a comprehensive socio-technical model of safe and effective health IT use to the formative evaluation of a novel tablet-based device designed to support primary care practice in rural India. Based on their conceptual model, they developed an assessment guide for the tablet system that was informed by literature review, interviews, and observations of health workers and supervisors. The assessment revealed and addressed both technical (functionality, content, usability, user interface) and non-technical (workflow, processes, and policies etc.) areas of improvement.

Part IV, titled "Clinical Decision Support" (CDS) interventions as integrated within an EHR, are designed to aid the clinician's decision-making process at the point of care. The current scope of CDS focuses primarily on medications, laboratory testing, radiology procedures, and providing access to clinical reference literature. There is substantial evidence to suggest that well-designed clinical decision support not only enhances the quality of care provided but directly impacts patient safety by decreasing common errors and reducing missed opportunities or omissions that result in patient harm. In spite of this, many electronic health records (EHRs) do not have robust or reliable decision support features, and poorly implemented HIT systems have been shown to adversely affect care by introducing errors. This section outlines overarching guidelines for effective, efficient, and reliable CDS systems and provides specific suggestions to improve the design, implementation, and use of these systems.

In Chapter 9, Bates and colleagues argue that while evidence-based medicine has increasingly broad-based support in health care, it remains difficult to get physicians to actually practice it. Across most domains in medicine, practice has lagged behind knowledge by at least several years. The authors believe that the key tools for closing this gap will be information systems that provide decision support to users at the time they make decisions, which should result in improved quality of care. Furthermore, providers make many errors, and clinical decision support can be useful for finding and preventing such errors. Over the last eight years the authors have implemented and studied the impact of decision support across a broad array of domains and have found a number of common elements important to success. The goal of this report is to discuss these lessons learned in the interest of informing the efforts of others working to make the practice of evidence-based medicine a reality.

Sittig and colleageus argue that a simple reminder is not always sufficient when it comes to encouraging various health reminders in Chapter 10. State-of-the-art electronic health record systems with advanced clinical decision support (CDS) capabilities can fundamentally improve quality and reduce costs of health care. However, these outcomes have not been universally achieved. They also argue that maximizing the potential of CDS for improving quality and safety of care requires attention to several factors, not all of which are related to the computer system.

Chapter 11, by Ash and colleagues, seeks to identify recommended practices for computerized clinical decision support (CDS) development and implementation and for knowledge management (KM) processes in ambulatory clinics and community hospitals using commercial or locally developed systems in the U.S. Guided by the Multiple Perspectives Framework, the authors conducted ethnographic field studies at two community hospitals and five ambulatory clinic organizations across the U.S. Using a Rapid Assessment Process, a multidisciplinary research team gathered preliminary assessment data; conducted on-site interviews, observations, and field surveys; analyzed data using both template and grounded methods; and developed universal themes. A panel of experts produced recommended practices. The team then identified ten themes related to CDS and

KM. These include: 1) workflow; 2) knowledge management; 3) data as a foundation for CDS; 4) user computer interaction; 5) measurement and metrics; 6) governance; 7) translation for collaboration; 8) the meaning of CDS; 9) roles of special, essential people; and 10) communication, training, and support. Experts developed recommendations about each theme. The original Multiple Perspectives Framework was modified to make explicit a new theoretical construct, that of Translational Interaction. These ten themes represent areas that need attention if a clinic or community hospital plans to implement and successfully utilize CDS. In addition, they have implications for workforce education, research, and national-level policy development. The Translational Interaction construct could guide future applied informatics research endeavors.

Chapter 12 seeks to detail what structures need to be put in place for EHS to be successful. Wright and colleagues describe clinical decision support (CDS) as a powerful tool for improving healthcare quality and ensuring patient safety. However, effective implementation of CDS requires effective clinical and technical governance structures. The authors sought to determine the range and variety of these governance structures and identify a set of recommended practices through observational study. Three site visits were conducted at institutions across the USA to learn about CDS capabilities and processes from clinical, technical, and organizational perspectives. Based on the results of these visits, written questionnaires were sent to the three institutions visited and two additional sites. Together, these five organizations encompass a variety of academic and community hospitals as well as small and large ambulatory practices. These organizations use both commercially available and internally developed clinical information systems. Characteristics of clinical information systems and CDS systems used at each site as well as governance structures and content management approaches were identified through extensive field interviews and follow-up surveys. Six recommended practices were identified in the area of governance, and four were identified in the area of content management. Key similarities and differences between the organizations studied were also highlighted. Each of the five sites studied contributed to the recommended practices presented in this paper for CDS governance. Since these strategies appear to be useful at a diverse range of institutions, they should be considered by any future implementers of decision support.

In Chapter 13, Wright and colleagues show that many computerized provider order entry (CPOE) systems include the ability to create electronic order sets, collections of clinically related orders grouped by purpose. Order sets, promise to make CPOE systems more efficient, improve care quality, and increase adherence to evidence-based guidelines. However, the development and implementation of order sets can be expensive and time-consuming, and limited literature exists about their utilization. Based on analysis of order set usage logs from a diverse purposive sample of seven sites with commercially and internally developed inpatient CPOE systems, the authors developed an original order set classification system. Order sets were categorized across seven non-mutually exclusive axes: admission/discharge/transfer (ADT), perioperative, condition-specific, task-specific, service-specific, convenience, and personal. In addition, 731 unique subtypes were identified within five axes: four in ADT (S = 4), three in perioperative, 144 in condition-specific, 513 in task-specific, and 67 in service-specific. Order sets (n = 1914) were used a total of 676,142 times at the participating sites during a one-year period. ADT and perioperative order sets accounted for 27.6% and 24.2% of usage respectively. Peripartum/labor, chest pain/acute coronary syndrome/myocardial infarction and diabetes order sets accounted for 51.6% of condition-specific usage. Insulin, angiography/angioplasty, and arthroplasty order sets accounted for 19.4% of task-specific usage. Emergency/trauma, obstetrics/gynecology/labor delivery, and anesthesia accounted for 32.4% of service-specific usage. Overall, the top 20% of order sets accounted for 90.1% of all usage. Additional salient patterns are identified and described.

Part V details the role of EHR in the referral process. Electronic health records are increasingly being used to facilitate referral communication in the outpatient setting. Outpatient referrals involve processes that include a transfer of responsibility for some aspect of patient's care from a referring provider to a secondary service or provider. They are an important but challenging aspect of primary care practice.

In Chapter 14, Esquivel and colleagues show that electronic health records are increasingly being used to facilitate referral communication in the outpatient setting. However, despite support by technology, referral communication between primary care providers and specialists is often unsatisfactory and is unable to eliminate care delays. This may be in part due to lack of attention to how information and communication technology fits within the social environment of health care. Making electronic referral communication effective requires a multifaceted "socio-technical" approach. Using an 8-dimensional socio-technical model for health information technology as a framework, the authors describe ten recommendations that represent good clinical practices to design, develop, implement, improve, and monitor electronic referral communication in the outpatient setting. These recommendations were developed on the basis of the authors' previous work, current literature, sound clinical practice, and a systems-based approach to understanding and implementing health information technology solutions. Recommendations are relevant to system designers, practicing clinicians, and other stakeholders considering use of electronic health records to support referral communication.

Section VI is about laboratory test result management and reporting practices, which include communication of test results from diagnostic services (e.g. radiology and laboratory) to the ordering clinical practitioners, are complex and vulnerable to breakdown. In the EHR-enabled healthcare environment, we rely upon technology to support and manage these processes. EHRs can incorporate standardized and automated features to improve the safety and effectiveness of how laboratory test result information is communicated.

Singh and Vij look at the reporting of abnormal test results in Chapter 15. Healthcare organizations continue to struggle to ensure that critical findings are communicated and acted on in a timely and appropriate manner. Recent research highlights the risks of communication breakdowns along the entire spectrum of test-result abnormality, including significantly abnormal but nonemergent findings. Evidence-based and practical institutional policies must uphold effective processes to guide communication of abnormal test results. Eight recommendations for effective policies on communication of abnormal diagnostic test results were developed based on policy refinement at the Michael E. DeBakey Veterans Affairs Medical Center (Houston), institutional experience with test result management, and findings from research performed locally and elsewhere. Research findings on vulnerabilities in existing policies and procedures were taken into consideration. The eight recommendations are based on important refinements to the policy, which clarified staff roles and responsibilities for test ordering, follow-up, and communication; defined categories of abnormal test results to guide appropriate follow-up action; and elaborated procedures for monitoring the effectiveness of test result communication and follow-up. Participation of key stakeholders is recommended to enhance buy-in from personnel and to help ensure the policies feasibility and sustainability. The proposed recommendations for ensuring safe test-result communication may be potentially useful to a wide variety of institutions and health care settings. These practical suggestions, based on research findings and experiences with a previous policy, may be a useful guide for designing or amending policies for safe test-result communication in both inpatient and outpatient settings.

Chapter 16, by Singh and colleagues, argues that early detection of colorectal cancer through timely follow-up of positive Fecal Occult Blood Tests (FOBTs) remains a challenge. In the authors' previous work, they found 40% of positive FOBT results eligible for colonoscopy had no documented response by a treating clinician at two weeks despite procedures for electronic result notification. They determined if technical and/or workflow-related aspects of automated communication in the electronic health record could lead to the lack of response. Using both qualitative and quantitative methods, they evaluated positive FOBT communication in the electronic health record of a large, urban facility between May 2008 and March 2009. They identified the source of test result communication breakdown and developed an intervention to fix the problem. Explicit medical record reviews measured timely follow-up (defined as response within 30 days of positive FOBT) pre- and post-intervention. Data from 11 interviews and tracking information from 490 FOBT alerts revealed that the software intended to alert primary care practitioners (PCPs) of positive FOBT results was not configured correctly and over a third of positive FOBTs were not transmitted to PCPs. Upon correction of the technical problem, lack of timely follow-up decreased immediately from 29.9% to 5.4% (p < 0.01) and was sustained at month 4 following the intervention. Electronic communication of positive FOBT results should be monitored to avoid limiting colorectal cancer screening benefits. Robust quality assurance and oversight systems are needed to achieve this. The authors' methods may be useful for others seeking to improve follow-up of FOBTs in their systems.

Part VII is titled "Bar Coded Medication Administration". Bar-Coded Medication Administration (BCMA) is a key component of a healthcare organization's inventory control system. A BCMA system consists of a barcode printer that adds a barcode label to each medication to be administered, a barcode reader used to scan the barcoded patient identification wristband attached to each patient, a mobile computer (with WiFi) that collects the information and transmits it to a central computer server that matches the patient identification information to the medication that was prescribed. These systems have the potential to improve medication safety by verifying that the right drug at the right dose via the right route is being administered to the right patient at the right time.

Chapter 17 gives some best practice recommendations. Patterson and colleagues show that since 2000, the Veterans Health Administration (VHA) has pioneered the development and deployment of a BCMA system. Based on VHA experience, 15 "best practices" for BCMA implementation, integration, and maintenance are recommended. Data were collected on potential barriers to the effectiveness of BCMA to improve patient safety by direct observation of medication administration, simulated BCMA use in a laboratory setting, a survey of nursing informatics specialists regarding policies and procedures, and 30 unstructured interviews with diverse stakeholders. Fifteen practices were proposed, categorized by implementation and continuous improvement, training, troubleshooting, contingency planning, equipment maintenance, medication administration, and maintenance of paper patient wristbands. For example, Recommendation 15 ("Periodic replacement of wristbands") advises weekly bar-coded wristband replacement in long-term care settings to improve the scanning reliability. Lessons learned about best practices to address challenges may offer insight to others considering implementation of bar-code technology.

The final section, Part VII, describes computer-based provider order entry; a module within an electronic health record system that allows the patient's healthcare provider (most often a physician, but a nurse practitioner or physician's assistant could also perform these tasks) to enter an order for a diagnostic procedure or therapeutic treatment. This order can then be sent electronically to the appropriate person or ancillary department (computer-based order communication) where it is carried out. In addition to eliminating the legibility problems that surround many hand-written orders and the need for repeated transcriptions and movement of the paper medical record, the system can also check for duplicate orders, potential drug-drug or drug-laboratory interactions, perform dosage checks, and ensure that all orders are complete. Computer-based provider order entry (CPOE) is the single most important clinical computing application that has been developed in terms of its ability to influence clinical decision-making and provider behavior at the point of care. While many informaticians, clinicians, and organizational leaders have recognized this and attempted to develop the clinical computing infrastructure and organizational culture that would allow such an application to be implemented over the past 30 years, to date, very few healthcare organizations have been successful.

Chapter 18, by Campbell and colleagues, attempts to identify and describe unintended adverse consequences related to clinical workflow when implementing or using computerized provider order entry (CPOE) systems. They analyzed qualitative data from field observations and formal interviews gathered over a three-year period at five hospitals in three organizations. Five multidisciplinary researchers worked together to identify themes related to the impacts of CPOE systems on clinical workflow. CPOE systems can affect clinical work by 1) introducing or exposing human/computer interaction problems, 2) altering the pace, sequencing, and dynamics of clinical activities, 3) providing only partial support for the work activities of all types of clinical personnel, 4) reducing clinical situation awareness, and 5) poorly reflecting organizational policy and procedure. As CPOE systems evolve, those involved must take care to mitigate the many unintended adverse effects these systems have on clinical workflow. Workflow issues resulting from CPOE can be mitigated by iteratively altering both clinical workflow and the CPOE system until a satisfactory fit is achieved.

The final chapter, Chapter 19, by Sittig and colleagues, is written in response to another article, "Unexpected Increased Mortality After Implementation of a Commercially Sold Computerized Physician Order Entry System" by Han et al. The authors are to be congratulated for their courage in bringing their compelling account of computerized physician order entry (CPOE) implementation problems to the medical literature as they tried to interpret their results concerning mortality. Their article is as much a search for answers as it is a recitation of the shortfalls in their implementation process and computer systems. It is critically important to understand that the types of problems described by Han et al. are not limited to their institution. In fact, setbacks and failures in the implementation of clinical information systems (CISs) and CPOE systems are all too common. Although it is tempting to focus solely on the role of new technology in the problems highlighted by this example, there are also important lessons to be learned about related organizational and workflow factors that affect the potential for danger associated with CPOE implementation.

PART I

INTRODUCTION

PART I

INTRODUCTION

CHAPTER 1

EIGHT RIGHTS OF SAFE ELECTRONIC HEALTH RECORD USE

DEAN F. SITTIG and HARDEEP SINGH

Computers can improve the safety, quality, and efficiency of health care.1 The pressure on hospitals and physicians to adopt electronic health records (EHRs) has never been greater. However, concerns have been raised about the safety of EHRs in light of the limitations of currently available software, the inexperience of clinicians and information technologists in implementation and use, and potential adverse outcomes associated with clinician order entry and other clinical applications.[2-4]

President Obama has referred to EHRs as a solution to reduce medical errors. To avoid medical errors resulting from EHR use and to achieve the promise of EHRs, this Commentary proposes 8 rights of safe EHR use. These rights are grounded in Carayon's Systems Engineering Initiative for Patient Safety, [5] a human factors engineering model that addresses work-system design for patient safety.

1.1 RIGHT HARDWARE OR SOFTWARE

An EHR system must be capable of supporting required clinical activities. If hardware or software is inadequately sized, configured, or maintained, the EHR will function poorly. Anything that slows or disrupts the clinician's workflow could negatively affect patient safety. [6] For example, an EHR should be able to calculate a medication dose, transmit the order to the appropriate department, and notify the nurse of a placed order. A medication error could easily follow a breakdown in any of these functions.

Local software oversight committees are a way to help ensure proper and safe functioning. [7] Another solution may be cloud computing, reliablecomputingservices that are accessible from remote locations via the Internet. Although the cloud may reduce hardware procurement, configuration, and maintenance burdens for health care organizations, its benefits hinge on the improvement of Internet speed, reliability, and access.

1.2   RIGHT CONTENT

Right content includes standard medical vocabularies to encode clinical findings and knowledge used to create specialty-specific features (eg, post transplant orders) and functions (eg, health maintenance reminders).Content must be evidence-based, carefully constructed, monitored, complete, and error free.

The federal government has taken a significant step toward advancing a controlled vocabulary with its support of Systematized Nomenclature of Medicine—Clinical Terms, the most comprehensive, multilingual clinical health care terminology in the world. The National Library of Medicine distributes it for free through an agreement with the International Health Terminology Standards Development Organization.Adoption of a standard vocabulary is prerequisite to implementing advanced clinical decision support (CDS).To increase access to a standards-based set of validated, evidence-based CDS, an open access clinical knowledge base of interventions should be developed, focusing on helping clinicians achieve the quality and safety targets for meaningful EHR use.

1.3   RIGHT USER INTERFACE

The right user interface allows clinicians to quickly grasp a complex system safely and efficiently. The interface should present all the relevant patient data in a format allowing clinicians to rapidly perceive problems, formulate responses, and document their actions. A key design consideration is the trade-off between clinicians' desire to see everything on 1 screen and limited screen space. Errors may follow when clinicians miss crucial information in applications that include too much information on 1 screen. Yet, systems with too many nested menu options or redundant pathways can be difficult to learn and time consuming to use. The physical aspects of the interface (eg, keyboard, mouse, or touch screen) may also contribute to error in the input or selection of information.

Another difficult problem facing clinicians is the requirement to navigate different interfaces safely and efficiently at different practice sites. Although remedying this problem is a complex undertaking, the federal government and EHR vendors should develop common user interface standards for health care applications.

1.4 RIGHT PERSONNEL

Trained and knowledgeable personnel are essential for safe use as are software designers, developers, trainers, and implementation and maintenance staff. System developers should have software engineering skills, be able to design effective user interfaces, use existing standardized clinical vocabularies, and have a sound understanding of clinical medicine. Trainers, implementers, and maintenance staff should have clinical experience, understanding of system capabilities and limitations, and excellent project management skills. [6] Clinicians should understand how to integrate the system into their workflows and how to function when it is unavailable. Close interaction among informatics experts, clinical application coordinators, and end users is essential for safe design and use.

In an attempt to create the right individuals, the American Medical Informatics Association has created the "1010 Training Programs" and has identified the knowledge and skills necessary for clinical informatics subspecialty fellowship programs. Such programs need to be implemented nationwide.

1.5　RIGHT WORKFLOW AND COMMUNICATION

Any disruption in workflow or information transfer is fertile ground for error. Prior to system implementation, a careful workflow analysis that accounts for EHR use could lead to identification of potential breakdown points. For example, vulnerabilities in hand-offs could be exposed in such an analysis, and communication tasks deemed critical could be required to have a traceable electronic receipt acknowledgment.

Errors may result from CDS interventions (ie, alerts and reminders) that are not well focused or not judiciously delivered at the point in the workflow that best supports the clinician's decision making or data entry. [8] Clinical decision support interventions should be streamlined with clinicians' electronically enabled workflow through a standard set of functions (eg, pop-up alerts, pick lists, or order sets).

1.6　RIGHT ORGANIZATIONAL CHARACTERISTICS

As with other safety models, a culture of innovation, exploration, and continual improvement are key organizational factors for safe EHR use. Organizations should actively facilitate reporting of errors or barriers to care resulting from EHR use, even if the findings are used only locally. Organizations must also carefully review their existing policies and procedures before implementation. For instance, although EHR systems can improve transmission of critical information through electronic notifications, this may do more harm than good if there are no policies for appropriate follow-up. [9] The Veterans Affairs health system exhibits many model organizational features, including a fair amount of central control, standardized procedures for collecting error data and implementing upgrades, and a recent emphasis on studying innovations from end users.

1.7　RIGHT STATE AND FEDERAL RULES AND REGULATIONS

State and federal regulations may act as barriers or facilitators for achieving safe use.

The American Recovery and Reinvestment Act stipulates that clinicians and health care organizations can receive incentive payments for "meaningful use" of EHRs. Depending on the definition and timeline for meaningful use, this legislation could result in a rush to implement suboptimal systems. Furthermore, the legislation includes patient privacy provisions, such as access to lists of all third-party data disclosures that will require significant modifications to existing systems. Regulations to safeguard patient privacy are clearly important but may also have the greatest unintended consequence on national EHR implementation. Policies must address the safety and effectiveness of health information exchange across organizational boundaries, which may reopen the debate about unique national patient identifiers. Currently used probabilistic patient matching algorithms, used to link patient information from disparate health care organizations, are prone to error, and many matches are never made. We recommend that state and federal governments should create a regulatory environment compatible with widespread use and interoperability, thereby enabling systems to continue evolving while maintaining appropriate safety and privacy oversight.

1.8 RIGHT MONITORING

The creation of the Certification Commission for Health Information Technology is a significant step toward accelerating adoption, but an equally detailed postimplementation usability inspection process is also needed. Several reports have described serious errors related to the use or misuse of EHR systems, many of which were the result of faulty system design, configuration, or implementation processes. [10] Organizations must continually evaluate the usability and performance of their systems after implementation, reliably measure benefits, and assess potential iatrogenic effects. Furthermore, the federal government should mandate use of a vendor-independent hazard reporting database and a national implementation accreditation test to help ensure that the systems are functioning as designed and are safe to use. The LeapFrog clinical decision support functionality test is an example of how such a test could be constructed.

EHR developers have encountered many roadblocks to achieving safe and effective EHRs for all. Success in the next 10 years will require a coordinated multidisciplinary research and development effort, much like the formation of National Aeronautics and Space Administration following President Kennedy's promise of a moon landing, to bring the best scientists, engineers, and clinicians together to address the problems and challenges in ensuring safe and effective use of EHRs. Efforts must move beyond the lone informatics researcher in an isolated laboratory if the complex interaction of organizational, technical, and cognitive factors that affect the safety of EHRs are to be understood and addressed and without this understanding, any solutions are certain to be far from optimal. Without high-quality, welldesigned, and carefully implemented EHRs, highly reliable, safe health care may never be achieved.

REFERENCES

1. Chaudhry B, Wang J, Wu S, et al. Systematic review: impact of health information technology on quality, efficiency, and costs of medical care. Ann Intern Med. 2006;144(10):742-752.
2. Han YY, Carcillo JA, Venkataraman ST, et al. Unexpected increased mortality after implementation of a commercially sold computerized physician order entry system. Pediatrics. 2005;116(6):1506-1512.
3. Koppel R, Metlay JP, Cohen A, et al. Role of computerized physician order entry systems in facilitating medication errors. JAMA. 2005;293(10):1197-1203.
4. The Joint Commission. Safely implementing health information and converging technologies. December 11, 2008. http://www.jointcommission.org/SentinelEvents/SentinelEventAlert/sea_42.htm. Accessed April 2009.
5. Carayon P, Schoofs Hundt A, Karsh BT, et al. Work system design for patient safety: the SEIPS model. Qual Saf Health Care. 2006;15(suppl 1):i50-i58.
6. Sittig DF, Ash JS. Clinical Information Systems: Overcoming Adverse Consequences. Sudbury, MA: Jones & Bartlett. In press.
7. Miller RA, Gardner RM. Recommendations for responsible monitoring and regulation of clinical software systems. J Am Med Inform Assoc. 1997;4(6):442-457.
8. Campbell EM, Guappone KP, Sittig DF, Dykstra RH, Ash JS. Computerized provider order entry adoption: implications for clinical workflow. J Gen Intern Med. 2009;24(1):21-26.
9. Singh H, Arora HS, Vij MS, Rao R, Khan M, Petersen LA. Communication outcomes of critical imaging results in a computerized notification system. J Am Med Inform Assoc. 2007;14(4):459-466.

10. Sittig DF, Ash JS, Jiang Z, Osheroff JA, Shabot MM. Lessons from "unexpected increased mortality after implementation of a commercially sold computerized physician order entry system." Pediatrics. 2006;118(2):797-801.

CHAPTER 2

TEN KEY CONSIDERATIONS FOR THE SUCCESSFUL IMPLEMENTATION AND ADOPTION OF LARGE-SCALE HEALTH INFORMATION TECHNOLOGY

KATHRIN M. CRESSWELL, DAVID W. BATES, and AZIZ SHEIKH

2.1 INTRODUCTION

Large-scale, potentially transformative, implementations of health information technology are now being planned and undertaken in multiple countries. [1 ,2] The hope is that the very substantial financial, human, and organizational investments being made in electronic health records, electronic prescribing, whole-system telehealthcare, and related technologies will streamline individual and organizational work processes and thereby improve the quality, safety, and efficiency of care. The reality is, however, that these technologies may prove frustrating for frontline clinicians and organizations as the systems may not fit their usual workflows, and the anticipated individual and organizational benefits take time to materialize. [3 ,4] In this article, we reflect on our mapping of the literature (see box 1) and complement this with our experiences of studying a range of national evaluations of various large-scale health information technology systems in the UK and USA to provide key pointers that can help streamline implementation efforts. [4 ,52–54] In so doing, we hope to inform policy and practice development to support the more successful integration of technology into complex healthcare environments. This is particularly timely given the US Health Information Technology for Economic and Clinical Health (HITECH) Act, which includes a \$19 billion stimulus package to promote the adoption of electronic health records and associated functionality. [55]

BOX 1: Factors associated with effective implementation identified in the literature [5–51]

Technical: usability, system performance, integration and interoperability, stability and reliability, adaptability and flexibility, cost, accessibility and adaptability of hardware

Social: attitudes and concerns, resistance and workarounds, expectations, benefits/values and motivations, engagement and user input in design, training and support, champions, integration with existing work practices

Organizational: getting the organization ready for change, planning, leadership and management, realistic expectations, user ownership, teamwork and communication, learning and evaluation

Wider socio-political: other healthcare organizations, industry, policy, professional groups, independent bodies, the wider economic environment, international developments

---

This paper complements a previous publication by Bates and colleagues on 'Ten commandments for effective clinical decision support', [11] which focused on lessons learned in relation to clinical decision support systems. We have developed a technology lifecycle approach to highlight key considerations at four stages: establishing the need for change, selecting a system, implementation planning, and maintenance and evaluation (figure 1).

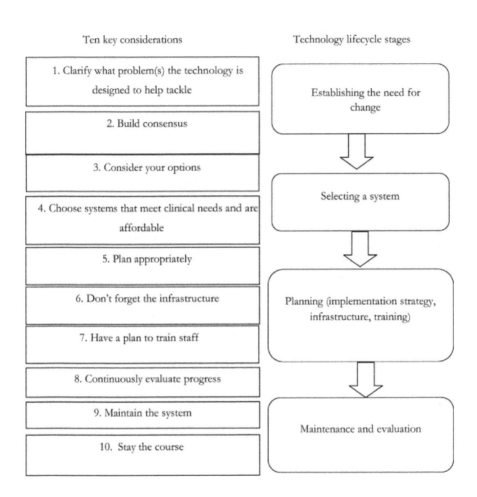

FIGURE 1: Summary of the lifecycle stages of health information technology and the ten key considerations.

2.2 TEN KEY CONSIDERATIONS FOR THE SUCCESSFUL IMPLEMENTATION OF HEALTH INFORMATION TECHNOLOGY

2.2.1 CLARIFY WHAT PROBLEM(S) THE TECHNOLOGY IS DESIGNED TO HELP TACKLE

Many health information technology procurements are based on assumed benefits, which are often poorly specified. This can result in difficulties agreeing on a shared vision across the healthcare organization. While terms like 'improved quality of care' and 'improved efficiency' are often used, detailed outcomes resulting from specific functionality are hard to measure and to anticipate as most implementations require fundamental changes to operational processes and many organizations do not even attempt this. [3 ,4 ,52–54] Thus, organizations often encounter difficulties conceptualizing the required short-, medium-, and long-term transformations.

A thorough mapping of existing local processes before implementation can mitigate this risk and help to identify existing problems as well as areas for improvement. In an ideal scenario, this groundwork would result in agreement on the problem(s) to be addressed by a specific functionality (eg, duplication of information) and, based on this, the development of a long-term strategic vision (eg, a common patient record that is populated by all health professionals). However, new technology may not always be the answer. It is therefore also important to assess if, and to what extent, existing/new health information technology can support these strategic goals and whether other approaches may also need to be considered.

2.2.2 BUILD CONSENSUS

Professional, managerial, and administrative consensus needs to be built around the strategic vision, in addition to creating the means to support the realization of this vision. [56] This may involve considering whether to aim for radical changes across the organization (eg, through implementing electronic health record functionality), or whether to focus on streamlining specific processes (eg, electronic prescribing) initially and then expanding functionality over time. Many authors in the field of organizational change have highlighted that high-level strategic leadership of senior management including both administrative and clinical leaders is vital, and this is accurate, but it is also essential to involve and get the buy-in of different professional stakeholder groups (eg, doctors, nurses, administrative staff, managers) in order to facilitate co-ownership and ensure commitment. [57, 58] From our experience, this balance is best achieved through the creation of a high-level strategic group that not only includes senior managers, but also clinical and administrative leads who represent different end-user groups.

An important factor to keep in mind is that attempts to align perspectives through, for example, consensus building activities, need to be skillfully handled with cognizance of the means to overcome rather than perpetuate existing professional hierarchies. One approach that we have successfully used is to identify domains in which there is already broad agreement versus those which need specific attention from different professional stakeholders. For the latter, efforts promoting the participation and empowerment of different groups by actively searching for inclusive solutions, have the highest potential to achieve coordinated implementation efforts. [59] Nurses, for instance, will have different needs to doctors, but all groups tend to agree that the provision of high standards of care should be the focus of activities. Patient-centered discussions could therefore be a point of convergence between different professional viewpoints.

2.2.3 CONSIDER YOUR OPTIONS

Once the need for a technological system has been established, it is important to commit adequate time and resources to thoroughly consider different options in terms of which system(s) to choose. We have found that this aspect of planning and the associated writing of business cases and procurement considerations are sometimes under-estimated and often rushed. [11, 52] It is, for example, important to be aware of the full range of system providers, and network with potential suppliers in order to understand the ethos and values of the companies with which the organization is considering embarking on a long-term relationship. Visiting other healthcare settings that have implemented similar technology can prove very helpful. [52]

Once available commercial systems have been appraised, it is appropriate to reflect on whether to build a customized system tailored to local needs, whether to customize an existing system, or whether to use an 'off-the-shelf' standardized solution. [58] The literature and our experiences indicate that there are inherent risks and benefits to each of these approaches. For example, although 'home-grown' customized systems tend to be better accepted by local users than standardized solutions, they are also not a cheap option and often do not easily integrate with other technological systems in the organization. [4, 52–54] In addition, considerable time is needed to customize systems, and such efforts are often led by individuals or small groups of enthusiasts and so may not have longevity. In the USA, for example, commercial systems have markedly improved in recent years and now dominate the marketplace. Internationally, most organizations will, we anticipate, also choose commercial systems in the future due to cost and interoperability considerations. Commercial systems are cheaper to purchase (as they are not customized to individual organizations and can therefore be produced in bulk) and they are also likely to be interoperable due to common data standards and architectures (such as, for example, the Health Level Seven International interoperability standards).

2.2.4   CHOOSE SYSTEMS THAT MEET CLINICAL NEEDS AND ARE AFFORDABLE

Once a decision on the basic type of system has been made, it is important to base the final choice not only on organizational, but also on clinical needs. [60] A system should be both fit for organizational purpose and fit for clinical practice. There are countless examples of systems that have been procured but never used (eg, if they are perceived to undermine professional values) or are deployed in unintended ways, which will then typically result in a failure to realize the hoped for improvements (see box 2, example 1). [4, 61]

BOX 2: Examples of 'failures' in implementation

Example 1: Rejection by users [61]
May and colleagues evaluated the implementation of a videophone, which was intended to be used by primary care physicians to refer patients to a community mental health facility. The team conducted qualitative interviews and observations with clinicians, managerial staff, and patients in order to explore the acceptability of the technology. They found that some professional groups, including community psychiatric nurses and occupational therapists, resisted using the system as they felt that it impacted adversely on the therapeutic relationship with their patients.

Example 2: Bandwidth undermining system performance (authors' own experience)
At one large hospital, operational management was told by the information technology leadership that the hospital's network was at maximal bandwidth at budget time. The management decided that the hospital would wait a year to upgrade the network, and instead purchased an expensive new imaging technology. However, several months later the institution's systems began to 'brown out,' and it was taking up to 30 minutes for a single screen change. Although the leadership immediately reversed field and authorized a network upgrade, this took several months to implement and care delivery was substantially impaired in the interim.

Example 3: The importance of user feedback (authors' own experience)
Getting an 'early fix' on how long a new system is taking to use is especially critical. At one hospital which was a pioneer in order entry, a system was implemented and users were told they had to use it. However, the leadership had no clear idea how long it was actually taking front-line clinical users to do their work—something that took an hour before implementation was now taking several hours, which resulted in an unworkable situation for front-line users. This eventually resulted in a computer monitor being thrown through a hospital window, and a work action by the clinical users. That got the leadership's attention and major changes were made.

Example 4: Tracking system performance (authors' own experience)
Maintenance includes tracking how the system is performing, and how the decision support within it is performing. Such tracking is much easier if it is built in from the beginning. At one large hospital, the allergy over-ride rates were initially very low. However, a series of apparently innocuous changes in the decision support system were made by the responsible committee with the result that several years later, large numbers of alerts were being delivered, with nearly all being over-ridden. After these data were reviewed, the system could be tuned, and the unimportant alerts were turned off.

A system therefore needs to fulfill a range of requirements on a variety of levels. It needs to be usable for end-users (not cumbersome for clinicians and beneficial for patients), cost-effective for organizations, and interoperable to allow secondary uses of data. These purposes are often difficult to align as requirements of different domains may result in trade-offs for others. [60] For example, it has repeatedly been found that many health information technologies slow down the work practices of users, despite improving overall organizational efficiency. [62] Speed is of the essence and any initiative that slows down key clinical tasks is likely to be strongly resisted by frontline staff. This issue can to some extent be addressed by purchasing systems that allow a large degree of customization, but these are often expensive to acquire and run, necessitating a careful balancing act between affordability and desired functionality. Our experiences suggest that the associated system costs are often under-estimated, particularly those relating to infrastructure, support, and maintenance.

2.2.5   PLAN APPROPRIATELY

It takes both targeted and reflective efforts to plan for transformative organizational ventures of any kind. Although flexibility in strategy is required, there are some general pointers that tend to characterize effective preparation across organizations and technologies. These include the aforementioned necessity to engage extensively with potential suppliers and other organizations who have already implemented, but also the decision to prioritize the implementation of functionality that can bring benefits to the greatest number of end-users as early as possible. [4, 52–54] Other factors relate to the avoidance of 'scope-creep' (ie, the tendency to increase the scope of a project when it is already underway) and maintaining open channels of communication between management and users.

Implementation strategies need to be tailored to organizational circumstances and systems, whether they involve 'phased' or 'big-bang' implementation approaches. The former relates to introducing incremental functionality slowly, while the latter relates to introducing functionality across the organization all at once. We suggest avoiding the running of parallel systems (both paper and electronic) wherever possible, as this tends to increase workloads for end-users and may inadvertently introduce new threats to patient safety. [4, 52–54]

2.2.6 DON'T FORGET THE INFRASTRUCTURE

Developing the right infrastructure is an essential part of planning activity. If this is not afforded sufficient attention, then software systems may perform sub-optimally (eg, if wireless networks are unavailable or bandwidth is too narrow), or may be inaccessible to users altogether (eg, if there is a lack of available hardware). Again, this increases the possibility that systems are not used at all or used in ways other than intended, potentially compromising benefits and increasing risks associated with technological systems. [4] We have repeatedly found that inappropriate infrastructure can negatively shape user attitudes towards software systems themselves, as it can impact on usability and performance. Inappropriate infrastructure, such as a slow wireless connection, may for example, reduce the speed of a system, which is an important (if not the most important) factor in determining adoption (box 2, example 2). [11]

2.2.7 TRAIN STAFF

Trained users tend to be more satisfied with new technologies than those who have not been adequately trained. [63] This may be due to a lack of understanding of system capabilities, which can in turn lead to work-arounds whereby the new systems are used in unintended ways—or worse still—avoided completely.

The most effective training is that which is tailored to the individual roles of users, without being too restrictive as this can undermine understanding of how the whole system functions. Training needs to allow users to practice 'hands-on' and as closely simulate the actual working environment as possible. [58, 64] It is also ideally conducted shortly before the implementation as otherwise staff may forget important functions. There may be a need for compulsory (eg, in relation to approaches to maintaining patient confidentiality) as well as voluntary components, and some individuals may need more training than others. For instance, older users may never have used a computer and may therefore require more basic training than younger individuals, who tend to be more accustomed to computers. For infrequent users and in relation to systems that are subject to regular upgrades, continuous training may be necessary. From our experience, training should typically total about 40% of an implementation budget, but is the area most often left short.

2.2.8 CONTINUOUSLY EVALUATE PROGRESS

Although it is now widely recognized that evaluation is important when considering new technologies, the reality is that it is still, more often than not, an afterthought as immediate implementation activities take priority. [65] Real-time, longitudinal data collection strategies providing formative feedback are desirable as emerging results can be incorporated in on-going implementation activity, but this is costly and time-consuming. However, it is essential to capture user feedback about problems that are identified and respond to it in a timely manner (box 2, example 3). In our experience, investments in evaluation activities are always worth it. These should begin with assessing existing and anticipated organizational and individual workflows, monitoring desired and undesired consequences, and tracking new innovative ways of working. [4, 52–54] It is also crucially important that this work is carried out over an appropriate length of time, as it may well take years for benefits and consequences to emerge. [60] Following developments over the long term can further help identify when systems have become obsolete and when there is a need for new solutions.

2.2.9 MAINTAIN THE SYSTEM

Maintenance is in many ways related to all of the above points as these issues need to be re-visited periodically throughout the technology lifecycle (see figure 1). Nevertheless, maintenance deserves particular attention as it is often under-estimated in relation to associated activities and cost. [66]

This is not only the case in relation to on-going costs (eg, pertaining to support, infrastructure, and system upgrades), but also costs relating to potential system changes as the strategic aims of organizations and therefore the capabilities of existing technological systems are likely to change over time (box 2, example 4).

2.2.10   STAY THE COURSE

The benefits of major transformative ventures are notoriously difficult to measure and may take a long time to materialize. [3, 4, 52–54] However, this is not to say that they are non-existent, rather they need to be tracked by appropriate evaluation work assessing how the new system is used and re-invented locally. This also requires an appreciation of the timelines surrounding the realization of expected benefits, allowing enough time for technologies to embed and data to be exploited for secondary uses. [60] Our work has shown that in many cases the expectations of organizations and individual users far exceed what is achievable in the short term. The managing of expectations is, therefore, important as otherwise there is a danger that stakeholders disengage with the initiative and negative attitudes may emerge. [4, 52–54]

2.3   CONCLUSIONS

Careful planning and on-going, critical evaluation of progress are central to the successful implementation of major health information technology. Taking a lifecycle perspective on the implementation of technological systems will, we hope, help organizations to avoid some of the all too commonly encountered pitfalls and improve the likelihood of successful implementation and adoption (see figure 1). It is, however, important to keep in mind that, although the stages and considerations discussed here were depicted in a linear manner, they may to some extent overlap. This is consistent with the complex nature of large-scale health information technology implementations, where a range of different inter-related factors are at play.

REFERENCES

1. Morrison Z, Robertson A, Cresswell K, et al. Understanding and contrasting approaches to nationwide implementations of electronic health record systems: England, the USA and Australia. J Healthc Eng 2011;2:25–42.
2. Bates D. Using information technology to reduce rates of medication errors in hospitals. BMJ 2000;320:788.
3. European Commission. Interoperable eHealth is Worth it. Securing benefits from Electronic Health Records and ePrescribing. Brussels: European Commission, 2010.
4. Sheikh A, Cornford T, Barber N, et al. Implementation and adoption of nationwide electronic health records in secondary care in England: final qualitative results from prospective national evaluation in "early adopter" hospitals. BMJ 2011;343:d6054.
5. Adler KG. How to successfully navigate your EHR implementation. Fam Pract Manag 2007;14:33–9.
6. Ammenwerth E, Iller C, Mahler C. IT-adoption and the interaction of task, technology and individuals: a fit framework and a case study. BMC Med Inform Decis Mak 2006;6:13.
7. Ash J, Berg M. Report of conference Track 4: socio-technical issues of HIS. Int J Med Inform 2003;69:305–6.
8. Austin CJ, Hornberger KD, Shmerling JE. Managing information resources: a study of ten healthcare organizations. J Healthc Manag 2000;45:229–38.
9. Bali RK, Wickramasinghe N. Achieving successful EPR implementation with the penta-stage model. Int J Healthc Technol Manag 2008;9:97–105.
10. Bates DW, Ebell M, Gotlieb E, et al. A proposal for electronic medical records in U.S. primary care. J Am Med Inform Assoc 2003;10:1–10.
11. Bates DW, Kuperman GJ, Wang S, et al. Ten commandments for effective clinical decision support: making the practice of evidence-based medicine a reality. J Am Med Inform Assoc 2011;10:523–30.
12. Beuscart-Zephir MC, Anceaux F, Crinquette V, et al. Integrating users' activity modeling in the design and assessment of hospital electronic patient records: the example of anesthesia. Int J Med Inform 2001;64:157–71.
13. Boonstra A, Broekhuis M. Barriers to the acceptance of electronic medical records by physicians from systematic review to taxonomy and interventions. BMC Health Serv Res 2010;10:231.
14. Bossen C. Test the artefact–develop the organization. The implementation of an electronic medication plan. Int J Med Inform 2007;76:13–21.
15. Callen JL, Braithwaite J, Westbrook JI. Contextual implementation model: a framework for assisting clinical information system implementations. J Am Med Inform Assoc 2008;15:255–62.
16. Chaudhry B, Wang J, Wu S, et al. Systematic review: impact of health information technology on quality, efficiency, and costs of medical care. Ann Intern Med 2006;144:742–52.
17. Clemmer TP. Computers in the ICU: where we started and where we are now. J Crit Care 2004;4:201–7.

18. Crosson JC, Stroebel C, Scott JG, et al. Implementing an electronic medical record in a family medicine practice: communication, decision making, and conflict. Ann Fam Med 2005;3:307–11.
19. Dagroso D, Williams PD, Chesney JD, et al. Implementation of an obstetrics EMR module: overcoming user dissatisfaction. J Healthc Inf Manag 2007;21:87–94.
20. Davidson E, Chiasson M. Contextual influences on technology use mediation: a comparative analysis of electronic medical records systems. Eur J Info Syst 2005;14:6–18.
21. De Mul M, Berg M, Hazelzet JA. Clinical information systems: careSuite from Picis. J Crit Care 2004;19:208–14.
22. Duggan C. Implementation evaluation. HIM professionals share their experiences bringing health IT online. J AHIMA 2006;77:52–5.
23. Fenton SH, Giannangelo K, Stanfill M. Essential people skills for EHR implementation success. J AHIMA 2006;77:60.
24. Ferneley E, Sobreperez P. Resist, comply or workaround? An examination of different facets of user engagement with information systems. Eur J Inf Syst 2006;15:345–56.
25. Giuse DA, Kuhn KA. Health information systems challenges: the Heidelberg conference and the future. Int J Med Inform 2003;69:105–14.
26. Goroll AH, Simon SR, Tripathi M, et al. Community-wide implementation of health Information technology: the Massachusetts eHealth collaborative experience. J Am Med Inform Assoc 2009;16:132–9.
27. Granlien MF, Hertzum M, Gudmundsen J. The gap between actual and mandated use of an electronic medication record three years after deployment. Stud Health Technol Inform 2008;136:419–24.
28. Halamka J, Aranow M, Ascenzo C, et al. E-Prescribing collaboration in Massachusetts: early experiences from regional prescribing projects. J Am Med Inform Assoc 2006;13:239–44.
29. Hendy J, Reeves BC, Fulop N, et al. Challenges to implementing the national programme for information technology (NPfIT): a qualitative study. BMJ 2005;331:331–6.
30. James D, Hess S, Kretzing JE Jr., et al. Showing "what right looks like"–how to improve performance through a paradigm shift around implementation thinking. J Healthc Inf Manag 2007;21:54–61.
31. Jones M. Learning the lessons of history? Electronic records in the United Kingdom acute hospitals, 1988–2002. Health Informatics J 2004;10:253–63.
32. Karsten H, Laine A. User interpretations of future information system use: a snapshot with technological frames. Int J Med Inform 2007;76:S136–40.
33. Keddie Z, Jones R. Information communications technology in general practice: cross-sectional survey in London. Inform Prim Care 2005;13:113–23.
34. Keshavjee K, Bosomworth J, Copen J, et al. Best practices in EMR implementation: a systematic review. AMIA Annu Symp Proc 2006;982.
35. Lium JT, Tjora A, Faxvaag A. No paper, but the same routines: a qualitative exploration of experiences in two Norwegian hospitals deprived of the paper based medical record. BMC Med Inform Decis Mak 2008;8.

36. Lorenzi NM, Smith JB, Conner SR, et al. The success factor profile for clinical computer innovation. Stud Health Technol Inform 2004;107:1077–80.
37. Lu Y-C, Xiao Y, Sears A, et al. A review and a framework of handheld computer adoption in healthcare. Int J Med Inform 2005;74:409–22.
38. Ludwick DA, Doucette J. Adopting electronic medical records in primary care: lessons learned from health information systems implementation experience in seven countries. Int J Med Inform 2009;78:22–31.
39. Mehta NB, Partin MH. Electronic health records: a primer for practicing physicians. Cleve Clin J Med 2007;74:826–30.
40. Miranda D, Fields W, Lund K. Lessons learned during 15 years of clinical information system experience. Comput Nurs 2001;4:147–51.
41. Moen A. A nursing perspective to design and implementation of electronic patient record systems. J Biomed Inform 2003;36:375–8.
42. Nikula RE. Why implementing EPR's does not bring about organizational changes– a qualitative approach. Stud Health Technol Inform 2001;84:666–9.
43. Ovretveit J, Scott T, Rundall TG, et al. Improving quality through effective implementation of information technology in healthcare. Int J Qual Health Care 2007;5:259–66.
44. Pagliari C. Implementing the national programme for IT: what can we learn from the Scottish experience? Inform Prim Care 2005;13:105–11.
45. Pare G. Implementing clinical information systems: a multiple-case study within a US hospital. Health Serv Manage Res 2002;15:71–92.
46. Pare G, Sicotte C, Jaana M, et al. Prioritizing the risk factors influencing the success of clinical information system projects. A Delphi study in Canada. Methods Inf Med 2008;47:251–9.
47. Pendergast DK, Buchda VL. Charting the course. A quality journey. Nurs Adm Q 2003;27:330–5.
48. Puffer MJ, Ferguson JA, Wright BC, et al. Partnering with clinical providers to enhance the efficiency of an EMR. J Healthc Inf Manag 2007;21:24–32.
49. Quinzio L, Junger A, Gottwald B, et al. User acceptance of an anaesthesia information management system. Eur J Anaesthesiol 2003;20:967–72.
50. Räisänen C, Linde A. Technologizing discourse to standardize projects in multi-project organizations: hegemony by consensus? Organization 2004;11:101–21.
51. Rose J, Jones M, Truex D. Socio-theoretic accounts of IS: the problem of agency. Scand J Info Syst 2005;17:133–52.
52. Cresswell K, Coleman J, Slee A, et al. Investigating and learning lessons from early experiences of implementing ePrescribing systems into NHS hospitals: a questionnaire study. PLoS One 2013;8:e53369.
53. Ash JS, Stavri PZ, Kuperman GJ. A consensus statement on considerations for a successful CPOE implementation. J Am Med Inform Assoc 2003;10:229–34.
54. Health Information Technology Evaluation Toolkit. http://www.healthit.gov/unintended-consequences/sites/default/files/pdf/ModuleIIpdf1.5.pdf (accessed 3 Jan 2013).
55. Blumenthal D. Stimulating the adoption of health information technology. New Engl J Med 2009;360:1477–9.

56. Markoczy L. Consensus formation during strategic change. Strategic Manage J 2001;22:1013–31.
57. Cresswell K, Morrison Z, Crowe S, et al. Anything but...engaged: user involvement in the context of a national electronic health record implementation. Inform Prim Care 2012;19:191–206.
58. Dagroso D, Williams PD, Chesney JD, et al. Implementation of an obstetrics EMR module: overcoming user dissatisfaction. J Healthc Inform Manage 2007;21:87–94.
59. Checkland P. Systems thinking, systems practice. Chichester: Wiley, 1981.
60. Cresswell K, Sheikh A. Effective integration of technology into health care needs adequate attention to sociotechnical processes, time and a dose of reality. JAMA 2012;307:2255.
61. May C, Gask L, Atkinson T, et al. Resisting and promoting new technologies in clinical practice: the case of telepsychiatry. Soc Sci Med 2001;52:1889–901.
62. Aarts J, Doorewaard H, Berg M. Understanding implementation: the case of a computerized physician order entry system in a Large Dutch University Medical Center. J Am Med Inform Assoc 2004;11:207–16.
63. Yusof MM, Kuljis J, Papazafeiropoulou A, et al. An evaluation framework for Health Information Systems: human, organization and technology-fit factors (HOT-fit). Int J Med Inform 2008;77:386–98.
64. Sicotte C, Pare G, Moreault M-P, et al. A risk assessment of two interorganizational clinical information systems. J Am Med Inform Assoc 2006;13:557–66.
65. Greenhalgh T, Stramer K, Bratan T, et al. Introduction of shared electronic records: multi-site case study using diffusion of innovation theory. BMJ 2008;337:1786.
66. McGowan JJ, Cusack CM, Poon EG. Formative evaluation: a critical component in EHR implementation. J Am Med Inform Assoc 2008;15:297–301.

Cresswell K.M., Bates D.W., and Sheikh A. Ten Key Considerations for the Successful Implementation and Adoption of Large-Scale Health Information Technology. Journal of the American Medical Informatics Association 18 April 2013. doi:10.1136/amiajnl-2013-001684. Reproduced with permission from BMJ Publishing Group Ltd.

PART II

IDENTIFYING AND PREVENTING EHR SAFETY CONCERNS

DEFINING HEALTH INFORMATION TECHNOLOGY-RELATED ERRORS: NEW DEVELOPMENTS SINCE TO ERR IS HUMAN

DEAN F. SITTIG and HARDEEP SINGH

3.1 INTRODUCTION

Two Institute of Medicine (IOM) reports have recommended the use of information technologies to improve patient safety and reduce errors in health care [1,2]. Broadly speaking, health information technology (HIT) is the overarching term applied to various information and communication technologies to collect, transmit, display, or store patient data. Despite HIT's promise in improving safety, recent literature has revealed potential safety hazards associated with its use, often referred to as e-iatrogenesis [3,4]. For example, Koppel et al. described 22 types of errors facilitated by a commercially-available EHR system's computerized provider order entry (CPOE) application [5]. In response to similar emerging concerns , the Office of the National Coordinator for HIT recently sponsored an IOM committee to "review the available evidence and the experience from the field" on how HIT use affects patient safety. Given the national impact of HIT, this initiative is a major step forward in ensuring safety and well-being of our patients. However, the field currently lacks acceptable definitions of HIT-related errors and it's unclear how best to measure or analyze "HIT errors".

The goal of this manuscript is to advance the understanding of HIT-related errors and explain how adverse events, near misses, and patient harm can result from problems with HIT itself or from interactions between HIT, its users, and the work system. HIT errors almost always jeopardize patient outcomes and have high potential for harm [6]. This is because many of these errors are latent errors that occur at the "blunt end" of the healthcare system [7], with potential to affect large numbers of patients if not corrected. Furthermore, if important structural or process-related HIT problems are not addressed proactively, care of millions of patients may be affected due to impending widespread adoption and implementation of EHRs [8]. We thus focus this manuscript heavily on errors related to the use of EHR systems.

3.2   GENERAL CRITERIA FOR A HIT ERROR

We define the HIT work system as the combination of the hardware and software required to implement the HIT as well as the social environment in which it is implemented. We thus propose that HIT errors should be defined from the sociotechnical viewpoint of end users (including patients, when applicable) rather than from the purely technical viewpoint of manufacturers, developers, vendors, and personnel responsible for implementation. Health information technology–related error occurs anytime the HIT system is unavailable for use, malfunctions during use, is used incorrectly, or when HIT interacts with another system component incorrectly resulting in data being lost or incorrectly entered, displayed, or transmitted. [10-11] Errors with HIT may involve failures of either structures or processes and can occur in the design and development, implementation and use, or evaluation and optimization phases of the HIT life cycle. [12] This approach is consistent with the currently recommended systems and human factors approaches used to understand and reduce error. [1]

The HIT system is considered to be unavailable for use if for any reason the user cannot enter, review, transmit, or print data (eg, patient's

TABLE 1: Examples of the types of errors that can occur within each dimension of the sociotechnical model [16] and corresponding suggested mitigating procedures

Socio-technical model dimension	Examples of types of errors that could occur in each dimension	Examples of potential ways to reduce likelihood of these errors
Hardware and Software – required to run the healthcare applications	Computer or network is not functioning [17]	Provide redundant hardware for all essential patient care activities
	Input data truncated (i.e. buffer overflow) – some entered data lost	Warn users when data entered exceeds amount that can be stored
Clinical Content – data, information, and knowledge entered, displayed, or transmitted	Allowable item can't be ordered (e.g. no "amoxicillin" in the antibiotic pick-list) [5]	Conduct extensive pre-release testing on all system-system data and human-computer interfaces to insure that new features are working as planned and that existing features are working as before
	Incorrect default dosage for given medication [5]	
Human Computer Interface – aspects of the system that users can see, touch, or hear	Data entry/review screen does not show patient name, medical record number, birthdate, etc.	Encourage and provide methods for clinicians to report when patient-specific screesn to not contain key patient demographics so that software can be fixed.
	Wrong decision about KCl administration based on poor data presentation on the computer screen [18]	Improve data displays and train users to routinely review and cross-validate all data values before making critical decisions
	Two buttons with same label, but different functionality	Pre-release inspection of all screens for duplicate button names
People – the humans involved in the design, development, implementation, and use of HIT	Two patients with same name; data entered on wrong patient [19]	Alert providers to potential duplicate patients and require re-confirmation of patient ID before saving data (e.g. display patient photo before signing)
	Incorrect merge of two patients' data [20]	Develop tools to compare key demographic data and calculate a probability estimate of similarity
	RNs scan duplicate patient barcode taped to their clipboard rather than barcode on patient to save time [21]	Improve user training, user interfaces, work processes, and organizational policies to reduce need for workarounds

TABLE 1: (*Continued*)

Workflow and Communication – the steps needed to ensure that each patient receives the care they need at the time they need it	Computer discontinues a medication order without notifying a human	Implement fail-safe communication (e.g. resend message to another hospital designee if no response from MD or RN) for all computer-generated actions [22]
	Critical abnormal test result alerts not followed up [23]	Implement robust quality insurance systems to monitor critical alert follow-up rates [24]; use "dual notification" for alerts judiciously [25]
Organizational Policies and Procedures – internal culture, structures, policies, and procedures that affect all aspects of HIT management and healthcare	Policy contradicts physical reality (e.g. required barcode med administration readers not available in all patient locations) [21]	Conduct pre- and post-implementation inspections, interviews, and monitor feedback from users in all physical locations
	Policy contradicts personnel capability (e.g. one pharmacist to verify all orders entered via CPOE in large hospital)	Conduct pre- and post-implementation interviews with all affected users to better gauge workload
	Incorrect policy allows "hard-stops" on clinical alerts, causing delays in needed therapy [26]	Disallow "hard-stops" on alerts; users should be able to override the computer in all but the most egregious cases (e.g. ordering promethazine as IV push by peripheral vein [27])
External Rules, Regulations, and Pressures – external forces that facilitate or place constraints on the design, development, implementation, use, and evaluation of HIT in the clinical setting	Billing requirements lead to inaccurate documentation in EHR (e.g. inappropriate copy and paste)	Highlight all "pasted" material and include reference to source of material
	Joint Commission required medication reconciliation processes [28] causing rushed development of new medication reconciliation applications that were difficult to use and caused errors [29]; rescinded safety goal [30] only to reinstate it 7/1/2011 [31]	Carefully considrer potential adverse unintentded consequences before making new rules or regulations; conduct interviews and observations of users to gauge effects of rules and regulations on patient safety, quality of care, and clinician work-life
System Measurement and Monitoring – of system availability	Incomplete or inappropriate (e.g. combining disparate data) data aggregation leads to erroneous reporting	Increase measurement and monitoring transparency by providing involved stakeholders with access to raw data, analytical methods, and reports

medication allergies or most recent laboratory test results). Reasons could include unavailable computer hardware (eg, missing keyboard or problems with the computer's monitor, network routers that connect the computer to the data servers and printers, or the server where data are stored), unavailable software (eg, missing components of the operating system that manages either the computer applications such as the internet browser and EHR or the interface between an EHR system and the information system of an ancillary service such as radiology or laboratory), and interruption of power sources (eg, a power outage that results in hospital-wide computer failure). [4]

The HIT system is considered to be malfunctioning (ie, available, but not working correctly) whenever a user cannot accomplish the desired task despite using the HIT system as designed. In this situation, error results from any hardware or software defect (or bug) that prohibits a user from entering or reviewing data or any defect that causes the data to be entered, displayed, transmitted, or stored incorrectly. For example, the clinician might enter a patient's weight in pounds, and the weight-based dosing algorithm might fail to convert it to kilograms before calculating the appropriate dose, resulting in a 2-fold overdose.

Finally, errors can occur even when hardware and software are functioning as designed. For instance, errors may result when users do not use the hardware or software as intended. For example, users might enter free-text comments (eg, "take 7.5 mg Mon-Fri only") that contradict information contained in the structured section of the medication order (eg, "Warfarin tabs 10 mg Q day"). [13] Errors may also arise when 2 or more parts of the HIT system (eg, CPOE application and the pharmacy's medication-dispensing system) interact in an unpredicted manner, resulting in inaccurate, incomplete, or lost data during entry, display, transmission, or storage. [14]

3.3   ORIGIN-SPECIFIC TYPOLOGY FOR A HIT ERROR

Leveson [15] proposes that new technologies have fundamentally altered the nature of errors and asserts that these changes necessitate new models

and methods for investigating technology-related errors. Thus, technological advances could potentially give rise to increasingly complex and
multifaceted errors in health care. In view of the resultant expanding and
evolving context of safe HIT implementation and use, we illustrate how a
recently developed sociotechnical model for HIT evaluation and use can
provide an origin-specific typology for HIT errors. [16] The model's 8
dimensions (Table 1) comprehensively account for the technology; its users and their respective workflow processes and how these 2 elements
interface with the technology; the work system context, including organizational and policy factors that affect HIT; and notably, the interactions
between all of these factors.[17] The Table lists examples of specific EHR-
related errors that can occur within each of the 8 dimensions of the socio-
technical model, along with examples of potential ways that the likelihood of each error could be reduced. Thus, the model not only illustrates
the complex relationships between active and latent errors but also lays a
foundation for error analysis.

3.4   CONCLUSION

Rapid advances in HIT development, implementation, and regulation
have complicated the landscape of HIT-related safety issues. Erroneous or missing data and the decisions based on them increase the
risk of an adverse event and unnecessary costs. Because these errors
can and frequently do occur after implementation, simply increasing
oversight of HIT vendors' development processes will not address all
HIT-related errors. Comprehensive efforts to reduce HIT errors must
start with clear definitions and an origin-focused understanding of
HIT errors that addresses important sociotechnical aspects of HIT use
and implementation. To this end, we provide herein a much needed
foundation for coordinating safety initiatives of HIT designers, developers, implementers, users, and policy makers, who must continue to
work together to achieve a high-reliability HIT work system for safe
patient care.

REFERENCES

1. Institute of Medicine. To Err Is Human: Building a Safer Health System. Washington, DC: National Academy Press; 1999.
2. Institute of Medicine. Patient Safety: Achieving a New Standard for Care. Washington, DC: National Academy Press; 2004.
3. Weiner JP, Kfuri T, Chan K, Fowles JB. "e-Iatrogenesis": the most critical unintended consequence of CPOE and other HIT. J Am Med Inform Assoc. 2007;14(3):387-389.
4. Myers RB, Jones SL, Sittig DF. Reported clinical information system adverse events in US Food and Drug Administration databases. http://aci.schattauer.de/en/contents/archive/issue/1349/manuscript/15776.html. Accessed May 17, 2011.
5. Koppel R, Metlay JP, Cohen A, et al. Role of computerized physician order entry systems in facilitating medication errors. JAMA. 2005;293(10):1197-1203.
6. Office of the National Coordinator for HIT. Patient safety and health information technology. http://www.iom.edu/Activities/Quality/PatientSafetyHIT.aspx. Accessed June 8, 2011.
7. Hofer TP, Kerr EA, Hayward RA. What is an error? Eff Clin Pract. 2000;3(6):261-269/
8. Reason J. Human error: models and management. BMJ. 2000;320(7237):768-770.
9. Stead W, ed, Lin H, ed. Computational Technology for Effective Health Care: Immediate Steps and Strategic Directions. Washington, DC: National Academies Press; 2009.
10. Mangalmurti SS, Murtagh L, Mello MM. Medical malpractice liability in the age of electronic health records. N Engl J Med. 2010;363(21):2060-2067.
11. Perrow C. Normal Accidents: Living With High-Risk Technologies. Princeton, NJ: Princeton University Press; 1999.
12. Walker JM, Carayon P, Leveson N, et al. EHR safety: the way forward to safe and effective systems. J Am Med Inform Assoc. 2008;15(3):272-277.
13. Singh H, Mani S, Espadas D, Petersen N, Franklin V, Petersen LA. Prescription errors and outcomes related to inconsistent information transmitted through computerized order entry: a prospective study. Arch Intern Med. 2009;169(10):982-989.
14. Kleiner B. Sociotechnical system design in health care. In: Carayon P, ed. Handbook of Human Factors and Ergonomics in Health Care and Patient Safety. Mahwah, NJ: Lawrence Erlbaum; 2007.
15. Leveson N. A new accident model for engineering safer systems. Saf Sci. 2004;42(4):237-270.
16. Sittig DF, Singh H. Eight rights of safe electronic health record use. JAMA. 2009;302(10):1111-1113.

17. Sittig DF, Singh H. A new sociotechnical model for studying health information technology in complex adaptive healthcare systems. Qual Saf Health Care. 2010;19(suppl 3) i68-i74.

18. Kilbridge P. Computer crash: lessons from a system failure. N Engl J Med. 2003;348(10):881-882.

19. Horsky J, Kuperman GJ, Patel VL. Comprehensive analysis of a medication dosing error related to CPOE. J Am Med Inform Assoc. 2005;12(4):377-382.

20. Shojania KG. Patient mix-up. http://www.webmm.ahrq.gov/case.aspx?caseID=1. Accessed May 17, 2011.

21. AHIMA MPI Task Force. Merging master patient indexes. http://www.cstp.umkc.edu/~leeyu/Mahi/medical-data6.pdf. Accessed May 17, 2011.

22. Koppel R, Wetterneck T, Telles JL, Karsh BT. Workarounds to barcode medication administration systems: their occurrences, causes, and threats to patient safety. J Am Med Inform Assoc. 2008;15(4):408-423.

23. Kuperman GJ, Teich JM, Tanasijevic MJ, et al. Improving response to critical laboratory results with automation: results of a randomized controlled trial. J Am Med Inform Assoc. 1999;6(6):512-522.

24. Singh H, Wilson L, Petersen LA, et al. Improving follow-up of abnormal cancer screens using electronic health records: trust but verify test result communication. BMC Med Inform Decis Mak. 2009;949.

25. Singh H, Thomas EJ, Sittig DF, et al. Notification of abnormal lab test results in an electronic medical record: do any safety concerns remain? Am J Med. 2010;123(3):238-244.

26. Singh H, Thomas EJ, Mani S, et al. Timely follow-up of abnormal diagnostic imaging test results in an outpatient setting: are electronic medical records achieving their potential? Arch Intern Med. 2009;169(17):1578-1586.

27. Strom BL, Schinnar R, Aberra F, et al. Unintended effects of a computerized physician order entry nearly hard-stop alert to prevent a drug interaction: a randomized controlled trial. Arch Intern Med. 2010;170(17):1578-1583.

28. Grissinger M. Preventing serious tissue injury with intravenous promethazine (phenergan). P T. 2009;34(4):175-176.

29. Joint Commission on Accreditation of Healthcare Organizations (JCAHO). JCAHO 2005 National Patient Safety Goals: Goal 8. http://www.fojp.com/Focus_2005_1.pdf. Accessed May 17, 2011.

30. Poon EG, Blumenfeld B, Hamann C, et al. Design and implementation of an application and associated services to support interdisciplinary medication reconciliation efforts at an integrated healthcare delivery network. J Am Med Inform Assoc. 2006;13(6):581-592.

31. Joint Commission on Accreditation of Healthcare Organizations. Approved: will not score medication reconciliation in 2009. http://www.jcrinc.com/common/PDFs/fpdfs/pubs/pdfs/JCReqs/JCP-03-09-S1.pdf. Accessed May 17, 2011.

32. Joint Commission Online. Revised NPSG on medication reconciliation is approved. http://www.jointcommission.org/assets/1/18/jconline_Dec_8_10.pdf. Accessed May 17, 2011.

CHAPTER 4

A RED-FLAG BASED APPROACH TO RISK MANAGEMENT OF EHR-RELATED SAFETY CONCERNS

DEAN F. SITTIG and HARDEEP SINGH

4.1 INTRODUCTION

Although electronic health records (EHRs) have a significant potential to improve patient safety, EHR-related safety concerns have begun to emerge. For instance, some unique risks of EHRs are inherent to the technologies themselves, whereas others are related to how these technologies are applied and used [1].

We previously participated in a web-based survey of the memberships of the American Society for Healthcare Risk Management and the American Health Lawyers Association between August and September 2012. A 17-item survey was developed to capture information about four content areas: (1) extent of EHR use at the primary facility of practice; (2) frequency of EHR-related serious safety events; (3) variables affecting EHR-related serious safety events; and (4) tracking of EHR-related safety measurements. Of 15,400 member e-mail invitations, the survey was completed by 369 respondents (2.4%), a majority of whom worked for large hospitals and healthcare systems. Based on this survey and supplemented by our previous work in EHR-related patient safety, we identified the following common EHR-related safety concerns:

1. Incorrect patient identification
2. Extended EHR unavailability (either planned or unplanned)
3. Failure to heed a computer-generated warning or alert
4. System-to-system interface errors

5. Failure to identify, find, or use the most recent patient data
6. Misunderstandings about time
7. Incorrect item selected from a list of items
8. Open or incomplete orders

Guidance for risk managers on how they should approach these safety concerns is limited. Many EHR-related safety concerns are not visible or apparent to end users. Others are distributed such that one user is often unaware of the broader significance of the safety concern (e.g., errors in system interfaces between the EHR and ancillary systems may not be visible since the person entering the order rarely sees what the ancillary system receives). Thus, voluntary detection and reporting of EHR-related safety problems may be an inadequate strategy. In this paper, we present a "red flag"-based approach that can be used by risk managers to identify potential EHR safety concerns in their institution. Red flags are indications that something may be wrong and should be given additional consideration or evaluation. In medicine, clinicians commonly look for red flags indicating that a seemingly minor problem may be more serious. For example, a 60-year-old patient who complains of a cough for a week may be given a diagnosis of upper respiratory infection and a prescription for cough syrup, whereas a 60-year-old patient who indicates he is coughing up blood warrants special attention, perhaps a chest x-ray [2], the red flag being that blood in sputum at that age could suggest another problem such as a lung cancer.

Risk managers routinely collect quality and safety data from multiple sources and are often privy to data from sources unavailable to information technology (IT) specialists or clinicians. Thus, risk managers are in a unique position to conduct a red-flag based analysis. In order to develop these red flags, we conducted an extensive literature search and relied heavily on our extensive experience in EHR-related patient safety research. In the following sections, we define each error type and list several "red flags" that risk managers or other interested parties can use to identify potential EHR-related safety issues within their organizations.

4.2 INCORRECT PATIENT IDENTIFICATION

There are two types of patient identification errors. A duplicate record exists when a single patient has more than one medical record. A co-mingled record exists when a single medical record contains information about two or more patients. Duplicate records are created when users create a new record for a patient with an existing record or when patient records from disparate systems are combined without checking for matching records. Co-mingled records result from incorrect patient selection and subsequent use [3]. The likelihood of such events is greatly increased when a) looking up patients in large, multi-institutional healthcare systems that may have over a million patient records; b) looking for patients with "common" names (e.g., Smith, Williams, Jones, Garcia, Rodriguez, etc.); c) attempting to merge patient records from two or more disparate systems without using state-of-the-art patient record matching algorithms; and d) allowing clinicians to open two or more patient records (i.e., either multiple tabs or windows) on the same device.

4.2.1 RED FLAGS FOR INCORRECT PATIENT IDENTIFICATION

- Key patient identifying information (i.e., first and last name, date of birth, gender, medical record number, inpatient location or home address, picture [4]) is missing from EHR screens or printouts [5].
- Absence of documented processes and procedures for checking patient ID at essential stages of a patient visit (e.g., when patients are called back for rooming, at entering of vital signs, prior to labs, procedures or medication administration, at checkout, etc.).
- A large number of clinician calls (e.g., > 1/1000 orders or notes entered) request "help desk" or IT support to move their erroneous EHR entries from patient A (the wrong patient) to patient B (the right patient). Incorrect entries could include orders, order sets, clinical notes, or test results.
- Nurses use copies of one or more patient barcode identification bands taped to their clipboard as a work-around when performing barcoded medication administration [6].
- A wrong site or wrong patient surgery or procedure was traced back to an order entered on the wrong patient.

- Greater than expected number of "erroneous notes" in the EHR (i.e., notes entered incorrectly on another patient) as identified by an automated scan of all notes in the system [7].

4.3   EXTENDED EHR UNAVAILABILITY (EITHER PLANNED OR UNPLANNED)

Extended (i.e., > 4 hours) EHR unavailability means that some portion, or more likely, all of the patient's medical records are unavailable for review. It results from total or partial failure or planned downtime in any part of the EHR computing infrastructure (e.g., electrical power, network connections, database servers, computer-to-computer interfaces, computer terminals on patient care units, software upgrades, etc.) [8]. These problems can lead to temporary, or even permanent, loss of data or inability to send or receive information from others [9]. The organization must do everything it can to reduce the likelihood of these events as well as prepare to continue providing care in the event a system failure does occur [10].

4.3.1   RED FLAGS FOR EXTENDED EHR UNAVAILABILITY

- Absence of documented EHR downtime and reactivation procedures.
- Absence of notification procedures for scheduled downtimes, suggesting poor preparedness for downtimes lasting longer than anticipated.
- No regular off-site backup of all data required to continue caring for patients (i.e., demographic, clinical, and financial).
- No pre-printed paper order sheets or clinical documentation forms in clinical care areas.
- Critical clinical computing hardware devices are not configured in a redundant manner (i.e., if one device fails, a backup device does not take over the work).
- Read-only summaries of recent (< 1 hour old) patient data are not available on a standalone computer connected to the "red" electrical plug in clinical areas.

4.4   FAILURE TO HEED A COMPUTER-GENERATED WARNING OR ALERT

Critical information, even if sent to the correct person at the right time and displayed prominently on the computer screen, can be overlooked amidst an overabundance of other false positive information (i.e., items that indicate a given condition exists, when it actually does not). Warnings or alerts can occur either synchronously (i.e., during the activity that the alert pertains to, such as a drug-drug interaction alert during order entry) or asynchronously (i.e., while the user is not engaged in the activity that generated the alert, such as an alert for an abnormal laboratory test result). These missed data can lead to erroneous or delayed diagnoses or treatments.

4.4.1   RED FLAGS FOR FAILURE TO HEED A COMPUTER-GENERATED WARNING OR ALERT

- Reports show widespread non-adherence to computer-generated alerts that are based on recommended guidelines [11].
- Clinicians report receiving too many irrelevant alerts during order entry or as asynchronous messages in their inboxes [12].
- Clinicians report intrusive alerts used to present information that is not critical (e.g., a pop-up message reading "Are you sure you want to send this prescription as an e-script?").
- Clinicians report working at home, staying late after work, or working on weekends to complete all the work in their inboxes (e.g., abnormal laboratory test results, prescription refills, orders to cosign) [13].
- EHR usage logs show that more than 20% of orders entered generate an alert.

4.5   SYSTEM-TO-SYSTEM INTERFACE ERRORS

Errors caused by miscommunication (or non-communication) between applications can result in data from one application (e.g., a laboratory system) failing to reach or being corrupted before reaching another application (e.g., the EHR). These errors can occur due to mistakes in the data translation tables (i.e., used to encode and decode orders and results) that are used to transmit information between components of an EHR or between disparate clinical systems. [14] Mismatched data fields may affect orders or results by introducing inadvertent changes (or outright data loss) that are virtually undetectable by the computer, or by the people not privy to the original sender's intentions.

4.5.1　RED FLAGS FOR SYSTEM-TO-SYSTEM INTERFACE ERRORS

- Orders or test results are reported to be missing for certain patients.
- The "error log" of the interface between components of an EHR contains orders or results that were not able to be transmitted automatically between different components of the EHR system.
- Laboratory reports in the EHR are reported to be incomplete (e.g., missing measurement units, reference ranges, date and time of result, or comments).
- Any report of patient receiving incorrect or unnecessary medications.
- Clinicians report errors or inconsistencies between the structured data fields and free-text comment fields or comments that fail to transfer from system-to-system. [15]
- The organization does not have a method for sending or receiving laboratory tests performed by an outside laboratory through a direct interface to the EHR, (i.e., requiring orders or results to be transmitted via mail or fax). [16]

4.6　FAILURE TO IDENTIFY, FIND, OR USE THE MOST RECENT PATIENT DATA

Failure to find or use the most recent patient data (e.g., medication orders, laboratory or radiology results) can cause clinicians to make erroneous clinical decisions and lead to incorrect, unnecessary, or delayed tests, procedures, or therapies. These failures often result from difficulties navigating, seeing, understanding or interacting with user interfaces.

4.6.1 RED FLAGS FOR FAILURE TO IDENTIFY, FIND, OR USE THE MOST RECENT PATIENT DATA

- EHR displays require either horizontal or vertical scrolling to see the most recent orders or results (i.e., data sorted chronologically [earliest to latest] rather than in reverse chronological order [most recent results first]).
- EHR displays require users to widen data display fields, or columns, to see the complete text of the order or result.
- Clinicians repeatedly order new diagnostic tests within a short time of the previous result. [17]
- Clinicians take inappropriate therapeutic actions due to missing recent test results (e.g., administering potassium when most recent potassium levels are high). [18]
- Diagnostic test results are displayed in multiple locations (i.e., different screens or tabs) in the EHR.

4.7 EHR TIME MEASUREMENT TRANSLATIONAL CHALLENGES

Translational challenges as a result of the inability of computers to properly translate time measurements as they are conceived and entered by users can lead to many different kinds of errors. For example, users may fail to understand how much time has passed since a displayed date (e.g., patient born 11/23/62 is now 50-years-old and due for a colonoscopy). Users often think and enter information in time relative to the current time. This can be difficult for others to interpret, especially at a later date (e.g., surgery scheduled for tomorrow), when historical information is entered with current time stamp, or when the computer is instructed to carry out a specific action at a future date and time without notifying the clinicians or patients affected.

4.7.1 RED FLAGS FOR EHR TIME MEASUREMENT TRANSLATIONAL CHALLENGES

- Routine tests, medications, or procedures ordered "daily" continue long after they are clinically indicated (i.e., no stop date is documented). Examples include daily chest X-rays for previously intubated patient and prophylactic antibiotics continued after 10 days with no sign of infection.

- Repeated delays in administration of time-sensitive medications (e.g., anti-biotics) ordered as "next routine administration time," or double doses are given when a multi-day course of medication is ordered to begin "now" and then inadvertently repeated when the "next routine administration time" occurs soon after the order time. [19]
- Clinicians report that critical medications have been cancelled automatically with no notice to clinicians. [20]
- Clinicians are unable to create reminders for future important actions within the EHR. [21]
- "Urgent" or "STAT" flags on orders are overused (e.g., more than 50% of orders placed as STAT on acute care hospital units) or any other evidence that clinicians are not confident in the EHR's ability to communicate their routine instructions in a timely manner.

4.8   INCORRECT ITEM SELECTED FROM A LIST OF ITEMS

Juxtaposition errors occur when an EHR user inadvertently selects a listed item that is directly adjacent to the item he or she intended to select. [22] These errors can occur if the user does not notice or understand the difference between items or simply selects the incorrect item. [23]

4.8.1   *RED FLAGS FOR INCORRECT ITEM SELECTED FROM A LIST OF ITEMS*

- Drop-down or static selection lists are too narrow to display the complete text of all items, include too many items, or items are too close together. [24]
- Drop-down or static selection lists are sorted alphabetically (i.e., rather than grouped by similarity of concept) or consist of all CAPITAL LETTERS.
- Clinicians or members of ancillary services report patient orders for wrong medications, diagnostic tests, or therapeutic procedures.
- A large number of orders are discontinued soon after they are entered.
- The EHR user interface has multiple cascading or fly-out sub-menus (i.e., secondary and tertiary menus displayed on demand from within the primary menu) [25].

4.9 OPEN OR INCOMPLETE ORDERS

Open or incomplete orders can result from failure to complete the order entry process including signing and submitting the order(s), or from failure of supervising physicians to co-sign orders that require co-signatures before becoming active. Although these errors may result from clinician oversight, they can also result from user interfaces that make it difficult to understand the current state of user actions.

4.9.1 RED FLAGS FOR OPEN OR INCOMPLETE ORDERS

- Orders requiring co-signature in a queue that are overdue according to the organization's policy (e.g., 24-48 hours old).
- A large number of incomplete tasks appear in various computer logs (e.g., unsigned orders, discharge summaries, dictated notes, etc.)
- Clinicians complain that the system is "losing" their orders (i.e., orders that they have entered are not carried out).
- Some providers use a high percentage of "verbal" orders, rather than entering them into the computer themselves.
- Referring providers do not receive notification back from specialists about consultations that are completed.

4.10 DISCUSSION

We have provided a list of red flags that risk managers can consider using in their ongoing activities to improve patient safety within the context of EHR-enabled healthcare delivery. Identifying that one or more common EHR-related safety concerns has occurred is only the first step in resolving a problem. In most cases, the risk manager or other responsible party should convene a multi-disciplinary group, including members of the IT department and affected clinicians, to investigate the causes of the problem. It may be necessary to work with the EHR vendor to identify the cause of the problem and potential solutions.

While we discussed many types of EHR-related safety concerns, these concerns likely represent only the tip of the iceberg. There might be other concerns we have missed. For instance, adoption of EHRs is still less than

50% of physicians [26] and currently, comprehensive closed claims analysis of EHR-related safety concerns is not available. Thus, the red flags listed could represent only a fraction of the possible factors that can be used to detect EHR-related problems. An organization that routinely conducts EHR-related surveillance activities, such as the ones proposed here, can significantly reduce the risks associated with EHR implementations.

4.11   CONCLUSION

EHRs represent one of the most important tools available to improve patient safety in healthcare organizations. Nevertheless, without careful and continuous surveillance of these systems as implemented, safety concerns can arise. Organizations can dramatically reduce both the number and severity of EHR-related serious safety events by addressing these red flags.

REFERENCES

1.   Sittig DF, Singh H. Electronic health records and national patient-safety goals. N Engl J Med. 2012 Nov 8;367(19):1854-60. doi: 10.1056/NEJMsb1205420.
2.   MedLinePlus. Coughing up blood. Available at: http://www.nlm.nih.gov/medlineplus/ency/article/003073.htm
3.   Henneman PL, Fisher DL, Henneman EA, Pham TA, Campbell MM, Nathanson BH. Patient identification errors are common in a simulated setting. Ann Emerg Med. 2010 Jun;55(6):503-9. doi: 10.1016/j.annemergmed.2009.11.017.
4.   Hyman D, Laire M, Redmond D, Kaplan DW. The use of patient pictures and verification screens to reduce computerized provider order entry errors. Pediatrics. 2012 Jul;130(1):e211-9. doi: 10.1542/peds.2011-2984.
5.   NHS CUI Programme Team, National Health Service Common User Interface (CUI) Design Guide Workstream – Design Guide Entry – Patient Banner v4.0.0.0 Baseline. Last modified on 25 June 2009 Available at: http://www.cuisecure.nhs.uk/CAPS/Patient%20Identification1/Patient%20Banner.pdf
6.   Koppel R, Wetterneck T, Telles JL, Karsh BT. Workarounds to barcode medication administration systems: their occurrences, causes, and threats to patient safety. J Am Med Inform Assoc. 2008 Jul-Aug;15(4):408-23. doi: 10.1197/jamia.M2616. Epub 2008 Apr 24.
7.   Wilcox AB, Chen YH, Hripcsak G. Minimizing electronic health record patient-note mismatches. J Am Med Inform Assoc. 2011 Jul-Aug;18(4):511-4. doi: 10.1136/amiajnl-2010-000068.

8. Hanuscak TL, Szeinbach SL, Seoane-Vazquez E, Reichert BJ, McCluskey CF. Evaluation of causes and frequency of medication errors during information technology downtime. Am J Health Syst Pharm. 2009 Jun 15;66(12):1119-24. doi: 10.2146/ajhp080389.

9. Sittig DF, Singh H. Defining health information technology-related errors: new developments since to err is human. Arch Intern Med. 2011 Jul 25;171(14):1281-4.

10. Nelson NC. Downtime procedures for a clinical information system: a critical issue. J Crit Care. 2007 Mar;22(1):45-50.

11. McCoy AB, Waitman LR, Lewis JB, Wright JA, Choma DP, Miller RA, Peterson JF. A framework for evaluating the appropriateness of clinical decision support alerts and responses. J Am Med Inform Assoc. 2012 May-Jun;19(3):346-52. doi: 10.1136/amiajnl-2011-000185.

12. Murphy DR, Reis B, Kadiyala H, Hirani K, Sittig DF, Khan MM, Singh H. Electronic health record-based messages to primary care providers: valuable information or just noise? Arch Intern Med. 2012 Feb 13;172(3):283-5.

13. Murphy DR, Reis B, Sittig DF, Singh H. Notifications received by primary care practitioners in electronic health records: a taxonomy and time analysis. Am J Med. 2012 Feb;125(2):209.e1-7.

14. Hamblin JF, Bwitit PT, Moriarty HT. Pathology results in the electronic health record. Electronic Journal of Health Informatics 2010;5(2):2010;5(2)e15. Available at http://www.ejhi.net/ojs/index.php/ejhi/article/view/131

15. Singh H, Mani S, Espadas D, Petersen N, Franklin V, Petersen LA. Prescription errors and outcomes related to inconsistent information transmitted through computerized order entry: a prospective study. Arch Intern Med. 2009 May 25;169(10):982-9. doi: 10.1001/archinternmed.2009.102.

16. Sittig DF, Singh H. Improving test result follow-up through electronic health records requires more than just an alert. J Gen Intern Med. 2012 Oct;27(10):1235-7.

17. Bates DW, Kuperman GJ, Rittenberg E, Teich JM, Fiskio J, Ma'luf N, Onderdonk A, Wybenga D, Winkelman J, Brennan TA, Komaroff AL, Tanasijevic M. A randomized trial of a computer-based intervention to reduce utilization of redundant laboratory tests. Am J Med. 1999 Feb;106(2):144-50.

18. Horsky J, Kuperman GJ, Patel VL. Comprehensive analysis of a medication dosing error related to CPOE. J Am Med Inform Assoc. 2005 Jul-Aug;12(4):377-82. Epub 2005 Mar 31.

19. FitzHenry F, Peterson JF, Arrieta M, Waitman LR, Schildcrout JS, Miller RA. Medication administration discrepancies persist despite electronic ordering. J Am Med Inform Assoc. 2007 Nov-Dec;14(6):756-64.

20. Institute for Safe Medication Practices (ISMP) Alert. Let's put a stop to problem-prone automatic stop order policies. August 9, 2000. Available at: http://www.ismp.org/newsletters/acutecare/articles/20000809_2.asp

21. Poon EG, Kuperman GJ, Fiskio J, Bates DW. Real-time notification of laboratory data requested by users through alphanumeric pagers. J Am Med Inform Assoc. 2002 May-Jun;9(3):217-22.

22. Walsh KE, Adams WG, Bauchner H, Vinci RJ, Chessare JB, Cooper MR, Hebert PM, Schainker EG, Landrigan CP. Medication errors related to computerized order entry for children. Pediatrics. 2006 Nov;118(5):1872-9.

23. Zhan C, Hicks RW, Blanchette CM, Keyes MA, Cousins DD. Potential benefits and problems with computerized prescriber order entry: analysis of a voluntary medication error-reporting database. Am J Health Syst Pharm. 2006 Feb 15;63(4):353-8.

24. Khajouei R, Jaspers MW. The impact of CPOE medication systems' design aspects on usability, workflow and medication orders: a systematic review. Methods Inf Med. 2010;49(1):3-19. doi: 10.3414/ME0630. Epub 2009 Jul 6. Review.

25. Tullis TS, Connor E, LeDoux L, Chadwick-Dias A, True M, Catani M. A Study of Website Navigation Methods. Usability Professionals Association (UPA) 2005 Conference in Montreal, Quebec. Available at: http://www.eastonmass.net/tullis/WebsiteNavigation/WebsiteNavigationPaper.htm

26. Wright A, Henkin S, Feblowitz J, McCoy AB, Bates DW, Sittig DF. Early results of the meaningful use program for electronic health records. N Engl J Med. 2013 Feb 21;368(8):779-80. doi: 10.1056/NEJMc1213481.

Sittig D.F., Singh H. A Red-Flag Based Approach to Risk Management of EHR-Related Safety Concerns. (in process). Journal of Healthcare Risk Management 2013. This article was originally published in the Q4 2013 Volume 33 No. 2 issue of the Journal of Healthcare Risk Management published by ASHRM and John Wiley & Sons, Inc. Used with permission.

CHAPTER 5

MATCHING IDENTIFIERS IN ELECTRONIC HEALTH RECORDS: IMPLICATIONS FOR DUPLICATE RECORDS AND PATIENT SAFETY

ALLISON B. MCCOY, ADAM WRIGHT, MICHAEL G. KAHN, JASON S. SHAPIRO, ELMER VICTOR BERNSTAM, and DEAN F. SITTIG

5.1 BACKGROUND AND SIGNIFICANCE

Increasing adoption of electronic health records (EHRs) and renewed emphasis on health information exchange (HIE) are leading to growing quantities of electronically available patient data that have the potential to reduce errors in a variety of ways, including improved clinical decision support. [1 ,2] However, health information technology (HIT) may also be associated with new errors. [3] One scenario that may lead to HIT-related errors is duplicate patient records. Three scenarios exist in relation to duplicate patient records: a correct registration exists when a single individual has a single medical record, a duplicate record exists when a single individual has more than one medical record, and a commingled record exists when a single medical record contains information about two or more individuals (figure 1).

When duplicate records occur, a clinician could easily miss important information that exists in a different record than the one that was initially accessed, and such gaps in information are associated with increased adverse outcomes. [4 ,5] One recent study found that duplicate records, even when empty, were associated with missed abnormal test results. [6] Prior research describes the occurrence of duplicate patient records in clinical datasets, frequently in the setting of creating master patient indexes (MPIs) for HIEs and data warehouses, and reports a number of methods

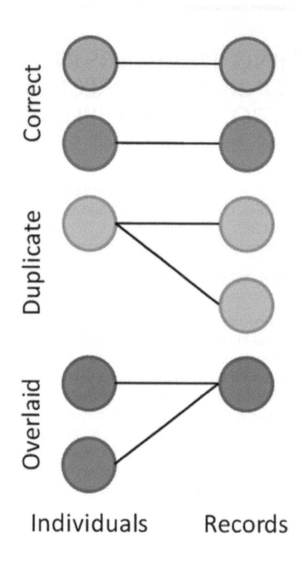

FIGURE 1: Scenarios for duplicate records.

for identifying and merging duplicate records that range from comparison of basic demographic data to probabilistic algorithms that include various spellings and forms of demographics or clinical data. [7–19]

A number of approaches to managing duplicate records have been described previously. The first approach is prevention, where institutions try to keep duplicate records from occurring. Prevention approaches include effective training, centralised registration, notifications to users when creating a new record that is similar to an existing record, and use of MPI technology. [10 ,20] When prevention is not implemented or is insufficient, institutions must have methods in place to detect duplicate records. Detection methods may include automated (eg, deterministic or probabilistic) and manual reviews for similarity. [7 ,11–13 ,17 ,21] After duplicate records have been detected, they must be removed. Finally, institutions should adopt error mitigation approaches, to prevent or reduce patient harm when duplicate or potentially duplicate patient records persist within systems. Methods for mitigating errors include notifying users who access a record that is similar to another record, alternating row colours in patient lists, requiring photo or biometric (eg, vein pattern matching) identification during patient registration and including an up-to-date picture of the patient in the record. [8 ,20 ,22–26]

One important indicator of a duplicate record is matching identifiers, for example, two records that have the same first and last names and dates of birth. However, two distinct individuals may have the same identifiers, especially when only first and last name are used. [27] These demographic collisions may be more common in settings with less heterogeneity among names, such as an institution with a larger percentage of minority patients.9 While potentially duplicate records are technically correct, they may leave patients at risk for misidentification, or a wrong patient error. Extensive previous literature describes these errors, which commonly include ordering or administration of medication or care to the wrong patient. [20 ,22–26 28–31] Duplicate records may also exist when the demographics are different; for example, a woman could have one record under her maiden name and one record under her married name. However, these scenarios are more difficult to detect and may require more complex, automated or manual approaches beyond matching first name, last name and date of birth.

In this paper, we quantify the number of patients at five institutions with identical first and last names and dates of birth as an indicator of duplicate or potentially duplicate records. We then identify solutions that may assist in detection, prevention and removal of duplicate records, reporting the rate of adoption of each method across the five institutions, and describing best practice recommendations for maximising patient safety related to records with matching identifiers.

5.2 METHODS

5.2.1 DATA COLLECTION

We performed a retrospective evaluation in five healthcare settings utilising EHRs: two large urban teaching hospitals with affiliated ambulatory practices across a variety of specialties using a locally developed EHR and Allscripts Enterprise EHR, a free-standing children's hospital using Epic, a regional HIE, and a large teaching hospital using Epic that is a member of the regional HIE. The study was approved by the institutional review board at each location.

5.2.2 QUANTIFICATION OF MATCHING PATIENT IDENTIFIERS

In each setting, we retrieved record counts, which were reported as the number of distinct medical record numbers (MRNs) having the matching identifier; individual elements of a patient's electronic medical record (eg, result reports, visit notes) were not counted separately, unless the patient had multiple MRNs. We first retrieved deidentified counts for records with exact matching first and last names, determining the occurrence of matching name pairs and the number of records associated with each matching name pair. We then repeated the process to retrieve counts for records with matching first name, last name and date of birth. Middle names or initials were not used, even if present. To depict the worst case for matching identifiers, we also retrieved the top 250 most common name pairs in each setting, determining the number of records occurring for each.

5.2.3 REVIEW OF METHODS FOR MANAGING DUPLICATE RECORDS OR RECORDS WITH MATCHING IDENTIFIERS

Through literature review and assessment of practices in place at each site of analysis, we identified methods for preventing, detecting and removing duplicate records in EHRs, in addition to methods for mitigating errors that may result from records with matching identifiers. For each site, we recorded whether the identified methods had been implemented.

5.3 RESULTS

5.3.1 QUANTIFICATION OF MATCHING PATIENT IDENTIFIERS

Table 1 depicts the occurrence of matching patient first and last names, and table 2 depicts the occurrence of matching patient first name, last name and date of birth. The number of total records and rates of matching identifiers varied across settings; Sites A and B had the highest percentage of patients having a matching identifier when using first and last names (40.07% and 40.66%, respectively) and when including date of birth (13.36% and 15.47%, respectively). Site C had the lowest percentage of patients having a matching identifier when using first and last name (16.49%), while Site D had the lowest percentage of patients having a matching identifier when including date of birth (0.16%). The rate of matches decreased substantially for each site when including the date of birth as an identifier.

Figure 2 illustrates the number of records having the same first and last name for the 250 most commonly occurring names in each setting. The most frequently occurring name pair for Sites A, B, C, D and E had 2552, 744, 41, 53 and 1634 distinct records, respectively.

TABLE 1: Patient records with matching first and last name

	Site A	Site B	Site C	Site D	Site E
Total records in the study setting database	4,256,844	2,678,033	1,014,969	1,012,059	779,736
Unique records identified by first and last name (%)	2,551,050 (59.93)	1,589,030 (59.34)	847,642 (83.51)	767,397 (75.83)	598,776 (76.79)
Records having one or more matching first and last name	1,705,794 (40.07)	1,089,003 (40.66)	167,327 (16.49)	244,662 (24,17)	180,960 (23.39)

TABLE 2: Patient records with matching first name, last name, and date of birth

	Site A	Site B	Site C	Site D	Site E
Total records in the study setting database	4,256,844	2,678,033	1,014,969	1,012,059	779,736
Unique records identified by first name, last name, and date of birth (%)	3,720,412 (87.40)	2,263,616 (84.53)	969,753 (95.55)	1,010,476 (99.84)	747,596 (95.88)
Records having one or more matching first name, last name, and date of birth	536,432 (13.36)	414,417 (15.47)	45,216 (4.45)	1,583 (0.16)	32,140 (4.35)

5.3.2 IMPLEMENTATION OF METHODS FOR MANAGING DUPLICATE RECORDS OR RECORDS WITH MATCHING IDENTIFIERS

Table 3 depicts the methods for each approach implemented by each institution to manage duplicate records or records with matching identifiers. The most frequently implemented approaches included those for prevention, with four sites implementing more than one method. Of the three sites having implemented MPI technology, two implemented technology from Initiate Systems (acquired by IBM) and one implemented Cerner Enterprise Master Patient Index. Detection and removal approaches were also frequently implemented, while only two sites implemented error mitigation approaches.

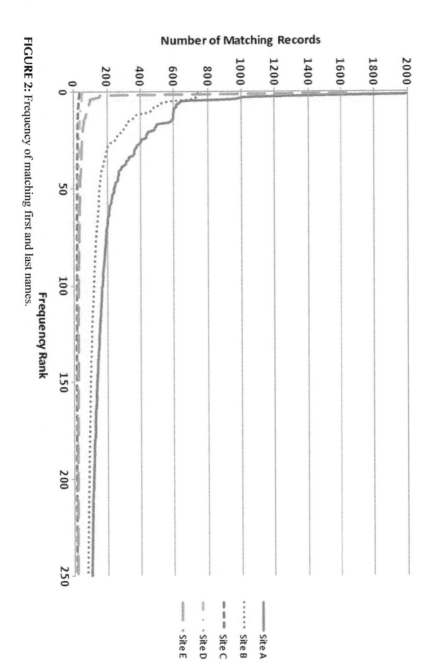

FIGURE 2: Frequency of matching first and last names.

TABLE 3: Methods for managing duplicate patient records or records with matching identifiers

	Site				
	A	B	C	D	E
Prevention					
Notifications to users when creating a record similar to an existing record	No	No	Yes	Yes	Yes
Centralised registration	No	No	Yes	No	No
Required training for registrars	Yes	No	Yes	Yes	Yes
Master patient index	Yes	No	Yes	No	Yes
Detection					
Automated demographics comparison	Yes	No	Yes	No	No
Name similarity comparison (e.g. Soundex, look-alike, common variations, common misspellings)	No	No	Yes	Yes	No
Automated chart comparison (e.g. clinical problems, labs, medications)	No	No	No	Yes	No
Manual reviews for similarity	Yes	No	Yes	Yes	No
Removal					
User ability to report duplicate records	No	Yes	No	No	No
Regularly scheduled institution efforts to merge records	No	No	Yes	Yes	No
Error mitigation					
Notification to users when accessing a record similar to other records	No	No	No	No	Yes
Photo identification during patient registration	No	No	No	Yes	No
Biometric identification during patient registration	No	No	No	No	No
Alternating row colours in patient lists	No	No	No	No	No
Total methods	3	1	8	7	3

5.3.3   DETAILED SITE ANALYSIS

Site C had the fewest records with matching patient identifiers and the most advanced methods for preventing, detecting and correcting duplicate patient errors. Thus, we present their methods in detail. Duplicate prevention starts at registration. At Site C, all registration is handled by a central phone registration service; clinics cannot register their own patients. To register a new patient, the registration clerk first searches for existing records using a variety of criteria, including name, insurance information, social security number and address. If an existing record for the patient is found, the registration clerk confirms that the record matches the patient and provides his or her existing MRN. If no record is found, the clerk queries a regional transaction clearinghouse to confirm the patient's insurance information and verify that there are no existing MRNs linked to that patient's identity in the clearinghouse. Only at this point will the clerk create a new record for the patient. The patient is then issued an identification card with their MRN, which they are encouraged to bring to all of their visits, and which is used to identify them; if the patient already has an MRN, they are issued a duplicate card with their previously issued MRN.

Although the initial central registration efforts prevent the creation of most duplicate records, there are still some cases where a duplicate record is created inadvertently. To manage these, a team in the Site C health information management department runs regular queries to find potentially duplicate records in their MPI. The query tool uses a variety of heuristics based on demographic information to identify potentially duplicate records, which are placed onto an action list for the team to investigate and, when necessary, merge records. The team also merges records in cases where a patient has to be temporarily registered without identifying information (eg, if the patient is not conscious and cannot be identified), with the goal of ensuring that there is always one record per patient.

5.4 DISCUSSION

We evaluated the number of matching patient identifiers and methods implemented for managing duplicate or potentially duplicate records at five unique sites. The rates varied across settings, from 16.49% to 40.66% of first and last name pairs having two or more records. With inclusion of patient date of birth in the search, the rates decreased, ranging from 0.16% to 15.47%. The number of records for the most frequently occurring name at each site ranged from 41 to 2552. Similarly, institutions varied widely in the implemented methods for managing duplicates or potential duplicates.

Previous work on duplicate patient records has most often focused on describing methods for identifying duplicate records or linking records in HIEs. [7–19] Our study is the first, to our knowledge, to quantify the rate of matching identifiers and the methods for managing duplicate records independently across multiple organisations. The rates we found are consistent with previous findings, [14 ,15] indicating there are potential patient safety problems across healthcare organisations despite various existing approaches for managing duplicate records.

Several factors may contribute to our observed rates of matching patient identifiers across sites. We anticipated that the number of matching identifiers would positively correlate with the number or type of implemented methods for managing duplicates; however, the data did not indicate any trends. Still, the fact that some institutions were very effective at preventing or removing duplicate records indicates that effective methods for managing duplicate records do exist. Further investigation is necessary to determine how effective these methods will be across institutions.

The large observed decrease in numbers of records with matching identifiers when including the date of birth in the search suggests that it is an important data element when identifying patients. It may also indicate that many of the first and last name pairs with two or more records belong to patients with common names (eg, John Smith, Maria Garcia), and those records with matching first name, last name and date of birth identifiers are more likely to be true duplicate records. The high number of records for the most frequently occurring names at each site confirms this theory, as it is more plausible that tens or thousands of different individuals have the same name than so many different records were created independently.

5.4.1 LIMITATIONS

We reported only the rates of identical patient identifiers and did not distinguish duplicates from potential duplicates, where different patients simply had the same demographic information. However, both these scenarios merit consideration as potential threats to patient safety. We also only used exact text matching, which did not account for typographical errors or variations in name spelling or form. More advanced methods for comparing the demographics would have likely found much higher rates of duplicates or potential duplicates. Finally, we did not evaluate how the approaches implemented for managing duplicate records at each site were implemented, possibly explaining our failure to detect an effect of the approaches. For instance, some methods of training registrars may be more effective than other methods; thus, the number of methods employed by a given institution may not be a good measure of effectiveness at preventing or eliminating duplicate records.

5.5 CONCLUSION

Despite a number of benefits that EHRs present for healthcare institutions, adoption of various methods for preventing, detecting and removing duplicate records, in addition to methods for mitigating errors in our sample was low; duplicate or potentially duplicate records persist, as indicated by high rates of matching patient identifiers in the evaluated institutions. Further efforts are necessary to improve management of duplicate or potentially duplicate records and minimise the risk for patient harm.

REFERENCES

1. Singh H, Naik AD, Rao R, et al. Reducing diagnostic errors through effective communication: harnessing the power of information technology. J Gen Intern Med 2008;23:489–94.
2. Sittig DF, Joe JC. Toward a statewide health information technology center (abbreviated version). South Med J 2010;103:1111–14.
3. Sittig DF, Singh H. Legal, ethical, and financial dilemmas in electronic health record adoption and use. Pediatrics 2011; 127(4):e10427.
4. Smith PC, Araya-Guerra R, Bublitz C, et al. Missing clinical information during primary care visits. JAMA 2005;293:565–71.
5. Stiell A, Forster AJ, Stiell IG, et al. Prevalence of information gaps in the emergency department and the effect on patient outcomes. CMAJ 2003;169:1023–8.
6. Joffe E, Bearden CF, Byrne MJ, Bernstam EV. Duplicate patient records—implication for missed laboratory results. AMIA Annu Symp Proc 2012;2012:126975.

7.   Achimugu P, Soriyan A, Oluwagbemi O, et al. Record Linkage system in a complex relational database—MINPHIS example. Stud Health Technol Inform 2010;160(Pt 2):1127–30.

8.   Arellano MG, Weber GI. Issues in identification and linkage of patient records across an integrated delivery system. J Healthc Inf Manag 1998;12:43–52.

9.   Duvall SL, Fraser AM, Kerber RA, et al. The impact of a growing minority population on identification of duplicate records in an enterprise data warehouse. Stud Health Technol Inform 2010;160(Pt 2):1122–6.

10. McClellan MA. Duplicate medical records: a survey of twin cities healthcare organizations. AMIA Annu Symp Proc 2009;2009:421–5.

11. Miller PL, Frawley SJ, Sayward FG. Exploring the utility of demographic data and vaccination history data in the deduplication of immunization registry patient records. J Biomed Inform 2001;34:37–50.

12. Sauleau EA, Paumier J-P, Buemi A. Medical record linkage in health information systems by approximate string matching and clustering. BMC Med Inform Decis Mak 2005;5:32.

13. Waien SA. Linking large administrative databases: a method for conducting emergency medical services cohort studies using existing data. Acad Emerg Med 1997;4:1087–95.

14. Thornton SN, Hood SK. Reducing duplicate patient creation using a probabilistic matching algorithm in an open-access community data sharing environment. AMIA Annu Symp Proc 2005;2005:1135.

15. Duvall SL, Fraser AM, Rowe K, Thomas A, Mineau GP. Evaluation of record linkage between a large healthcare provider and the Utah Population Database. J Am Med Inform Assoc 2012;19(1e):e549.

16. Grannis SJ, Overhage JM, Hui S, et al. Analysis of a probabilistic record linkage technique without human review. AMIA Annu Symp Proc 2003;2003:259–63.

17. Grannis SJ, Overhage JM, McDonald C. Real world performance of approximate string comparators for use in patient matching. Stud Health Technol Inform 2004; 107(Pt 1):43–7.

18. Jurczyk P, Lu JJ, Xiong L, et al. FRIL: a tool for comparative record linkage. AMIA Annu Symp Proc 2008;2008:440–4.

19. Márquez Cid M, Chirlaque MD, Navarro C. DataLink record linkage software applied to the cancer registry of Murcia, Spain. Methods Inf Med 2008;47:448–53.

20. Bittle MJ, Charache P, Wassilchalk DM. Registration-associated patient misidentification in an academic medical center: causes and corrections. Jt Comm J Qual Patient Saf 2007; 33:25–33.

21. DuVall SL, Kerber RA, Thomas A. Extending the Fellegi-Sunter probabilistic record linkage method for approximate field comparators. J Biomed Inform 2010;43:24–30.

22. Henneman PL, Fisher DL, Henneman EA, et al. Patient identification errors are common in a simulated setting. Ann Emerg Med 2010;55:503–9.

23. Lee ACW, Leung M, So KT. Managing patients with identical names in the same ward. Int J Health Care Qual Assur Inc Leadersh Health Serv 2005;18:15–23.

24. O'Neill KA, Shinn D, Starr KT, et al. Patient misidentification in a pediatric emergency department: patient safety and legal perspectives. Pediatr Emerg Care 2004;20:487–92.

25. Ranger CA, Bothwell S. Making sure the right patient gets the right care. Qual Saf Health Care 2004;13:329.
26. Sideli RV, Friedman C. Validating patient names in an integrated clinical information system. Proc Annu Symp Comput Appl Med Care 1991;1991:588–92.
27. Yancey WE. Expected Number of Random Duplications Within or Between Lists. JSM 2010;2010:2938–46.
28. Gray JE, Suresh G, Ursprung R, et al. Patient misidentification in the neonatal intensive care unit: quantification of risk. Pediatrics 2006;117:e43–47.
29. Henneman PL, Fisher DL, Henneman EA, et al. Providers do not verify patient identity during computer order entry. Acad Emerg Med 2008;15:641–8.
30. Schulmeister L. Patient misidentification in oncology care. Clin J Oncol Nurs 2008;12:495–8.
31. Magrabi F, Ong M-S, Runciman W, Coiera E. Using FDA reports to inform a classification for health information technology safety problems. J Am Med Inform Assoc 2012; 19(1):4553

McCoy A.B., Wright A., Kahn M. G., Shapiro J. S., Bernstam E.V., and Sittig, D.F. Matching Identifiers in Electronic Health Records: Implications for Duplicate Records and Patient Safety . Quality and Safety in Health Care 2013; 0:1–6. doi:10.1136/bmjqs-2012-001419 Reproduced with permission from BMJ Publishing Group Ltd.

PART III

EHR USERS AND USABILITY

CHAPTER 6

RIGHTS AND RESPONSIBILITIES OF USERS OF ELECTRONIC HEALTH RECORDS

DEAN F. SITTIG and HARDEEP SINGH

Over the last 10 years the governments of Australia, [1] Belgium, [2] Canada, [3] Denmark, [4] the United Kingdom [5] and most recently the United States, [6] have all made long-term, multibillion dollar investments in health information technologies, including electronic health records. Although the definition of electronic health records might vary across countries, most systems are widely accessible across a health care network and provide a computer-based user interface that replaces the paper chart. The primary goal of these initiatives in health information technologies is to transform the collection, display, transmission and storage of patient data with the aim of improving health. A secondary goal is to use patient data to improve the system of health care delivery. The rationale for these investments stems from numerous concerns of quality and safety related to paper-based systems, which include problems with legibility, access limited to a single provider at a single location, difficulties with aggregating information from multiple records, and problems maintaining confidentiality of records and accurate backup copies. [7] Comprehensive, well-implemented electronic health records with advanced clinical decision support interventions have potential to reduce errors with medications [8] and to increase the quality, efficiency and reliability of information transfer. [9,10]

Despite progress in the use of electronic health records, [11] their adoption has resulted in larger than expected challenges in day-to-day clinical processes. [12] For example, processing electronic information can reduce the productivity of clinicians and increase their workloads, [13–15] and other disruptions of workflow can result in safety concerns owing to loss of attention and situational awareness. [16] Thus, clinicians may perceive that the costs of electronic health records (e.g., in time or money, or from required changes in workflow) outweigh direct benefits to themselves, whereas patients and payers appear to benefit more readily. [17] Clinicians require assurances that electronic health records will deliver the features and functions they need and that the regulatory environment will support them.

Based on recent literature and our research in informatics and health care quality and safety, we identified 10 emerging topics that, if addressed, could overcome some of these challenges. Topics were based on our recently developed eight-dimension sociotechnical model of safe and effective use of electronic health records. [18] These topics were circulated among several colleagues, including practising clinicians, informaticists and computer scientists, who offered their feedback. This was followed by presentations at four international scientific meetings with multidisciplinary audiences who gave additional feedback. We used this input to refine the topics and generate 10 "rights" and responsibilities of clinicians with a goal of making them as universally acceptable and applicable as possible.

6.1   CONTEXTUALIZING TOPICS AS RIGHTS AND RESPONSIBILITIES OF CLINICIANS

Some disruption of workflow is inevitable with the implementation of electronic health records, which requires modification of long-standing work processes derived from paper-based systems. In addition, clinicians' use of electronic health records often results in loss of autonomy because of increased external oversight (i.e., clinician profiling) and control (i.e., orderable medications limited to formulary) facilitated by the features and functions of electronic systems. Concomitantly, practising clinicians are often at a relative disadvantage when negotiating issues related to electronic health records with other stakeholders (e.g., health care administrators, vendors of health information technologies, governments, insurance companies or other payers, and policy-makers). To preserve a balance and to encourage debate between clinicians and other stakeholders involved, we discuss these topics in the context of what front-line practising clinicians would want as professional rights (i.e., not merely desirable but must-have electronic health record features, functions and user privileges that are important to provide the highest quality, safest and most cost-effective care). Each right is accompanied by a corresponding responsibility of clinicians, without which the ultimate goal of improving the quality of health care might not be achieved. [19]

We acknowledge that contextualizing these topics as rights of clinicians has important implications for other stakeholders, but these issues must be addressed to move forward in the adoption of electronic health records. Although these rights are clearly not of the same magnitude or universal importance as the World Health Organization's human rights–based approach to health [20] or the Hippocratic Oath, [21] recognition of these rights could reduce unintended adverse consequences on patient care and clinicians' livelihoods. These rights could be a foundation upon which designers, developers, implementers, policy-makers and, most importantly, users of health information technologies can co-create a new age of computer-assisted health care. [22]

6.2 TEN RIGHTS AND RESPONSIBILITIES

6.2.1 UNINTERRUPTED ACCESS TO RECORDS

Extended outages of electronic health records pose a substantial risk to patient care. Therefore, clinicians have the right to have a system they can continuously access via a secure, organizationally approved, network-attached device. Although no device or system can be 100% reliable, vendors of electronic health records, institutions and physicians must work together to design, develop, implement and use fail-safe equipment and processes for downtime to ensure that patient care continues in the event of an outage.

Clinicians have the responsibility to protect their passwords, log off the system when done, and access only records of patients under their care or within their administrative purview.

6.2.2   NO MISSING DATA

Clinicians have the right to see all clinical data that were captured in the normal course of care for each of their patients. [23] Amid concerns about patient privacy, some argue that patients or clinicians should be able to "hide" specific data (e.g., records of psychiatric or substance-abuse treatment) [24] or even to "opt out" of having their data available to other clinicians. [25,26] This withheld data unnecessarily increases the liability of clinicians.

Clinicians have the responsibility to ensure that the availability of all patient data on their desktops does not replace the time-honoured tradition of observing, listening to and examining patients. [27]

6.2.3   SUCCINCT PATIENT SUMMARIES

Current electronic health records contain a wealth of clinical data. As more community-wide health information systems come online, the amount of data available for review will grow exponentially, increasing the likelihood that relevant information will be overlooked. Clinicians thus have the right to electronic health records that provide succinct summaries of their patients' medical problems, medications, laboratory results, vital signs and progress notes. [23] Some systems currently have "summary" views that arrange data by type (e.g., all laboratory results together) and time (e.g., most recent data first) on different screens. However, future innovations in this area are needed. For example, problem-oriented summaries that integrate data from different sources on one screen could potentially facilitate better information processing and exert a lower cognitive load. [7]

Clinicians conversely have the responsibility to maintain accurate, up-to-date problem lists using a controlled clinical terminology (e.g., SNOMED CT [Systematized Nomenclature of Medicine — Clinical Terms]) and link them with corresponding diagnostic and treatment elements through the electronic system to prevent "incomplete care." [28]

6.2.4 ABILITY TO OVERRIDE COMPUTER-GENERATED INTERVENTIONS

Clinicians receive a large number of computer-generated alerts, many of which are considered unnecessary. [29] These alerts can cause cognitive overload and fatigue. Even more troublesome, some alerts cannot be overridden because of institutional configuration decisions requiring "hard stops" (i.e., the computer prohibits completion of the task). [30] Clinicians should have the right to override, but not permanently disable, any computer-generated clinical intervention. In the event of an exceptionally hazardous scenario or when the organization's clinical leadership decides that a particular order should never occur, clinicians should be required to obtain a co-signature from a higher-ranking or more experienced clinician before completing the task of overriding an alert. Disallowing overrides through hard stops implies that computers have access to more accurate data and greater medical knowledge and expertise than clinicians. In reality, computers are often not able to interpret or convey the clinical context for many reasons: unavailable or inaccurate data, errors in logical processing (e.g., software bugs) and situation-specific clinical exceptions (e.g., user request for blood transfusion denied by a computer-generated intervention that did not capture active bleeding since last hemoglobin result).

Clinicians have the responsibility to justify overrides and be accountable for decisions by agreeing to have their actions reviewed. Additionally, they must participate on clinical decision support oversight committees and work with other stakeholders to review, redesign, test, re-implement or remove clinical decision support interventions that are judged ineffective. [31]

6.2.5   RATIONALE FOR CLINICAL DECISION SUPPORT

Advanced clinical decision support interventions are necessary if electronic health records are to generate expected improvements in the quality, safety and effectiveness of health care. Nevertheless, clinicians have the right to request and receive a clear, evidence-based rationale at the point of care for all computer-generated interventions (e.g., alerts or reminders).

Physicians have the responsibility to carefully consider computer-generated interventions. Blindly following or ignoring clinical decision support interventions can lead to errors. [32]

6.2.6   RELIABLE PERFORMANCE MEASUREMENT

Performance measurement based on electronic health records is inevitable. Current methods of data collection and measurement are not fail-safe and often measure what is easy to measure. [33] To correct discrepancies, clinicians have the right to review all processes based on electronic health records used to generate reports that inform policy decisions or performance measurement. [34] All computer-based measurements should have unambiguous exclusion criteria and allow clinicians to identify patients to whom the measure does not apply (e.g., no diabetic foot examinations on patients with bilateral below-the-knee amputations). If needed, clinicians should have access to queries, data extracts and statistical methods used. Proactive collaboration with stakeholders such as organizational leaders will help ensure that performance measurements are valid.

To ensure continuous quality improvement, physicians have the responsibility to review the performance feedback they are provided and act on it.

6.2.7   SAFE ELECTRONIC HEALTH RECORDS

Software errors and usability issues in electronic health records are increasingly linked to safety hazards that can lead to patient harm ("e-iatrogenesis").

[35,36] Clinicians have the right to expect that all errors related to electronic health records will be reported, investigated and resolved in a timely manner. [37] Vendors and health care organizations responsible for maintaining the electronic health records should make these reports, along with their responses, publicly available so that others can learn from them. [38]

Clinicians have the responsibility to report, help investigate and learn from safety hazards related to electronic health records.

6.2.8 TRAINING AND ASSISTANCE

State-of-the-art electronic health records are complex tools designed to facilitate the entry, storage, review, interpretation and transmission of patient data. Clinicians have the right to receive training — either from their vendor or their health care organization — in all features of electronic health records. Ongoing training and support should include access to online instruction and availability of real-time assistance while caring for patients, preferably in person. [39]

Clinicians have the responsibility to maintain a high level of user proficiency with the same level of diligence as for other clinical skills. To improve efficiency and safety, clinicians must learn to type, complete training in electronic health records and show competence in use of all functions required to care for patients (e.g., enter orders, add problems and initiate referrals). Finally, clinicians are responsible for asking for help when they reach limits of their proficiency.

6.2.9 COMPATIBILITY WITH REAL-WORLD CLINICAL WORKFLOWS

Clinicians have the right to safe, effective and usable electronic health records that contain evidence-based, problem- and task-specific order sets, documentation templates and information displays designed to be compatible with their clinical workflows. [40]

Clinicians have the responsibility to work with vendors and local information technologists to design, develop and implement data entry, data review and clinical decision support tools, and to modify previous paper-based workflows to overcome limitations of electronic health records.

6.2.10   FACILITATION OF COMMUNICATION, COORDINATION AND TEAMWORK

Electronic health records fundamentally change the way clinicians coordinate their work activities, communicate and collaborate to deliver high-quality, safe and effective health care. [41] Most current electronic health records are not optimal for team-based care that includes patients and their caregivers. [42] Clinicians have the right to future innovations in electronic health records that facilitate complex communication and coordination tasks across time, space and people.

Clinicians have the responsibility to use electronic health records in ways that foster teamwork. They must document their findings, decisions and actions succinctly, avoid reckless copy and paste, and respond to human- and computer-generated requests for information and action in a timely manner.

6.3   NEXT STEPS

Although our article lays the groundwork for future debate, it has several limitations. First, we do not specifically outline who might enforce these clinician rights and responsibilities or what alternatives could be pursued if these conditions are not met. However, we believe it is premature for us to do so at this stage of conceptualization without further debate and agreement. Second, we recognize that even with consensus regarding the necessity of these rights, delivering them in the short term will be difficult using today's technology and in today's sociopolitical and economic environments. Our goal, however, is to lay the foundation for a long-term agenda for providing clinicians access to safe, effective and easy-to-use electronic health records that support their cognitive and physical work processes. Finally, we recognize that achieving high-quality and affordable health care is a complex, sociotechnical endeavour. Thus, these clinician rights might not be the perfect solution because there are many competing and often opposing views of the best way to accomplish this endeavour.

A competing view is that other stakeholders in this debate, including payers, administrators, policy-makers and patients, are also entitled to an equally important and valid set of rights, which may conflict with one or more of the clinicians' rights. Payers, administrators and policy-makers, for example, have the right to mandate use of functions related to electronic health records that promote patient safety (e.g., order entry), prohibit use of functions that jeopardize patient safety (e.g., use of a non-secure, Web-based calendar to facilitate clinician workflow [43] or use of text messaging for order entry [44]), enforce specific rules and regulations (e.g., reprimanding users for unauthorized access to patient data), create new clinical decision support interventions to encourage efficient, effective, evidence-based care, and evaluate clinicians' performance using data from electronic health records. Likewise, patients have the right to access their data, have any errors of data entry corrected, obtain a list of everyone who has viewed their data, confidentially communicate electronically with their providers, and request that certain data not be used for purposes other than research or public health benefit without their written consent (e.g., no selling of data). [45]

In the event that one group's rights infringe upon those of another group, we are optimistic that organizations and the constituents they represent will participate in an open, constructive debate on these rights and reach consensus. [46] If this consensus were formalized and ratified, then relevant stakeholders (e.g., vendors, implementers, professional boards, hospital committees, users, patients and government agencies) could work together to design and implement electronic health records and the corresponding policies, procedures and regulations required to ensure these rights.

6.4 SUMMARY

The 10 key issues discussed here form a set of features, functions and user privileges of electronic health records that clinician users require to deliver high-quality, safe and effective care. Issues discussed are generalizable to clinicians and electronic health records across the globe. Addressing these rights and responsibilities comprehensively will be challenging but can make the care delivered through the electronic health records–based work system safer and more efficient.

Key points:

- Despite the potential benefits of electronic health records, clinicians have experienced several challenges in their adoption and use.
- To encourage debate on strategies to overcome these challenges, we developed a set of 10 "rights" of clinicians that represent important features, functions and user privileges of electronic health records that clinicians need to provide safe, high-quality care.
- Each right is accompanied by a corresponding responsibility of clinicians, without which the ultimate goal of improving quality of health care might not be achieved.

REFERENCES

1. HealthConnect Implementation Strategy. Version 2.1. Canberra (Australia): Commonwealth of Australia; 2005. Available: www.health.gov.au/internet/hconnect/publishing.nsf/Content/archive-docs/$File/implementation.pdf (accessed 2012 Jan. 25).
2. France FR. eHealth in Belgium, a new "secure" federal network: role of patients, health professions and social security services. Int J Med Inform 2011;80:e12–6.
3. Blueprint EHRS: an interoperable EHR framework. Version 2. Canada Health Infoway; 2006. Available: https://knowledge.infoway-inforoute.ca/EHRSRA/doc/EHRS-Blueprint.pdf (accessed 2012 Jan. 25).
4. Protti D, Johansen I. Widespread adoption of information technology in primary care physician offices in Denmark: a case study. Issue Brief (Commonw Fund) 2010;80:1–14.
5. House of Commons Public Accounts Committee. The National Programme for IT in the NHS: progress since 2006. Second report of session 2008–09. London (UK): The Stationery Office; 2009. Available: www.publications.parliament.uk/pa/cm200809/cmselect/cmpubacc/153/153.pdf (accessed 2012 Jan. 25).
6. Blumenthal D. Wiring the health system — origins and provisions of a new federal program. N Engl J Med 2011;365:2323–9.
7. Powsner SM, Wyatt JC, Wright P. Opportunities for and challenges of computerisation. Lancet 1998;352:1617–22.

8. Bates DW, Leape LL, Cullen DJ, et al. Effect of computerized physician order entry and a team intervention on prevention of serious medication errors. JAMA 1998;280:1311–6.

9. Singh H, Arora HS, Vij MS, et al. Communication outcomes of critical imaging results in a computerized notification system. J Am Med Inform Assoc 2007;14:459–66.

10. Singh H, Naik AD, Rao R, et al. Reducing diagnostic errors through effective communication: harnessing the power of information technology. J Gen Intern Med 2008;23:489–94.

11. Protti D. Comparison of information technology in general practice in 10 countries. Healthc Q 2007;10:107–16.

12. Westbrook JI, Braithwaite J. Will information and communication technology disrupt the health system and deliver on its promise? Med J Aust 2010;193:399–400.

13. Poissant L, Pereira J, Tamblyn R, et al. The impact of electronic health records on time efficiency of physicians and nurses: a systematic review. J Am Med Inform Assoc 2005;12:505–16.

14. Magrabi F, Ong MS, Runciman W, et al. An analysis of computer-related patient safety incidents to inform the development of a classification. J Am Med Inform Assoc 2010;17:663–70.

15. Committee on Patient Safety and Health information Technology Board on Healthcare Services. Health IT and patient safety: building safer systems for better care. Washington (DC): The National Academies Press; 2011.

16. Singh H, Giardina TD, Petersen LA, et al. Exploring situational awareness in diagnostic errors in primary care. BMJ Qual Saf 2012;21:30–8.

17. Sprivulis P, Walker J, Johnston D, et al. The economic benefits of health information exchange interoperability for Australia. Aust Health Rev 2007;31:531–9.

18. Sittig DF, Singh H. A new sociotechnical model for studying health information technology in complex adaptive healthcare systems. Qual Saf Health Care 2010;19(Suppl 3):i68–74.

19. Good medical practice: the duties of a doctor registered with the General Medical Council. Med Educ 2001;35(Suppl 1):70–8.

20. World Health Organization. A human rights-based approach to health. Available: www.who.int/hhr/news/hrba_info_sheet.pdf (accessed 2011 Nov. 27).

21. The Hippocratic Oath [Translated by North Michael]. Bethesda (MD): US National Library of Medicine; 2002. Available: www.nlm.nih.gov/hmd/greek/greek_oath. html (accessed 2011 Apr. 7).

22. Stead WW, Searle JR, Fessler HE, et al. Biomedical informatics: changing what physicians need to know and how they learn. Acad Med 2011;86:429–34.

23. Committee opinion no. 472: Patient safety and the electronic health record. Obstet Gynecol 2010;116:1245–7.

24. Popovits RM. Confidentiality law: Time for change? Behav Healthc 2010;30:11–3.

25. Watson N. Patients should have to opt out of national electronic care records: FOR. BMJ 2006;333:39–40.

26. Halamka JD. Patients should have to opt out of national electronic care records: AGAINST. BMJ 2006;333:41–2.
27. Verghese A. Culture shock — patient as icon, icon as patient. N Engl J Med 2008;359:2748–51.
28. Gandhi TK, Zuccotti G, Lee TH. Incomplete care — on the trail of flaws in the system. N Engl J Med 2011;365:486–8.
29. Isaac T, Weissman JS, Davis RB, et al. Overrides of medication alerts in ambulatory care. Arch Intern Med 2009;169:305–11.
30. Strom BL, Schinnar R, Aberra F, et al. Unintended effects of a computerized physician order entry nearly hard-stop alert to prevent a drug interaction: a randomized controlled trial. Arch Intern Med 2010;170:1578–83.
31. Wright A, Sittig DF, Ash JS, et al. Governance for clinical decision support: case studies and recommended practices from leading institutions. J Am Med Inform Assoc 2011;18:187–94.
32. McCoy AB, Waitman LR, Lewis JB, et al. A framework for evaluating the clinical impact of computerized medication safety alerts. J Am Med Inform Assoc 2011; Aug. 17 [Epub ahead of print].
33. Ofri D. Quality measures and the individual physician. N Engl J Med 2010;363:606–7.
34. Department of Health and Human Services Centers for Medicare & Medicaid Services. 42 CFR Part 401, CMS-5059-F, RIN 0938-AQ17. Availability of Medicare data for performance measurement. Available: www.gpo.gov/fdsys/pkg/FR-2011-12-07/html/2011-31232.htm (accessed 2012 Jan. 25).
35. Myers RB, Jones SL, Sittig DF. Review of reported clinical information system adverse events in US Food and Drug Administration databases. Appl Clin Inform 2011;2:63–74.
36. Institute of Medicine. Health IT and patient safety: building safer systems for better care. Washington (DC): The National Academies Press; 2012. Available: http://iom.edu/Reports/2011/Health-IT-and-Patient-Safety-Building-Safer-Systems-for-Better-Care.aspx (accessed 2011 Dec. 16).
37. Singh H, Classen DC, Sittig DF. Creating an oversight infrastructure for electronic health record-related patient safety hazards. J Patient Saf 2011;7:169–74.
38. Walker JM, Carayon P, Leveson N, et al. EHR safety: the way forward to safe and effective systems. J Am Med Inform Assoc 2008;15:272–7.
39. Ash JS, Stavri PZ, Dykstra R, et al. Implementing computerized physician order entry: the importance of special people. Int J Med Inform 2003;69:235–50.
40. Karsh B-T. Clinical practice improvement and redesign: how change in workflow can be supported by clinical decision support. Rockville (MD): Agency for Healthcare Research and Quality; 2009.
41. Campbell EM, Guappone KP, Sittig DF, et al. Computerized provider order entry adoption: implications for clinical workflow. J Gen Intern Med 2009;24:21–6.
42. Thomas EJ. Improving teamwork in healthcare: current approaches and the path forward. BMJ Qual Saf 2011;20:647–50.
43. Monthly report to congress on data incidents. Nov 1–28, 2010. Washington (DC): United States Department of Veterans Affairs; 2010. Available: www.va.gov/ABOUT_VA/docs/monthly_rfc_nov2010.pdf (accessed 2011 Nov. 27)

44. The Joint Commission. Texting orders. Oakbrook Terrace (IL): The Commission; 2011. Available: www.jointcommission.org/standards_information/jcfaqdetails.asp x?StandardsFaqId=401&ProgramId=1 (accessed 2011 Nov. 27).
45. Smith M. Patient's Bill of Rights — a comparative overview (PRB 01-31E). Ottawa (ON): Library of Parliament; 2002. Available: http://dsp-psd.pwgsc.gc.ca/Collec-tion-R/LoPBdP/BP/prb0131-e.htm

Sittig D. F., and Singh H. Rights and Responsibilities of Users of Electronic Health Records. Canadian Medical Association Journal. 2013 Feb 13. PMID: 22331971. Reprinted with permission.

CHAPTER 7

A HUMAN FACTORS GUIDE TO ENHANCE HER USABILITY OF CRITICAL USER INTERACTIONS WHEN SUPPORTING PEDIATRIC PATIENT CARE (NISTIR 7865)

SVETLANA Z. LOWRY, MATTHEW T. QUINN, MALA RAMAIAH, DAVID BRICK, EMILY S. PATTERSON, JIAJIE ZHANG, PATRICIA ABBOTT, and MICHAEL C. GIBBONS

7. 1 BACKGROUND: USABILITY AND CRITICAL USER INTERACTIONS

Adoption of electronic health record (EHR) systems in hospitals and physician practices is accelerating. [1] At the same time, however, the lack of usability of EHRs has been identified as an important factor impacting patient safety, [2] and national guidelines have been released to evaluate, test, validate, [3] and document summative usability testing results. [4] In addition, recommendations have been made to improve the usefulness, [5,6,7,8] interoperability, [9] and ability to conduct research [10] of EHRs for pediatric patients.

Pediatric patients have unique characteristics that translate into higher complexity for providing care with both paper-based charts and EHRs. As such, EHRs have the potential to reduce complexity with advanced decision support features, and thus improve patient safety. Meeting this potential will likely require a specialized assessment of the unique challenges in providing pediatric care with EHRs, and in particular, unique usability issues associated with critical user interactions. [11,12,13] It is not surprising, then, that the adoption of EHRs by pediatric providers has lagged behind adoption for general population providers. [14] In this document, we highlight user interactions that are unique to or especially salient for pediatric care. As such, these interactions impact EHR usability in particular and user-centered design (UCD) in general.

User-centered design (UCD) is an approach to designing systems; the approach is informed by scientific knowledge of how people think, act, and coordinate to accomplish their goals.[15] UCD design practices employ both formative and summative practices in order to achieve systematic discovery of useful functions grounded in an understanding of the work domain. Particularly for systems used in high-risk environments, where mistakes can result in fatalities, ensuring system usability is an important objective. Usability has traditionally been defined as "The extent to which a product can be used by specified users to achieve specified goals with effectiveness, efficiency and satisfaction in a specified context of use." [16] In healthcare settings implementing EHRs, an emerging consensus is that many of the critical risks for the care of pediatric patients associated with the use of the EHR are related not just to the system's user interfaces, but also to the system's functionality and workflow. Therefore, for the purposes of this document, we use a unified framework for defining EHR usability: "how useful, easy to use, and satisfying a system is for the intended users to accomplish goals in the work domain by performing certain sequences of tasks" [17]

The focus of this document is not on all aspects of EHR usability, but rather on those that are part of critical user interactions. Critical user interactions are interactions between a user, such as a physician, nurse, pharmacist, caregiver, or patient, and the EHR, which can potentially lead to errors, workarounds, or adverse events that are associated with patient harm. Critical does not imply level of clinical care, such as critical care, but rather the highest-priority interactions to consider with respect to usability and patient safety in the context of his or her associated pediatric care. In other words, these are safety-critical interactions with the EHR. In safety-critical environments (hospitals, emergency departments, etc.), the importance of well-designed, usable interfaces is increased precisely because of the potential for catastrophic outcomes. The importance is further increased in the presence of time pressure, [18] as is the case in much of healthcare. Time pressure reduces a user's opportunity to detect signals in the face of noise and may also lead to inadvertent confirmation bias, so appropriate user interface design is all the more important in such environments.

Several usability-related concerns are not addressed in this report and considered outside the scope of this document. These include challenges associated with supporting collaborative work and shared situation awareness among interdisciplinary team members, transitions across care settings, interoperability between systems, integration with bar code point of care and other medical devices, quality improvement and research using data pulled from EHRs, integration with social media and handheld devices, and software designed exclusively for use by caregivers or nontraditional healthcare providers. The user interactions and associated recommendations described in this report were identified by consensus during a series of teleconferences. Participating experts represented the disciplines of human factors engineering, usability, informatics, and pediatrics in ambulatory care and pediatric intensive care. In addition, extensive peer review was provided by experts in pediatric informatics, emergency medicine, neonatology, pediatrics, human factors engineering, usability engineering, and software development and implementation.

The notion of critical user interactions takes on special importance with pediatric patients. As is explained in the next section, pediatric patients are unique. Their uniqueness creates at least two important consequences with respect to EHR usability. First, the young and very young pediatric patients may be more physiologically vulnerable to even small mistakes or care delays. Second, pediatric patients have unique care challenges, which can create additional physical and/or mental demands on pediatric clinicians. Both of those observations reveal that user interactions with EHRs that might not be deemed critical in other environments become critical with pediatric patients. The unique pediatric factors are explained next.

7.2   SPECIAL CONSIDERATIONS FOR PEDIATRIC PATIENTS

7.2.1   GENERAL PEDIATRIC CONSIDERATIONS

Pediatric patients have been identified as a high-priority, high-risk population for patient safety due to differences in physical characteristics, developmental issues, and issues relating to the legal status of minor age children and complicated custody and guardianship situations. [19] Even within pediatric patients, there is much variability in clinical needs based upon 1) age group (prenatal, neonatal/infant, preschool child, school-age child, adolescent, and young adult); 2) health issues (health maintenance and preventive care [well child, including newborn care], critical and emergency care, chronic disease management, behavioral care); and 3) site and process of care (birth, delivery and neonatal/newborn care, inpatient care, primary ambulatory care, specialty care). Providing care in general, and medication management in particular, is more complex and has higher patient safety risks for pediatric patients for at least three reasons: 1) patient physiology, 2) the complex nature of common or routine tasks, and 3) patient limited communication ability. [20]

First, in terms of physiology, children undergo dramatic developmental changes from birth to adulthood. Disease states in children are dynamic and change over a continuum with age. Specific disease states, symptoms, exam findings, laboratory findings, and treatments vary with gestational age, actual age, weight, length, Body Surface Area, Body Mass Index, and other variables. In the first month alone, each organ system in the body (e.g., neurological, cardiac, pulmonary, hematologic, renal, hepatic, hematologic, and immune) transitions from fetal life to postnatal life; organ system changes happen in hours and days in the Neonatal Intensive Care Unit (NICU). The range of physical characteristics in pediatrics is much larger than for adults – for example, from a 500 gram premature infant to a 100 kilogram 12-year-old.

These unique pediatric characteristics influence the clinician's selection of: (a) factors to consider for appropriate care, (b) parameters on which to base decisions, (c) goals to attempt to achieve, and (d) tasks to implement that are required to achieve these goals. In turn, these characteristics and the clinician's preferred course of action influence how the user interface of an EHR must be designed to accommodate and support the cognitive and decision-making requirements of the clinician. This is why the unique aspects of pediatric care make selection and arrangement of information displays, definition of "normal" ranges and thresholds for alerts, among many other display and user interface considerations, more challenging to design and implement. In particular, for example, the norms which define "normal," "standard," and "wrong" dosages for pediatric patients change rapidly over time and the clinical parameters upon which "normal" pediatric doses are defined (age, Body Surface Area, and/or weight) also change with time. The user interface must be designed to flexibly and reliably accommodate the realities of the rapidly changing pediatric patient and relevant clinical parameters and settings. A one-sizefits-all user interface design will not accommodate the clinical needs of pediatric patients or support the cognitive and decision-making requirements of their care providers. Ideally, the user interface will provide tools to support the configurability of the clinical parameters and setting that permits the clinician to modify those clinical parameters or settings over which they should have control (e.g., entering the body weight of the pediatric patient) while limiting or restricting access to other clinical parameters or settings (e.g., definition of "normal" dosages), which presumably should not be modified by a single care provider without careful consideration.

Second, there is immense complexity even for standard daily tasks such as ordering medications and vaccinations and administering breast milk that are not pertinent to adult patient care. The complexity stems from added burdens of calculations, individual tailoring, and patient identification not typically present in adult care. If designed properly, the EHR will provide the functions and features for advanced decision support in these areas.

Third, young and very young children may not be able to communicate at all or sufficiently to direct a clinician to important information, raise questions, correct errors, complain, or articulate symptoms. This may seem similar to the situation with very sick adults, but may be different in one important way. Very sick adults may at least have family and care providers that are able to help fill in gaps of information for current clinicians based on communications with the patient prior to them becoming sick. Clinicians caring for the young and especially very young may not be able to rely as much on past medical history or even family members, since the young and very young can no more communicate with their family than they can with clinicians. This lesser ability to communicate, like the aforementioned physical and physiological changes, translates into different EHR design needs to support care. If clinicians cannot rely as much on the patients, they may need to rely more on the EHR. Data that support clinical decision should be available, easily accessible, and customizable by groups of end users. All important information should be viewable with one click or "hover over" capability to minimize navigation burdens. Seeing more of what one might need is especially important for users who must rely more on the display and less on the patient.

Taken together, the unique physiology, task complexity, and patient communication abilities for pediatric patients create unique physical and cognitive burdens on care providers that must be accommodated by the design of EHRs. We suggest that flexible designs that accommodate the rapidly changing physiologic realities of these unique patients, pediatric-specific decision support, and well organized displays are high-level goals to help achieve more usable pediatric EHRs. Next we review specific pediatric considerations.

7.2.2   SPECIFIC PEDIATRIC CONSIDERATIONS

The medication use process, specifically weight-based dosing, is more complex and difficult to standardize. [21] Additional complexities with medication orders include the use of alternative liquid, nasal, or partial-tablet formats, combinations of prescriptions. For example, Amoxicillin Clavulanate will typically be used in one or two dose forms for adults, whereas there are 13 different formulations from which a pediatric provider may choose. With low-weight patients, sophisticated rounding strategies and accurate weight measurements are particularly critical to avoid over-dosing or under-dosing.

Caregivers are another special consideration that must be factored. The role of pediatric caregivers is larger than with other populations, with the possible exception of the elderly. When caring for children, lay caregivers calculate and administer medications (e.g., breathing treatments to cystic fibrosis patients) instead of medical personnel in some hospitals, which creates the need to support nontraditional EHR users.

Risks for misidentification are different for pediatric patients, and generally higher. Although these risks are not new, many paper-based systems had evolved to have additional protections that are not available in most EHRs, such as filing charts of siblings together in the same location with handwritten cross-references to sibling chart numbers, which provided an intuitive indication for how many siblings were in a family. [22] Pediatric siblings are the only cohort of patients which share outpatient visits with a primary care provider on a routine basis, and usually have the same last name (although not always). In the case of multiple births, patients additionally share the same date of birth. In the case of newborns, many patients on the same unit will have the same birth date, and which is sometimes the same date as the current date.

Newborn children are more likely to have identical birthdays in a labor and delivery unit than other parts of the hospital. As genetic information becomes more readily available and integrated into patient-centered care, it will be important to link updated information across patient records for patients who are genetically related, such as parents, children, and siblings.

There are sources of information that are unique to pediatric care. Growth charts are critically important and should be depicted in internationally accepted formats. There is a greater need to access information across multiple-birth patients, including the infant/child, parents, siblings, and other family members, particularly for genetic information and for information related to the labor and delivery process. High-risk patients, particularly low-birth-weight neonates, are often transferred to institutions that support higher levels of complex care, injecting further difficulty into information exchange. While a date of birth may seem quite straightforward in an adult EHR, a premature infant can have gestational age, postnatal age, and a date of birth. The phrase "days of life" is often used in neonatal ICUs (NICUs) and pediatric ICUs (PICUs) to prevent confusion.

Alerts for crossing normative thresholds are particularly challenging for the pediatric population, due to the need to do both age-based and weight-based tailoring with respect to medication doses and vaccination schedules. That is, what is perceived as "normal" changes rapidly, and so what is an appropriate alert changes too.

Finally, there is immense complexity even for standard daily tasks such as ordering medications and vaccinations and administering breast milk that are not pertinent to adult patient care. If designed properly, the EHR will provide the functions and features for advanced decision support in these areas.

7.3   A CONCEPTUAL MODEL OF UNIQUE USE-RELATED RISKS OF EHR SYSTEMS FOR PEDIATRIC PATIENTS

Many of the critical risks for the care of pediatric patients associated with the use of the EHR are related not just to the system's user interfaces but also to the system's functionality and workflow. The Task, User, Representation, and Function (TURF) framework for EHR usability was developed by the National Center for Cognitive Informatics and Decision Making in Healthcare. [23] The TURF framework integrates user interfaces, functionality, and workflow into a coherent structure. A conceptual model of unique use-related risks of EHR systems that can be applied to the pediatric population is provided in Figure 1, building upon the TURF framework.

TURF outlines usability as how useful, usable, and satisfying a system is for the intended users to accomplish goals in the work domain by performing certain sequences of tasks. In this case, primary users are anticipated to include pediatricians, pediatric trainees (resident physicians and fellow physicians in pediatric training programs), physicians' assistants, registered nurses, licensed practical nurses, nurse practitioners, school-based health personnel, home nursing personnel, including for hospice care, and community-based pediatric health caregivers.

Additional users include respiratory care providers, physical therapists, social workers, lactation consultants, religious support persons, lay caregivers, play therapists, and subspecialty consultants, including neurologists, radiologists, and others. Secondary users are anticipated to include parents and nontraditional caregivers, adolescent and young adult patients, administrators, quality improvement personnel, and public health officials monitoring outbreaks and immunizations.

In order for an EHR system to be useful, it should have functions that enable providers to meet the complex needs of their work domain, providing care to pediatric patients. Usefulness is to address the intrinsic complexity of the work domain, and it is determined by the functions of the system. "Usable" addresses the extrinsic difficulty of user interactions with the system, and it reflects the difficulty when a user uses a specific representation or user interface to perform a specific task. Extrinsic

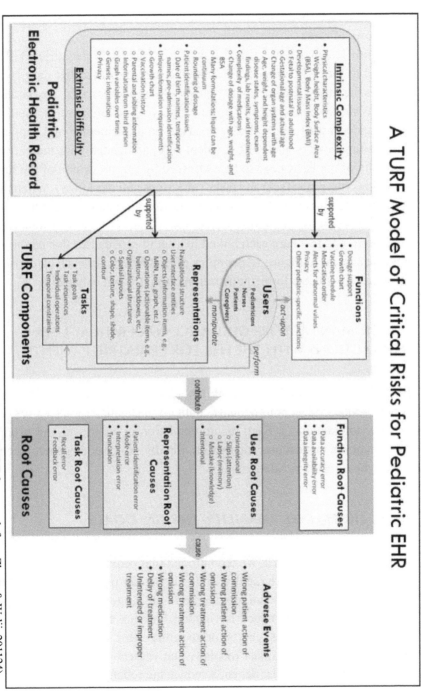

FIGURE 1: TURF model of unique use-related risks for pediatric patients (based on the TURF framework from Zhang & Walji, 2011[24])

difficulty is mainly determined by the formats of representations and the workflows of tasks.

Figure 1 shows how critical risks associated with pediatric EHR are mapped to the TURF model. The unique nature of pediatric care is captured as the intrinsic complexity that should be addressed by any pediatric EHR, as shown on the left of Figure 1. To avoid adverse events, the list of items under intrinsic complexity needs to be implemented and supported as core functions of the EHR. Critical risks associated with the extrinsic difficulty of the EHR need to be addressed by careful design of the representations (user interface) and tasks (task steps and workflow). When there is a mismatch between the intended workflow with an EHR and the actual workflow, risks for pediatric patients are higher. Functions, users, representations, and tasks are each linked to a set of root causes that can lead to adverse events. In Figure 1, examples of root causes for each category are provided. This list is for demonstration only; it is not exhaustive.

7.4   HUMAN FACTORS GUIDANCE FOR CRITICAL USER INTERACTIONS WITH THE EHR FOR PEDIATRIC PATIENTS

First, we provide high-level usability design goals and specific design considerations relevant to pediatric patients ("Detailed guidance for critical user interactions"). Each recommendation is numbered and grouped by category of critical user interaction. Finally, we provide general themes across these recommendations.

7.4.1   HIGH-LEVEL USABILITY DESIGN GOALS

As explained in Section 2, we recommend that pediatric EHRs be flexible enough to accommodate rapid changes in patient physiology and related changes in relevant parameters and provide targeted decision support. EHR displays should reduce navigation burdens when complete views of critical graphs, tables, charts, or structured text are displayed without needing to scroll. Additional displays that present together data that are considered for a particular decision reduce the reliance on human memory when needing to access separate tabs or screens. [25] As is common when human factors design guidance is applied to special populations, when one designs to accommodate users with the greatest need for usable systems, generally everyone else benefits too. If a door is designed to accommodate the tallest among us, then everyone else can fit through. Similarly, many of our design recommendations for pediatric patients likely would benefit all patients. The specific recommendations below are consistent with these high-level goals.

7.4.2   DETAILED GUIDANCE FOR CRITICAL USER INTERACTIONS:

7.4.2.1   PATIENT IDENTIFICATION

When assigning and/or verifying patient identification numbers and names, the risk profile for pediatric care differs from the adult care population. Human factors engineering has a long history of employing systematic methods to conduct risk assessments of the potential for human error in a given setting. Recognized methods include: Human Reliability Analysis (HRA), Probabilistic Risk Assessment (PRA), Accident Sequence Eval ation Program (ASEP), and Standardized Plant Analysis Risk (SPAR). [26] Some of these methods were used to assess the potential for "wrong patient" errors for adult populations in healthcare settings. [27] Based upon the unique risks for pediatric patients, we make the following recommendations to employ multiple means of identification criteria:

Use unique patient identification numbers that are not based upon social security numbers.

Most EHRs already follow this practice by using either unique patient identification (UPI) numbers or Globally Unique Identifiers (GUID). This is a prior recommendation for all patient populations due to a number of considerations. [28] Nevertheless, this recommendation is particularly important for newborn patients who have not yet received a social security number yet require care and documentation of care in the EHR. In addition, newborn infants sometimes have changes to last names in the first days of life (e.g., BG Jones for Baby Girl Jones changes to Sara Smith). In addition, it is recommended that identification numbers/medical record numbers not be sequential in order to reduce the risk of confusing multiple birth patients as well as newborns born on the same day in the same hospital. Utilization and maintenance of master patient indexes, particularly across multiple hospital organizations, could aid in reconciling temporary and permanent identifiers for newborn patients. [29]

Include photographs of newborns with primary caregivers for patient identification.

Photographs of newborn infants with their primary caregivers in the EHR would reduce the risks for wrong patient identification. At a minimum, warnings could be employed when patients with the same last name and same date of birth are in the same unit. For labor and delivery units, patients cannot be distinguished by birth date. In addition, particularly for cultures that have many common last names, unrelated patients can be located next to each other and have the same last name and same date of birth.

Include age, gender, and weight on constant-identification banner headers on all screens

Based upon the unit's population, the following variables might be included: name, gender, weight, age, gestational age, post-conceptual age, and date of birth. For pediatric patients, it is common practice for family members with the same last name to be cared for by the same providers and/or same organizations during the same appointment. In order to prevent "wrong patient" errors, constant-identification banner headers should include gender, weight (in kilograms), and age as well as the units for age, which can range from "days of life" to "months" to "years" in scale. Note that for same age siblings due to multiple births, first name, medical record number, and unique medical events, such as birth time in minutes, can be the main distinguishing elements, and therefore should be easily accessible if not included on the banner header. Finally,there is information that is of little interest for pediatric care that can be distracting to users, such as information about smoking, drinking, and vaccinations that are only given to elderly patients.

Distinguish between newly generated and copied information

When taking care of multiple birth patients and patients in the same family, it is often important to have multiple charts open simultaneously in order to reduce reliance on human memory, reduce navigation burdens, and reduce the risks for missing or duplicate tasks that are the same for multiple patients. Nevertheless, having multiple charts open at the same time increases the risk for "wrong patient" errors where documentation is copied and pasted into the wrong chart. Providing the ability to track where information was copied from can aid in detecting these types of errors. For example, subtle background color can be used behind any text that is copied and as data is entered, the background becomes clear (normal) behind the written text. In addition, the source of the copied information can be displayed upon mouse rollover or other interaction to request the information. An additional protection against "wrong patient" errors in this context is to be able to return to the system configuration including automatically saved information that was being worked on when a user was automatically logged out when interrupted to do another task.

7.4.2.2   MEDICATIONS

When ordering medications for pediatric patients, there are unique factors that increase the risks for mode errors. Mode errors are actions performed in one mode that were intended for another mode. [30] A mode error example could be ordering a dose that would be appropriate for a weight in kilograms, but is incorrect for a weight in pounds, and vice versa. Mode errors have been reported due to confusion of prescribing a medication as the volume in milliliters (mL) rather than milligrams (mg). This common mode error results in tenfold iatrogenic overdoses in hospitalized young children receiving intravenous acetaminophen for pain relief. [31] Unique pediatric risks for mode errors are created by childspecific formats for calculating medication doses, including mg/kg/dose, mg/kg/day, mg/M^2, mg, ml, and dose intervals based on gestational and postnatal age. The last mode, "dose intervals," is particularly complex because it is temporally sensitive. For example, vancomycin has a recommended dosing interval of 18 hours for patients with a gestational age less than 30 weeks old and a postnatal age less than 15 days, but shifts to every 8 hours for a patient with gestational age from 37 to 44 weeks with a postnatal age of more than 8 days. In order to protect against unique risks with mode errors, the following recommendations are made:

Protect against mode errors for mg/kg dosing and ml dosing

For infant care, EHRs should support ordering expressed by volume of drug and by mass of a drug. [32] In the best case, EHRs would be designed to recognize inappropriate dosing based on the unit of measure it is displaying and the specific patient characteristics. In this way, if a clinician accidentally entered a value based on the wrong mode, the EHR could recognize it, prevent it, and warn the clinician. A weaker solution would be to highlight the distinction between these two modes (e.g., terms never truncated on the menu, mode risk items not placed near each other, units highlighted on the order form).

Flag that an intended dose is unusual

For example, when a 10 mg/kg dose is delivered with an every-18-hour (Q18) schedule, the attention of the user can be brought to the unusual dose regimen either through passive graphical or text displays of dose ranges or with alerts. A detailed discussion of alert design is beyond the scope of this report. Human factors alert design recommendations have been made for adult populations that are likely also relevant for pediatric patients. [33]

Support high-precision dosing for low-weight patients

Low-weight patients can experience toxicity if medications are rounded to the nearest digit. [34] In particular, medications with narrow therapeutic indices such as digoxin or insulin have a great potential for adverse consequences if dosed improperly. For example, for a 575-gram infant, kilogram units need to be accommodated to three decimal points. Therefore, a higher resolution for precision during medication dosing needs to be supported and encouraged with the interface design fields for patients below a particular weight for a particular medication. At a minimum, automated rounding based upon needs for adult patients which cannot be overridden should not be permitted for low-weight patients. This is particularly true for neonatal infants (e.g., 0.016 mg digoxin is the accurate dose needed). Note that this issue also exists for body weight. The weight of infants who weigh less than one kilogram should not be rounded up to one kilogram.

Do not permit automated defaults to adult doses

Some EHRs employ defaults for standard doses in the event of what appears to be an erroneous dose entry since it is much lower than the adult normal dose. This practice is extremely risky for low-weight patients, particularly if no warning is provided to the provider of the change. For pediatric patients, errors due to "automation surprises" [35] where the system makes unexpected, automated changes to medication orders can have higher patient safety impacts than for adult populations.

Support custom formulations for liquid medications

With pediatric patient care, a common task is ordering medication in liquid form. Custom formulations, such as "mg/ml," should be available as an option.

Support documentation of incomplete medication information.

With pediatric patient care, it is not uncommon for medications to be prescribed by other providers and for caregivers to have incomplete information about the medication. For example, if a parent describes that the patient is on "some antibiotic," that information needs to be captured even if the medication is not ordered in the EHR. For example, if a medication is ordered to address arrhythmia, a disorder of the heart rate or rhythm, it needs to be verified that the ordered medication does not negatively interact with the specific antibiotic. Similarly, if a caregiver reports that a patient is allergic to "an over-the-counter fever medicine." there should be a way to document that information without having to select a specific one.

Reduce displayed options for medication orders

Medication prescribing for children is a more complex process than for adult patients, particularly in intensive care. [36] With most paper-based ordering systems, medications are ordered by physicians without the specificity used in pharmacies. When pharmacy-specific information is displayed to physicians, there can be 17 choices for a common medication, creating complexity that can lead to erroneous selection of medications. For medications for children, medications are often given together or with complex dosing regimens, thereby increasing the number of potential options for ordering. Fewer and simpler options are recommended, which would then require support for nurses or pharmacists to correctly translate the order into the level of detail required during the dispensing process.

Display where the ordered dose (in mg or mg/kg or mg/kg/day) is with relation to the recommended dose range

One protection against mode errors is to display the expected dose range for a selected amount, particularly in order to prevent errors on the scale of ten times the amount. A stronger protection would be afforded by using "guardrails" technology which alerts when medication orders are outside pre-specified ranges. This type of technology would require a low rate of false alarms and pediatricspecific information in order to be usable.

Display "input masks" for data entry to clarify type of data

A technique to standardize data entry is to control the format that is allowed, including the format and number of digits allowed, with input masks (e.g., 0.0 mL for volume-based dosing of preschool-age children and 0.00 mL for volume-based dosing of neonates).

Avoid truncation of medication names and dosages in menus

Users should be able to view the full name of the medication and dose without having to select the item to see the full text. The full text should be viewable without additional interactions. When display space is too limited, at a minimum, rollover interactions that show the full text when the user moves their mouse or other input device over the items are recommended rather than requiring an item to be actively selected to view all of the information.

7.4.2.3 ALERTS

For pediatric patients, there is much specialized expertise that is taken into account when determining a "normal" range for medications, lab results, and other variables. In theory, clinical decision support systems can be extremely useful in aiding especially novice providers with an order that falls outside the normal range. On the other hand, even for adult patient populations, warnings about potential drug interactions are overridden about 90 percent of the time, [37] primarily due to very high false alarm rates and associated "alert fatigue." [38] Other types of alarms have similar override rates, including in a pediatric intensive care unit. [39] Recommendations to improve effectiveness of alerts, reminders, and warnings follow

Support flexibility in unit-based settings for alarms, warnings, and alerts based upon weight and age

Specialized units focusing on pediatric care including pediatric intensive care units, pediatric emergency departments, labor and delivery, and pediatric outpatient clinics need to be able to adapt threshold settings appropriate for their patient demographics, particularly with respect to weight and age. A committee is recommended to be responsible for determining these settings for groups rather than for individuals in collaboration with staff members, including pharmacists, physicians, nurses, and administrators, and with periodic updates to thresholds and underlying logic.

Ensure that adult-based thresholds do not replace pediatric-specific thresholds following a system-wide crash

Pediatric-specific thresholds can be designed to apply wherever indicated and maintained locally by units that specialize in pediatric care. In the event that local adaptations are used rather than embedded in the system settings that are used upon start-up of a system, an important consideration is how to recover after a system-wide shutdown, planned or unplanned. Although reasonable for systems providing care to adult patients to put in place system-wide generic default settings for alarms after a system crash, this practice could be dangerous for pediatric patients, particularly if providers are not alerted to the changes in default range settings. For this situation, no system defaults are preferable to defaults for adult populations.

Do not permit "hard stops" for changes to medication orders

"Hard stop" alerts are pop-up alerts which block the ability for clinicians to complete an intended action with potentially serious consequences. Instead, alerts that permit users to override a recommendation in exceptional situations are recommended. Even when warnings are effective in preventing dangerous drug combinations such as the anti-clotting drug warfarin and certain antibiotics that can produce hazardous effects in combination, somewhat rare but critical situations where exceptions need to be made will be critically delayed. [40] Therefore, alerts with override features are recommended rather than "hard stops."

Cap the dose at the standard adult dose and allow override with justification.

When an order is entered for a child less than 14 years of age that exceeds the standard adult dose, provide a real-time alert that the adult dose has been exceeded. Alerts should not be "hard stops" in that they should be allowed to be overridden with a justification, particularly for obese adolescent patients.

Display normal ranges for medication doses and lab values based upon weight and age information

Even in cases when EHRs do not have normal ranges for medications based upon weight and age information available, the systems could support ways for organizations to incorporate this additional information and display it.

Display together parameters that are continuously monitored to facilitate rapid interventions

It is particularly important to rapidly intervene for premature infants based upon a defined set of pre-identified parameters that are displayed together on a single screen. Parameters to support monitoring of respiratory distress, hypoglycemia, nutrition, muscle tone, circulation, and perfusion are particularly important. [41] Navigating to other areas of the EHR for real-time monitoring is inefficient and may lead to delays and potential errors. A common example is accessing glucose levels in a labs report screen, plus the feeding schedule on a different screen, with additional information about timing documented in nurses' notes on yet another screen.

7.4.2.4   GROWTH CHART

For patients between the ages of 0 and 24 months, the World Health Organization (WHO) international growth standard is a critical tool for nearly every pediatric diagnosis. The Centers for Disease Control (CDC) growth chart is recommended for patients older than 2 years old. [42] Training for pediatricians is standardized for these representations for quick and effective clinical care. When nonstandard representations are used, there is a risk of creating the "representation effect." This human factors phenomenon refers to the fact that expertise when using cognitive artifacts is contextualized such that the specialized knowledge is difficult to apply when information is not represented in the way in which professionals were trained to use it. [43] Therefore, to best support cognitive strategies based upon clinical expertise, the following recommendations are made:

Change measurement units (e.g., lb vs. kg) only when initiated by the user.

For infants, it is somewhat common to use the English pound measurement system for data collection and then convert to the metric system when ordering medications. In order to reduce mode error risks from working in different measurement systems, displays should not automatically default to a different measurement system. In addition, displaying units of measure along with data values reduces risks for confusion about the current measurement system and scale.

Support accurate conversion from pounds to kilograms

A frequent task is converting weights for children from pounds to kilograms, and vice versa for communicating with caregivers, and can be supported by the EHR to increase the usefulness of the system.

Ensure visibility of chart data and axes

Axes should be clearly labeled and the values for plotted data should be easily visible. Plotted data points should not overlap or otherwise obscure information about other data points. Vertical (age) axes should be in 1-month increments (rather than 2-3 month increments for the first year of life). A useful feature would be providing additional information when "hovering" over a plotted data point, such as a percentile. For some functions, it is also useful to have this information for parts of the graph that are not plotted, such as for determining a target body weight for a particular length.

Display units accurately in standard notation

Standard "shorthand" notation for units such as "kg" for kilogram or "lb" for pounds should be employed. Age information needs to be clearly denoted as whether it is the current age or age at the time of the last visit.

Support selection of particular weight data value to display

Although an important function of growth charts is to see trends, there are situations in which an exact weight data are needed, such as when dosing medications. Therefore, retrieving the exact number plotted on a graph quickly is an important feature.

Display age-based percentiles for weight, height, head circumference, and BMI data

Percentiles are critically important indicators for tracking whether growth trajectories are stable or changing. Changes in percentiles in weight and height (length or stature) can be a signal of poor health. Extreme ends of percentiles might be considered healthy as long as the percentile values remain relatively constant over time. Therefore, displaying this information as a temporal trend over hours, days, weeks, or years is highly useful; the timeline scale is context-dependent.

Single-click navigation to access growth chart display

Growth charts should be easily accessible with little navigational burden to access the chart (e.g., one click on an easily recognizable icon or menu item).

Single-click interaction to view complete growth chart

The most frequently used growth charts should be easily viewed in their entirety with little navigational burden (e.g., no scrolling to view the entire chart).

Display height and weight on the same chart

Pediatricians are trained to visualize growth charts that display height and weight on the same chart; the visual representation points quickly to various types of growth abnormalities that have diagnostic importance. The CDC and the WHO growth standard charts are available online.

Support custom views with custom time ranges

For some diagnostic tasks, it is important to look closely at a narrow point in time, such as ages 3 to 6 months. Similarly, it is helpful to look at an enlarged segment of a chart when there are many points plotted on a chart. Therefore, supporting the ability to focus on specific time periods or otherwise expand a portion of the chart is a useful feature.

Support corrections to plotted data

There are a number of reasons why plotted data may be inaccurate and need to be corrected in order to aid decision making. One common reason is when a premature infant's chronological age is evaluated based upon a younger age group. One technique is to "move back" data points by a time period (e.g., two months) in order to assess growth given the premature birth. Data quality issues might also arise based upon where measurements were taken, how the data were collected, and errors in data entry.

7.4.2.5   VACCINATIONS

Delivering vaccinations is a scheduling task, which has been a muchresearched task in human factors engineering. [44] The scheduling task complexity is greatly increased when there is interdependency among tasks, otherwise known as task coupling. [45] Recommended vaccination schedules from the Centers for Disease Control are available for children from 0 to 6 years old and 7 to 18 years old. [46] In situations where multiple care providers coordinate ordering and administering vaccinations, vaccinations are received at more than one organization (e.g., child attending college), vaccinations are missed or children did not follow a typical schedule (such as children adopted from other countries), modifying the schedule is an extremely challenging cognitive task. To reduce errors in vaccine tracking and ordering processes, the following recommendations are made:

Allow ordering vaccination via reminder

Reminders that suggest ordering a vaccine can facilitate the process by allowing direct ordering via the reminder's dialog box, rather than requiring navigation to an area dedicated for orders or vaccinations.

Allow data entry for vaccinations given at other institutions

In the event that systems are not completely integrated across institutions, at a minimum, it should be possible to document vaccinations given at other institutions. Displaying the origin of the information upon demand would be extremely useful, particularly when there are discrepancies. For example, a child attending a university might receive a vaccination at the student clinic, and this should be able to be documented by the primary care provider at home. The same goes for children who switch providers because of a move. This ability would reduce the risk of double vaccinations. Similarly, printouts of vaccination records should incorporate data from all institutions where vaccinations were given.

Support display and tracking of components of combination vaccines

In the event that vaccinations are administered in combination format rather than individually, the system should support tracking what has been administered and when. Ideally, there would be support for evaluating whether vaccination intervals satisfy requirements for both regular schedules and catch-up schedules. Vaccination scheduling requirements can be partially based on whether a vaccine is live (activated) as opposed to inactivated, so EHRs supporting tracking and alerting based on that information would be useful. For example, two live vaccinations could be administered the same day.

Display the days on which prior vaccinations were given and support alerts for recommended minimum/ideal/maximum intervals between vaccinations. Information about recommended intervals between vaccinations is publicly available and infrequently hanges. [47] A useful feature would be to support scheduling when to give vaccines when the recommended schedules were not previously followed for any number of reasons, including waiting until school to receive vaccinations and adoptions from other countries with different schedules.

Allow sorting of vaccination data by multiple fields
Information about vaccinations is used to support a variety of clinical decisions. Sorting displayed information alphabetically, by time, by component, and in a shot record format should all be supported.

7.4.2.6   LABS

For pediatric patients, the definition of "normal ranges" is extremely complex and based upon data that are often only relevant for pediatric patients, such as body surface area. In addition, the definitions of "normal" ranges vary based upon the source of the definition. Therefore, to increase the chances of accurately depicting findings against useful "normal" ranges and support effective communications among the relevant personnel, the following are recommended:

Support communications to change inaccurate normal ranges
It is recommended that one contact person be designated to receive requests to change inaccurate normal ranges for medications and labs. Requests for change are recommended to be facilitated by EHR features, which automatically direct the request for change to the designated person.

Enable seeing where normal ranges originated from

For example, normal ranges in pediatrics could be based on adult normal, pediatric normal, weight-based normal, age-based normal, or body surface area normal, depending on which entity generated the ranges.

Enable integrated view of test results from different sources

EHRs provide the ability in principle to improve reliability and efficiency of the management of electronic test results, such as lab results. In adult patient care, one survey found that 83 percent of responding physicians reviewing at least one test result in the previous two months reported "they wished that they had known about earlier." [48] For the care of pediatric patients, concerns have been raised that electronic results management systems were not designed explicitly for use in pediatric purposes and thus might pose a threat to patient safety. In particular, there can be delays in diagnosis, missed diagnoses, and delays in the receipt of appropriate care. [49] In one study, a primary barrier to adoption was found to be lack of inclusion of all ordered tests in the system. [50] When labs are received from multiple locations, there should be a way to track trends over time despite originating from different institutions. For example, International Normalized Ratio (INR) levels from a blood test need to be tracked carefully over time for patients who have had cardiac valves replaced and are thus treated with Coumadin. When integrating information, it will be important to identify differences in measurement units (e.g., molar vs. concentration values) and normative ranges.

7.4.2.7   NEWBORN CARE

Newborn infants require special considerations as a category where many of the standard assumptions for adult patients do not apply. In particular, more and unique information is needed for much quicker decision-making cycles by highly specialized physician, nursing, and other care providers. Particularly for premature infant care, it is appropriate to have distinct workflows and information displays since the care needs are sufficiently distinct to warrant unique support for high-stakes tasks. It is possible that the recommendations made below will not be sufficient to truly meet the unique needs of this vulnerable population, and that specialized products might be required for safe and effective systems. In the situation where newborn care is supported by existing EHRs, the recommendations are:

Enable efficient creation of newborn records

Newborns should be able to receive urgent care immediately upon birth regardless of whether there is an EHR-based requirement for services such as providing blood for a transfusion. For example, there could be an efficient means for creating a new record for a newborn that automatically pulls relevant data from the mother's record that is accomplished with a single selection of a menu item or push of a button.

Support updating information that is initially inaccurate or unknown

Information is often not immediately available in the NICU or labor and delivery, such as last names, sex, and weight.

Support the use of gestational age and corrected age for patient care (in addition to chronologic age)

Care decisions are often made based upon nonstandard age formats in the NICU and for care of premature infants.

Support efficient processes for administration of breast milk, including labeling and matching mother to baby to milk

Inefficient processes for verifying matches between mothers, babies, and milk can be frustrating and time-consuming, particularly in the NICU where it is a frequent and potentially error-prone activity.

Support connecting prenatal data (e.g., fetal imaging procedure) with post-birth data

Prenatal data is often available in the EHR chart for the parent, but it would be helpful to explicitly link these data with the child's EHR chart. Of particular importance is information about maternal infections, blood type, and pregnancy complications, including substance abuse.

Support efficient documentation of blood type

Newborns can receive more appropriate blood transfusions than O negative blood if the information can be efficiently entered based upon information obtained during birth.

Support the use of alternative weights for dosing

Newborn weights can vary dramatically in the first days of life. In some cases, birth weight or "dry weight" (weight before surgery) is used to dose medications rather than current weight, referred to as a "dosing weight."

For example, when weight is automatically populated in medication ordering, the wrong weight could result in ineffective or toxic amounts. This is exacerbated when equipment such as an "arm board," a board to which the arm is taped in order to deliver medications intravenously, is included in the weight measure.

Support conversion from Days of Life (DOL) to Days Old (DO) during care transitions

Some healthcare organizations use "Days of Life" and some use "Days Old" to denote the age of a newborn infant. During transitions of authority and responsibility across organizations, it is critically important to be accurate with this information. Since all EHRs can be expected to have accurate birthdate and current date information, it should be possible to allow hospitals to use either convention and support this conversion from one system to the other.

7.4.2.8   DISPLAY WEIGHTS IN GRAMS AND AGES IN DAYS, WEEKS, OR MONTHS UNDER THRESHOLDS

For newborns, the appropriate unit is often different given the young age and low weight. Under 3 kilograms, it may be preferable to display weights in grams. During patient rounds and other verbal communications between neonatologists, grams are often used, and supporting this convention, as well as supporting accurate conversions to kilograms for dosing, may reduce conversion errors. Under thirty days, it is preferable to view age in days, weeks, and months. In addition to better support decision making and communications with caregivers, having an age such as "0.005 years old" could lead to erroneous assessments.

7.4.2.9   PRIVACY

Ensuring patient privacy and allowing sufficient support for communications to provide effective care is challenging for any patient. For pediatric patients, there are special considerations due to the unique nature of the transfer of care responsibility based upon age and maturity from the parent or nontraditional caregiver to the child for responsibility for care, particularly with respect to mental health and sexual information. The following recommendations are made:

Support documenting consent agreements for nontraditional parents

It is important to support privacy for nontraditional caregiving arrangements such as children in foster or custodial care, adults who are not parents, adoptive parents, and guardians.

Support "break the glass" privacy law violations for urgent care situations.

In urgent care scenarios, it might be necessary to access critical health information that is available in an EHR yet restricted for privacy or security purposes. In the event this is needed, the system should support access as long as documentation is made by the user logging the event, who accessed the information, and the reason for getting access.

Make easily visible what information can be viewed, printed, and transferred with different levels of privacy or security

Many levels of confidentiality for different notes can make it difficult for users to understand what privileges are provided with each level, particularly if the distinctions are not well-defined in the online help documentation. For example, systems can have confidential notes, sticky notes, private notes, and internal notes, each of which has different definitions regarding access for viewing and transferring to other systems. Access issues are particularly complicated for adolescent patients based on age, assent status, and nontraditional caregiving arrangements.

7.4.2.10   RADIOLOGY

Radiology is a particularly important specialty in pediatric care. Knowing which test to order is an important decision because the risk associated with exposure to radioactivity is particularly high for infant patients whose cell division is very active and whose cumulative exposure over a lifetime is just beginning. For adult patient populations, consultations between a physician and a radiologist about which test is appropriate to order are important communications. For pediatric patients, the stakes are much higher. Sedation, intubation, and radiation for pediatric patients are much higher-risk activities than for adult patients. Having multiple scans due to inaccurate selection of correct procedures from physician-radiologist communications conducted only through EHR orders and poor usability of the interface can have many negative clinical implications for pediatric patients. Therefore, the following recommendations are made:

Support physician-radiologist communications to clarify which scan variation to order for high-stakes sedation and intubation procedures

A useful feature would be supporting real-time communications between an ordering physician and a radiologist about which procedure to order in order to reduce delays in care and redundant procedures. In order to ensure that the correct test has been ordered, a narrative including a diagnostic, short history and indication for the reason for the test is needed. It is also important to include information about who can be contacted in real time in order to answer a radiologist's questions. In addition, this support could meet The Joint Commission's (TJC) recommendation to "Create and implement processes that enable radiologists to provide guidance to and dialogue with referring physicians regarding the appropriate use of diagnostic imaging using the American College of Radiology's Appropriateness Criteria." [51] For example, this communication could avert an erroneous order of "chest CT" when a "chest and abdomen CT" is needed. In the event that realtime communications cannot be supported, support could be provided for quality improvement reports to facilitate quality improvement by interdisciplinary teams of physicians and radiologists.

Support alerts for contraindicated procedures

There is often information electronically available from the chart that, in theory, could inform alerts about procedures potentially being contraindicated during the ordering process. In the event that the current level of technology cannot support this with an acceptable rate of false alarms, reports could be printed to support manual review by assigned personnel prior to the date of a procedure.

Monitor cumulative radiation exposure over time

A listing in one location of all radiology tests, done at any location, for each patient would help to monitor and reduce exposure to ionizing radiation. Over the past two decades, the U.S. population's total exposure to ionizing radiation has nearly doubled. [52] For newborn patients, it is possible that new sources of radiation will emerge in future decades, further raising the cumulative exposure over a lifetime. High cumulative radiation exposures create cancer and other undesirable consequences. As such, The Joint Commission has recommended that dose information be captured in the patient's EHR. [53] Once the dose information is captured, a highly useful feature would be a cumulative plot of radiation exposure over time for physicians, nurses, radiologists, and ideally caregivers and patients.

7.4.3 SUMMARY OF HUMAN FACTORS THEMES IN RECOMMENDATIONS

In addition to the detailed recommendations described above, there are several overall recommendations that apply across multiple categories to enhance usability in general. These are:

- Facilitate smart rounding of the dose of the medication based on actual formulation of drugs. For example, digoxin is 50 mcg/mL, 10 mcg/kg/day. For a baby with a low weight, an order of 0.4553 mL is too specific, but the ability to order 0.46 mL and not 0.5 mL is important to avoid toxicity. Systems must take into account the correct amount of arithmetic precision needed in values.
- Avoid truncation of displayed information. This includes medication names for ordering medications, units for displayed data, names of vaccinations, and information for points plotted so closely together that the information was obscured.
- Support notations on data. Much of the numeric information used by pediatric clinicians is influenced by data quality issues. Being able to notate "fussy" on a blood pressure medication reading, information such as "6-week preemie" on growth chart data, and "needs booster shot at next visit" for vaccinations would be extremely helpful. In addition, it is very important to know where information originated from, particularly when there are unusual data values or discrepancies to resolve.
- Support local display options for age and weight. Age and weight do not have the same meaning, units, or ranges for pediatric patients as for adult populations. In addition, there are multiple variations on these measures. Having the ability to locally select display options (e.g., g vs. kg, Days of Life [DOL] vs. Days Old [DO], dosing weight vs. current weight) would be useful.
- Support the use of customized forms, charts, graphs, and reports. There are many specialized tasks that some pediatric providers perform routinely that are supported by specialized forms, graphs, charts, and other tools. In general, these tools require graphing and analyzing quantitative data where the interpretation is based on other dynamic factors. For example, if a patient

has a dilated aortic root, their dimensions are tracked based on Z-score, which is a measure of standard deviation from the mean based on the Body Surface Area. When an adult has an aortic root being tracked, you simply follow the absolute value of the dimension (e.g., 4 cm, 4.1 cm, 4.2 cm). For pediatric patients, the variables that are tracked change with age, weight, height, and other factors. Another example is tracking INR data to see what the dose of an anticoagulation should be. With paper-based records, physicians typically made flowsheets and graphs that were pasted into the chart. With electronic records, most EHRs currently lack flexibility to provide support for data entry, graphing, or documentation of paper graphs.

- Support optimizing alerts. Alerts are particularly important in pediatrics given the extreme complexity of providing care, particularly for vaccination scheduling and medication ordering. On the other hand, designing threshold settings for alerts is particularly challenging in pediatrics given high variability and the need for specialized information that may change quickly over time. Being able to optimize the alert settings locally, particularly for particular units and levels of experience, would be highly useful. In general, in pediatrics, the variability is so high that it is strongly recommended that all alerts can be overridden at the discretion of the provider.

7.5 OPPORTUNITIES FOR INNOVATION

Developers interested in developing specialized "child modules" for pediatric patient care that can be used in conjunction with established EHR systems might consider the following areas that we believe would be viewed as useful features:

- "Normal" dose ranges, lab, and vital sign values for pediatric patients. Complex factors are used in each of these calculations. For example, vital signs and blood pressure ranges depend on height and age but not weight, whereas dosing is based on weight.
- Support seeing all variations on a medication order (e.g., amoxicillin) or procedure (e.g., CT scan) without clicking on them, and view which ones have most frequently been selected.
- Support selecting the necessary billing codes and generating the associated documentation to receive the appropriate financial reimbursement from third parties (e.g., insurance companies).
- Support innovations in "smart alerts," including expertise-based adjustments and escalations of who receives alerts based on values and combinations of variables with Boolean logic.
- Provide smart vaccine support, such as verifying vaccine combinations, catch-up doses, and missed doses.

- Support locally adding charts for specific conditions (e.g., Down syndrome). The growth chart is not the only chart that is useful for pediatric patient care.
- Support tracking and graphing medical data, where the interpretation is based on other dynamic factors. For example, if a patient has a dilated aortic root, their dimensions are tracked based on Z-score, which is a measure of standard deviation from the mean based on the Body Surface Area. When an adult has an aortic root being tracked, you simply follow the absolute value of the dimension (e.g., 4 cm, 4.1 cm, 4.2 cm). For children, the variables that are tracked change with age, weight, height, and other factors. With paper-based records, physicians typically made flowsheets and graphs that were pasted into the chart. With electronic records, most EHRs currently lack flexibility to do this strategy.
- Support role-based access control for sensitive portions of the note. As responsibility for care is transferred from parents to children, there is an increased need to protect sensitive portions of the note from parents, such as psychology notes and suicide flags. Provide support for communications to add medications to the formulary, reduce false alarms for alerts, reminders, and warnings, and address sources of inaccurate data. It is recommended that one contact person be designated to receive requests to change inaccurate settings or undesirable settings. Requests for change are recommended to be facilitated by EHR features, which automatically direct the request for change to the designated person.
- Provide support for identifying areas for quality improvement by displaying clinical data for cohorts of patients against benchmarks. A useful feature, particularly for quality improvement or administrative personnel, is to have reports and dashboard displays to see how patient care measures relate to national benchmarks. Pediatric subspecialties are continuously advancing local, state, and hopefully eventually national standards for care and associated measures, few of which are currently captured with existing or future requirements for quality improvement measures for adult patients. For example, all infants with a fever within the last 28 days treated in the hospital might want to be reviewed for quality improvement or research purposes.
- Drug dictionaries with pediatric-specific dose ranges and alerts that include single-dose, daily-dose, and cumulative-dose decision support, including lifetime cumulative dose for chemotherapies. [54]
- Support physician-radiologist communications to clarify which scan variation to order for high-stakes sedation and intubation procedures. A useful feature would be supporting real-time communications between an ordering physician and a radiologist about which procedure to order in order to reduce delays in care and redundant procedures. In addition, it is important to track the frequency of radiology procedures to assess the cumulative patient safety risk.
- Support warnings for contraindicated procedures. There is often information electronically available from the chart that could inform the system

notifying the user that a procedure is contraindicated during the ordering process. For pediatric patients, procedures often are more challenging than for adult patients due to small sizes and resistance to staying still during intubation and other critical activities. On the other hand, some procedures occur more often, such as lumbar punctures for young infants since they have a higher risk of meningitis and do not reliably show signs of meningeal irritation. Patients with increased intracranial pressure (ICUP) are contraindicated for receiving a lumbar puncture.

- Accommodate critical information exchange for patient facility transfers (particularly for premature neonates). Extremely sick premature neonates will frequently be transferred to receive care at institutions with the most specialized knowledge to provide care. Having an efficient way to get an overview of critical information is critical to meet the needs of these patients. In most cases, no social security number will yet be available for these patients; therefore, additional support for accurate identification is needed.
- Display the origin of medication, lab, and procedure information. Knowledge of where information originates is critical to determining what information to consider when there are discrepancies. As EHRs begin to incorporate more information originating from other systems designed for other purposes, such as insurance companies, billing services, and personal health records, this ability will be even more important.

7.6   CONCLUSION

Usability of EHR systems has been identified as an important factor in patient safety. The adoption of EHRs by providers specializing in pediatric patient care has lagged behind adoption for general population providers. Pediatric patient care has unique features and some aspects of care are more complex and have higher stakes. In this document, we highlighted unique user interactions important for providing pediatric care with the support of an EHR and provided guidance from the human factors literature to increase usability. Of particular importance in the provided recommendations are:

- Display information in menu items and on charts/graphs without truncating critical information, including doses and measurement units;
- Support one-click access to the growth chart in the standard display format;
- Eliminate automated changes to adult doses for medication orders; and

- Protect against ordering medications in the wrong units, which could result in tenfold or higher dosing errors.

REFERENCES

1. Jha, A.K., Desroches, C.M., Campbell, E.G. et al., "Use of electronic health records in U.S. hospitals," The New England Journal of Medicine, 2009;360(16) :1628–1638.
2. IOM. Health IT and Patient Safety: Building Safer Systems for Better Care. Washington, DC: The National Academies Press; 2012.
3. (NISTIR 7804) Technical Evaluation, Testing and Validation of the Usability of Electronic Health Records
4. (NISTIR 7742) Customized Common Industry Format Template for Electronic Health Record Usability Testing.
5. Spooner, A. and Council on Clinical Information Technology. Special Requirements of Electronic Health Record Systems in Pediatrics. Pediatrics. 2007;119(3): 631-637.
6. Shiffman et al. Information Technology for Children's Health and Health Care: Report on the Information Technology in Children's Health Care Expert Meeting, September 21-22, 2000. J Am Med Inform Assoc 2001;8:546-551.
7. Grace, E., Kahn, J., Finley, S. Model Children's EHR Format. HIMSS 2011 Annual Conference. February 23, 2011.
8. United States Pharmacopoeia. Error-Avoidance Recommendations for Medications Used in Pediatric Populations. Available at: http://www.usp.org/hqi/patientSafety/resources/pedRecommnds2003-01-22.html (Accessed March 22, 2011).
9. Hinman, A.R., Davidson, A.J. Linking Children's Health Information Systems: Clinical Care, Public Health, Emergency Medical Systems, and Schools. Pediatrics 123 Supplement 2 January 1, 2009; S67 - S73.
10. Stiles, P.G., Boothroyd, R.A., Robst, J., Ray, J.V. Ethically Using Administrative Data in Research Medicaid Administrators' Current Practices and Best Practice Recommendations. Administration & Society March 2011:43(2):171-192.
11. Scanlon, M. C. Human factors and ergonomics in pediatrics. In: Carayon P, ed. Handbook of Human Factors and Ergonomics in Patient Safety: Lawrence Erlaum and Associates; 2006.
12. Scanlon, M.C., Karsh, B., Densmore E. Human Factors and Pediatric Patient Safety. Pediatric Clinics of North America. 2006;53:1105-19.
13. Spooner, A. and Council on Clinical Information Technology. Special Requirements of Electronic Health Record Systems in Pediatrics. Pediatrics. 2007:119(3):631-637.
14. Nakamura, M.M., Ferris, T.G., DesRoches, C.M., Jha, A.K. Electronic health record adoption by children's hospitals in the United States. Arch Pediatr Adolesc Med. 2010 Dec;164(12):1145-51.

15. Flach, J.M., Dominguez, C.O. Use-centered design: Integrating the user, instrument, and goal. Ergonomics in Design: The Quarterly of Human Factors Applications, July 1995;3(3):19-24.

16. ISO/IEC. 9241-14 Ergonomic requirements for office work with visual display terminals (VDTs) - Part 14 Menu dialogues, ISO/IEC 9241-14: 1998 (E), 1998.

17. Zhang, J., Walji, M. TURF: Toward a unified framework of EHR usability. Journal of Biomedical Informatics, 2011: 44 (6):1056-1067.

18. Hancock, P.A., Szalma, J.L. Operator stress & display design. Ergonomics in Design. 2003;11(2):13-8.

19. Steering Committee on Quality Improvement and Management and Committee on Hospital Care. Principles of Pediatric Patient Safety: Reducing Harm Due to Medical Care. Pediatrics Vol. 127 No. 6 June 1, 2011 , pp. 1199 -1210.

20. Hughes, RG,Edgerton, EA. (2005). First, Do No Harm: Reducing Pediatric Medication Errors. American Journal of Nursing, 105(5), 79-84.

21. Caldwell, N, Power B. (2012). The pros and cons of electronic prescribing for children. Archives of Diseases in Childhood 2012;97 (2):124-128.

22. Ross Koppel. Commentary on EMR Entry Error: Not so Benign. http://www.webmm.ahrq.gov/case.aspx?caseID=199.

23. Zhang, J., Walji, M. TURF: Toward a unified framework of EHR usability. Journal of Biomedical Informatics, 2011; 44 (6):1056-1067.

24. Ibid.

25. Koch, S.H., Weir, C., Haar, M., et al. Journal of the American Medical Informatics Association (2012). Intensive care unit nurses' information needs and recommendations for integrated displays to improve nurses' situation awareness. 2012 Mar 21 [Epub ahead of print].

26. Lyons M, Adams S, Woloshynowych M, Vincent C. Human reliability analysis in healthcare: A review of techniques. International Journal of Risk & Safety in Medicine 16 (2004) 223–237.

27. DeRosier J, Stalhandske E, Bagian JP, Nudell T. Using Health Care Failure Mode and Effect Analysis™: The VA National Center for Patient Safety's Prospective Risk Analysis System. The Joint Commission Journal on Quality Improvement Volume 27 Number 5:248-267, 2002.

28. Hildebrand, Richard, James H. Bigelow, Basit Chaudhry, et al. "Identity Crisis: An Examination of the Costs and Benefits of a Unique Patient Identifier for the U.S. Health Care System." 2008. www.rand.org/pubs/monographs/MG753.html.

29. www.himss.org/ASP/topics_privacy.asp.

30. Sarter, N.B., Woods, D.D. How in the world did we ever get into that mode? Mode error and awareness in supervisory control. Human Factors, 37(1):5–19.

31. Cooper, W.O., Habel, L.A., Sox, C.M., et al. ADHD drugs and serious cardiovascular events in children and young adults. New England Journal of Medicine, 2011; 365:1896.

32. Spooner, A. and Council on Clinical Information Technology. Special Requirements of Electronic Health Record Systems in Pediatrics. Pediatrics. 2007;119(3): 631-637.

33. Handbook of Human Factors in Medical Device Design Boca Raton, FL: CRC Press, 2010.

34. Johnson, K.B., Lee, C.K., Spooner, S.A., Davison, C.L., Helmke, J.S., Weinberg, S.T. Automated doserounding recommendations for pediatric medications. Pediatrics. 2011 Aug;128(2):e422-8.

35. Sarter, N.B., Woods, D.D. Pilot Interaction with Cockpit Automation: Operational Experiences with the Flight Management System. International Journal of Aviation Psychology, 1992;2(4): 303-321.

36. van Rosse, F., Maat, B., Rademaker, C.M., van Vught, A.J., Egberts, A.C., Bollen, C.W. The effect of computerized physician order entry on medication prescription errors and clinical outcome in pediatric and intensive care: a systematic review. Pediatrics. 2009 Apr;123(4):1184-90.

37. Isaac, T., Weissman, J.S., Davis, R.B., Massagli, M., Cyrulik, A., Sands, D.Z., Weingart, S.N. Overrides of Medication Alerts in Ambulatory Care. Archives of Internal Medicine. 2009;169(3):305-311.

38. Van der Sijs, H., Aarts, J., Vulto, A., Berg, M. Overriding of drug safety alerts in computerized physician order entry. Journal of the American Medical Informatics Association. 2006; 13(2):138-47.

39. Lawless, S.T. Crying Wolf: false alarms in a pediatric intensive care unit, Critical Care Medicine. 1994:22;981-5.

40. Strom, B., M.D., M.P.H. ,Schinnar, R, et. al. Unintended Effects of a Computerized Physician Order Entry Nearly Hard-Stop Alert to Prevent a Drug Interaction. Archives of Internal Medicine. 2010;170(17):1578-1583.

41. http://clinicaltrials.gov/ct2/show/NCT01478711.

42. http://www.cdc.gov/growthcharts/clinical_charts.htm.

43. Woods, D. D., Roth, E. M. Cognitive engineering: Human problem solving with tools. Human Factors, 1988;30(4): 415-430.

44. Emmett, J., Lodree, E., Geigerb, C., Jiangc, X. Taxonomy for integrating scheduling theory and human factors: Review and research opportunities. International Journal of Industrial Ergonomics, January 2009;39(1): 39-51.

45. Snoo, C., Wezel, W. Coordination and task interdependence during schedule adaptation. Human Factors and Ergonomics in Manufacturing & Service Industries. Online 12 Dec 2011.

46. http://www.cdc.gov/vaccines/recs/schedules/.

47. Gardner, P., Pickering, L.K., Orenstein, W.A., Gershon, A.A., Nichol, K.L. Guidelines for Quality Standards for Immunization. CID 2002:35 (1 September 2002): 503-511.

48. Poon, E.G., Gandhi, T.K., Sequist, T.D., Murff, H.J., Karson, A.S., Bates, D.W. "I wish I had seen this test result earlier!": dissatisfaction with test result management systems in primary care. Archives of Internal Medicine. 2004;164(20):2223–2228.

49. Wahls, T.L., Cram, P.M. The frequency of missed test results and associated treatment delays in a highly computerized health system. BMC Family Practice. 2007;8:32.

50. Ferris, T.G., Johnson, S.A., Co, J.P., Backus, M., Perrin, J., Bates, D.W., Poon, E.G. Electronic results management in pediatric ambulatory care: qualitative assessment. Pediatrics. 2009 Jan;123 Suppl 2:S85- 91.

51. Recommendation 2. http://www.jointcommission.org/assets/1/18/SEA_471.PDF.

52. National Council on Radiation Protection and Measurements: Ionizing radiation exposure of the population of the United States (2009). NCRP Report No. 160, Bethesda, Md.:142-146.

53. Recommendation 19. http://www.jointcommission.org/assets/1/18/SEA_471.PDF.

54. Kim, G.R., Lehmann, C.U., Council on Clinical Information Technology. Pediatric Aspects of Inpatient Health Information Technology Systems. Pediatrics. December 1, 2008;122(6):e1287 e1296.

Lowry, S. Z., Quinn M.T., Ramaiah, M., Brick D., Patterson, E. S., Zhang, .J, Abbot, P., and Gibbons, M. C.. A Human Factors Guide to Enhance EHR Usability of Critical User Interactions when Supporting Pediatric Patient Care (NISTIR 7865) Available at: http://dx.doi.org/10.6028/NIST.IR.7865. June 28, 2012.

CHAPTER 8

SOCIOTECHNICAL EVALUATION OF THE SAFETY AND EFFECTIVENESS OF POINT-OF-CARE MOBILE COMPUTING DEVICES: A CASE STUDY CONDUCTED IN INDIA

DEAN F. SITTIG, KANAV KAHOL, and HARDEEP SINGH

8.1 INTRODUCTION

Several countries are aiming to transform their health care delivery systems with unprecedented economic investments in their health information technology (IT) infrastructures. Concurrently, policy initiatives in India and elsewhere have called for technology implementation to enhance health care quality and access [1]. Despite this momentum and commitment of resources, the pace of health IT adoption initiatives has been slower and more variable than expected [2]. Globally, only a few organizations have achieved successful transformation of their systems [3,4]. Many health care settings are just now beginning their health IT journey while others are using health IT partially and still modifying their work processes to make health IT fit[5,6]. The unexpected slower pace of health IT adoption could partially be explained by challenges to successful health IT implementation within the workflow of a complex health care system. For example, a number of unanticipated problems, including issues with patient safety and provider productivity [7-10] have occurred with IT adoption.

In view of the challenges that clinicians and organizations face with implementation of health IT, we previously developed an 8-dimension, socio-technical model of safe and effective IT use[11]. This model (see Figure 1) offers a comprehensive framework for evaluating the design, development, implementation, use, and monitoring of health IT within complex health care systems and was recently applied to electronic communication [12]. We are also using this model as a guide to proactively identify risks and opportunities to improve new and existing health IT systems [13]. Using this model to guide our current project, we sought to evaluate a mobile computing device in rural Indian healthcare settings.

8.2 BACKGROUND

To reform India's highly fragmented healthcare system, one essential prerequisite is a safe and effective "health IT-enabled clinical work system" [14] that has potential to reach and improve the health of over one billion patients. In October 2010, the Planning Commission of India convened a High-Level Expert Group (HLEG) on Universal Health Coverage (UHC) and charged this Group to develop a framework for providing easily accessible and affordable health care to all Indians.1 One of HLEG's recommendations was to develop a national health information technology network based on uniform standards to ensure inter-operability between all healthcare stakeholders. More than two-thirds of the population in India lives in rural areas where health care access is limited, technology penetration is low and physicians are scarce. Nevertheless, one possible method of outreach is through front-line non-physician health care workers who are technology-enabled and use mobile devices to collect/interpret basic clinical data. Globally, informaticians, and clinicians have always anticipated a small, inexpensive portable device that is capable of collecting, interpreting, storing, and transmitting patient data from the point-of-care (POC) for clinical and administrative functions. The widespread availability of tablet computers with Bluetooth and 3G/4G networking capabilities has brought such tools within closer reach.

With this vision, the Public Health Foundation of India, Division of Health Technologies, developed the "Swasthya Slate," [15] a state-of-the-art Android-based tablet computer that is designed to collect and process administrative, demographic, and physiologic data relevant to all aspects of primary care, including maternal and child care [16]. The Swasthya Slate system was designed primarily to empower frontline health work-

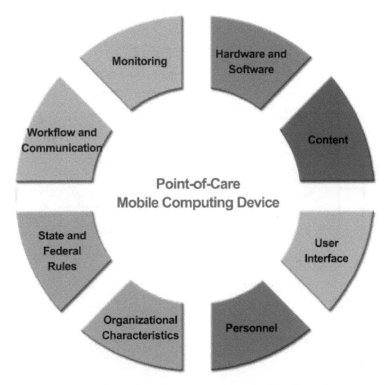

FIGURE 1: 8-dimension socio-technical model used to identify and categorize the items in the guide

ers to deliver high quality care. This system provides a seamless inter-face to the electronic medical record, which, when combined with cloud computing technologies, can automate data reporting to central authorities, reducing the burden of secondary data entry. Additionally, using global positioning satellites (GPS) and images, it is possible to validate and authenticate care delivery. For example, a supervisor who oversees 5-6 providers at different primary health centers can review the GPS locations at which visit data were entered and review pictures for authentication.

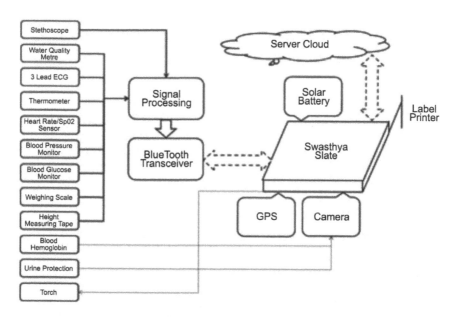

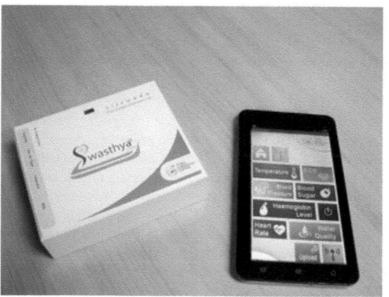

FIGURE 2: Swasthya Slate Hardware Block Diagram and system (see www.swasthyaslate.org)

8.2.1   SWASTHYA SLATE FUNCTIONALITY

In addition to supporting manually entered information, Swasthya Slate enables digitization of test data and point-of-care-diagnostics. For example, Bluetooth-enabled blood pressure monitors and blood sugar monitors can transmit data directly to the device [17]. The tablet can also image and analyze reactive test strips to diagnose, for instance, high levels of blood glucose and anemia [18].

The system further facilitates the provision of high-quality healthcare by including clinical decision support (CDS) systems as part of the tablet. CDS systems use artificial intelligence algorithms or basic logical flow-charts that encode guidelines from governmental health agencies to provide healthcare workers with on-the-spot help in delivering care. These systems can also provide logistical support to the healthcare workers, for example, by enabling them to easily access daily plans, plot their care delivery routes, get reminders, and access emergency services and learn about resources at nearest care facilities to properly guide the patient.

The peripherals used with the Swasthya Slate are equivalent to those used in standard practice in the Indian public health system and include: 1. stethoscope; 2. water quality meter; 3. 3-lead ECG; 4. digital thermometer; 5. heart rate and Sp02 sensor (for oxygen saturation); 6. blood pressure monitor; 7. hemoglobin color scale; 8. urinalysis test strips; 9. blood glucose monitor; 10. digital weight scale; 11. flashlight; and 12. measuring tape. Thus, the device could enable a non-physician health care worker to collect many of the basic parameters for a medical assessment of common conditions.

To ensure that the robust functionality of this system fits within the social context of India's health system, we developed a sociotechnical assessment tool for its formative evaluation. Our study objective was to apply our sociotechnical model to develop a comprehensive evaluation strategy for the Swasthya Slate and use this evaluation to address both technical and non-technical areas of improvement during the all-important design, development, and usability testing phases of user-centered design. Our ultimate goal was to ensure the device's safe and effective, large-scale use in rural India.

8.3   MATERIALS AND METHODS

8.3.1   DEVELOPMENT OF A "SOCIOTECHNICAL" ASSESSMENT GUIDE

First, we developed an itemized assessment guide to identify potential risks or challenges to safe and effective use of the tablet under realistic clinical practice conditions. Item content was derived from several sources: 1. an extensive review of the literature, 2. interviews with experts in clinical care and health IT implementation, 3. surveys of challenges and opportunities to user acceptance of these types of devices, and 4. field observations of primary care workers with various levels of clinical and computing expertise working with these and similar devices.

8.3.1.1   LITERATURE REVIEWS

We reviewed the literature relevant to each of the eight dimensions of our model to identify items that were applicable to safe and effective use of IT, particularly those which were directly applicable to tablet devices.

8.3.1.2   INTERVIEWS

We conducted interviews in both the US and India with experts in public health, medicine, and health IT. We focused to a large degree on frontline health workers, who bear the burden of delivering most clinical care in rural India. Interviews with health workers were important to identify potential improvements to the system in terms of usability (user interface), training requirements, compliance with local, regional and national laws and reporting requirements for specific clinical conditions (e.g. pregnancy), workflow and communication, and supervision and monitoring by physicians. We interviewed administrators to further understand legal, moni-

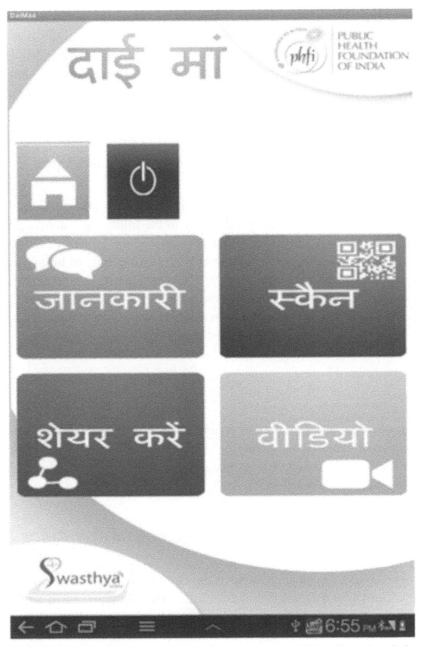

FIGURE 3: Health maintenance reminders for maternal and child health are installed and working

toring, and workflow issues which could pose as barriers and facilitators to implementation of such a device. Finally, we interviewed physicians regarding issues of clinical content (knowledge, rules and logic embedded into the device) and whether the communication and reporting channels under development and supervision mechanisms of front-line personnel collecting data would be aligned with their expectations.

8.3.1.3   DOCUMENTING/OBSERVING USER ACCEPTANCE

We administered the IsoMetrics Usability Inventory [19] to frontline healthcare workers to document usability in the following 7 domains: 1. suitability for the task; 2. self-descriptiveness of the system (e.g. functions of the system are self-explanatory); 3. controllability of the system; 4. conformity with user expectations; 5. error tolerance; 6. suitability for individualization; and 7. suitability for learning. We also administered a custom developed questionnaire to evaluate how well the system fulfilled the reporting requirements of selected conditions such as pregnancy.

8.3.1.4   FIELD OBSERVATIONS

Field observations were used to examine the effectiveness of training of trainers and evaluate the durability of the tablet. It also helped us study how environmental factors (e.g., temperature, rain, direct sunlight) affect the usability of the system.

8.3.2   MOBILE COMPUTING DEVICE EVALUATION GUIDE

An initial set of evaluation items from each of the eight sociotechnical dimensions was created from the results of the literature search and interviews. The items were then refined based on additional expert opinion, user acceptance testing, and observations. The following items (under each dimension) were determined to be most relevant to the safety and effectiveness of the device (and potentially other similar devices) and were included in the final draft of the guide.

8.3.2.1   HARDWARE AND SOFTWARE

Reliable hardware and software is essential for any mobile POC mobile device. The following items were found to be most relevant for safety and effectiveness of POC devices.

- The tablet will run the required software applications for at least 4 hours on battery power.
- The device has a protective case to reduce breakage or damage and prevent entry of dust into the system.
- The device is water-resistant; the screen can be cleaned with liquid disinfectant.
- The device has up-to-date virus protection software.
- The device's hardware interfaces have been tested with all external, ancillary devices (i.e., thermometer, water quality gauge, blood glucose monitor, etc.).
- The device is password protected.
- The device's hard drive is encrypted and can be erased by remote command in the event the device is lost or stolen.
- The device can connect to the Internet through a variety of means (e.g., either a wireless LAN or 3G/4G connection) and has a way to store data locally and then upload it at a later time in the event that Internet connections are not available.

8.3.2.2   CLINICAL CONTENT

Up-to-date clinical content (i.e., data, information, and knowledge) is required to encode the user entered information as well as provide clinicians with reference information at the point of care.

- Required clinical content has been loaded on the device.
- Clinical content can be updated remotely.
- Clinical guidelines and CDS content are up to date.
- Clinical content is available in one of the native languages of the user. (An example of the system in Hindi appears in Figure 3.)

8.3.2.3   HUMAN-COMPUTER USER INTERFACE

The user interface enables users to interact with the data, information, and knowledge required to understand the patient's physiologic state and document their findings and intended actions.

- Users can see the information on the screen in direct sunlight.
- The fonts are large enough for middle-aged and older health care workers to read without difficulty.
- The touch screen is properly registered (i.e., when the user touches an item on the screen, the device recognizes that object has been touched).
- The device cannot be used with gloves on.
- The required software applications can be used with a finger or a stylus.
- The application allows both freehand and keyboard-based data entry.
- The device and key software applications provide multi-language support.
- Using the applications on the device requires limited text interface with audio support.
- The applications are easy to learn and text-based, audio, or video support is readily available.
- The software does not create tasks that are superfluous to the user's normal daily routine.
- The software adds value to the user's daily life.
- The software automatically produces reports and letters of discharge and referrals to minimize administrative work.

8.3.2.4   PERSONNEL

People are required to design, develop, implement, use, and manage all aspects of the IT-enabled healthcare system.

- All health care workers have had at least 2 hours of training on how to use the tablet in their native language.
- Centralized IT support personnel are accessible via cellphone or Voice-over-IP to health care workers.
- Health care workers are able to answer healthcare questions that are frequently asked by patients in rural areas who are unfamiliar with similar types of data collection instruments.

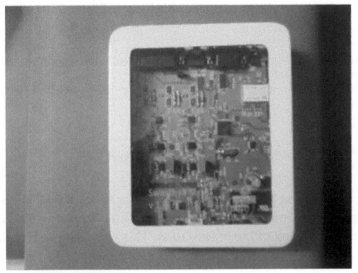

FIGURE 4: Earlier box design

8.3.2.5 WORKFLOW AND COMMUNICATION

Modern healthcare requires extensive collaboration between disparate members of the healthcare team. Meeting the needs of various healthcare workers continues to be a challenge.

- Workflow observations are conducted and recorded prior to local implementation of the tablet.
- Indications for referral are clearly specified and sent to the referring provider either via paper, fax, email, etc. [20].

8.3.2.6 ORGANIZATIONAL POLICY, PROCEDURE, CULTURE, & ENVIRONMENT

In organizations that are involved with implementing and using the mobile device, policies and procedures and the culture and physical environment should empower workers and not burden them with constraints. Items that address this include:

- Standard operating procedure documents specify the scope and indications for use of the tablet.
- Procedures for maintenance and technical problem-solving are clearly delineated.

8.3.2.7   EXTERNAL RULES AND REGULATIONS

Local, regional and federal rules and regulations (i.e. those that originate outside of the organization) also have a significant impact on the safe and efficient functioning of the organization. This was addressed by the following items:

- Laws and provisions created by the government are adequate to protect the use of the tablet for its intended purposes and to prevent fraud and theft.
- Regulations create mechanisms to strictly reinforce the delivery of expedited clinical care and referrals for patients who are found to need urgent medical attention.

8.3.2.8   MEASUREMENT AND MONITORING

The key to improving the safety and efficiency of the IT-enabled healthcare system is to measure and monitor important details. This was addressed by the following items:

- The demographics interface is able to validate patient identity through a legitimate source such as user identification (UID), ration card, etc.
- Calibration of all physiologic or chemical sensors is performed every 3 months.
- 5% of data collected are validated for accuracy (e.g., 5% of automated EKG interpretations should be verified by a clinician).
- Outcome assessments are conducted using random samples of 5% of patients should be conducted to ensure that the tablet is serving its intended purpose (e.g., a positive diabetes screening should consistently prompt a referral or treatment).

8.4 RESULTS

Use of the guide for formative evaluation of the Swasthya Slate system resulted in several product enhancements and considerations of how the device fit within the larger social context of the health system. For instance, the tablet case was redesigned in response to feedback generated from these items (see Figure 4). The initial design emphasized the technology focus, but the final design aims to provide a more robust look with better protection against environmental factors.

Software reliability was significantly improved as well. The user interface was also improved by focusing on both affect (i.e., making it look more "sophisticated") and functionality. We utilized Microsoft's new "metro interface" design language emphasizing typography and large text on large buttons to catch the user's eye. This allowed users with limited education to use the tablet easily. We developed the reporting system to be in line with the reporting requirements of the government. For example, one of the requirements was that health workers complete a registry with a list of mothers. We interfaced the Slate with a label printer to automatically generate stickers for applicable cases, which the health worker could in turn simply stick on the register to save time and reduce omission or transcription errors. Following the ethnographic observations, the workflow was modified so that the upfront diagnostics were performed before the checkup which fit the user's workflow better as well as minimizing the time the kit needed to be turned on, maximizing the battery life. To comply with legal directives (external rules and regulations), our decision support system (content) was designed to limit interventions by frontline health workers to those that are non-pharmacological, i.e. so they didn't receive specific CDS interventions about prescribing medications beyond their expertise. We also identified skill sets specific to the types of personnel that would be using the device.

Quantitative data were also collected and analyzed with a specific focus on improving the usability of the tablet. To date, we have surveyed 100 community health workers, 50 nurse midwives, and 50 equivalent health workers in the private sector for our usability study. A composite scoring system was developed for each of the 7 usability domains. The mean usability rating across all of the domains was 8.9/10 (SD = 0.6). The lowest domain score was for user customization (mean 7.8/10, SD 1.1), although this was not unexpected because, by design, customization was limited to avoid potential interference with best practices. The highest domain score was suitability for the task (mean 9.2/10, SD 0.6).

Average learning time to first correct execution of the software was 10 minutes, and by 45 minutes users were able to use the apps with less than 1% "slip" errors (e.g., accidental pressing of buttons, etc.). Our training, which lasts 1 day, has been very successful in ensuring the full use of the system.

As the device is implemented more widely, we will continue to conduct additional iterative evaluation to inform device use as well as add additional items to the guide if needed for its subsequent use in other types of settings.

8.5   DISCUSSION

We developed a "sociotechnical" assessment guide for safe and effective use of a mobile computing health care device in India. A sociotechnical assessment can be used to help prevent unintended consequences of using mobile IT and for helping proactively detect, mitigate, and ameliorate unintended consequences and potential failures associated with the use of such devices. Our evaluation was grounded in our previously used multifaceted socio-technical model of health IT implementation and use. Based upon the work we conducted, others planning to collect and interpret data at the point of care in rural settings could consider similar formative evaluation methods to ensure successful design, development, implementation and use of these devices.

Health information technology is changing the way we deliver health care and can be used in reforming health care and improving health care access especially in developing countries. In India, there is a large deficit of physicians in rural settings, and thus point of care mobile devices that can be used by trained non-physician health care workers to collect data can assist with providing primary health care needs. However, there might be little benefit of data collection and point of care devices unless the data is used successfully to improve clinical care in terms of improving quality, safety and efficiency. Thus, these devices must be integrated within the social context of the health system where they are implemented and used. We envision that stakeholders planning to use such devices would assemble multidisciplinary assessment teams to conduct such a comprehensive evaluation which will ensure that the device fits within the broader context of health care delivery and improvement.

Our study limitations include absence of outcome data on how Swasthya Slate impacts care processes or outcomes of clinical conditions. Nevertheless, the Slate is being pilot tested in several rural settings in India and data on impact will be available in the future. In addition, our evaluation might only be generalizable to certain types of rural healthcare settings.

8.6   CONCLUSION

To better leverage health IT, a sociotechnical approach is necessary to avoid unexpected challenges and failures [21]. This includes both technical and non-technical formative and summative evaluations of health IT devices to ensure that they fit within the social context. Our evaluation strategy facilitated a comprehensive sociotechnical assessment and improvement of a promising point of care computing device in India. Our assessment revealed and addressed both technical (functionality, content, usability, user interface) and non-technical (workflow, processes and policies etc.) areas of improvement.

REFERENCES

1. Thakur J. Key recommendations of high-level expert group report on universal health coverage for India. Indian Community Med. 2011 Dec;36(Suppl 1):S84-5. http://www.ncbi.nlm.nih.gov/pmc/articles/PMC3354908/.
2. Sittig D, Ash J. Clinical information Systems: Overcoming adverse consequences. Sudbury, MA: Jones and Bartlett Publishers, LLC; 2009.

3. Chaudhry B, Wang J, Wu S etal. Systematic review: impact of health information technology on quality, efficiency, and costs of medical care. Ann Intern Med 2006;144:742-52.

4. Protti D. Comparison of information technology in general practice in 10 countries. Healthc Q. 2007;10:107-116.

5. Sittig DF, Ash JS, Zhang J, et al. Lessons from "Unexpected increased mortality after implementation of a commercially sold computerized physician order entry system". Pediatrics. 2006;118:797-801.

6. Blumenthal D, Tavenner M. The "Meaningful Use" Regulation for Electronic Health Records. New England Journal of Medicine. 2010;363:501-504.

7. Campbell EM, Sittig DF, Ash JS, et al. Types of Unintended Consequences Related to Computerized Provider Order Entry. J Am Med Inform Assoc. 2006;13:547-556.

8. Metzger J, Welebob E, Bates DW, et al. Mixed results in the safety performance of computerized physician order entry. Health Aff (Millwood). 2010;29:655-663.

9. Magrabi F, Ong MS, Runciman W, et al. Using FDA reports to inform a classification for health information technology safety problems. J Am Med Inform Assoc. 2011.

10. Harrington L, Kennerly D, Johnson C. Safety issues related to the electronic medical record (EMR): synthesis of the literature from the last decade, 2000-2009. J Healthc Manag. 2011;56:31-43.

11. Sittig DF, Singh H. A New Socio-technical Model for Studying Health Information Technology in Complex Adaptive Healthcare Systems. Quality & Safety in Healthcare, 2010 Oct;19 Suppl 3:i68-74.

12. Singh H, Spitzmueller C, Petersen NJ, et al. Primary care practitioners' views on test result management in EHR-enabled health systems: a national survey. J Am Med Inform Assoc. 2012 doi:10.1136/amiajnl-2012-001267

13. Singh H, Ash JS, Sittig DF. Safety Assurance Factors for Electronic Health Record Resilience (SAFER): study protocol. BMC Med Inform Decis Mak, 2013; (in press).

14. Sittig DF, Singh H. Electronic health records and national patient-safety goals. N Engl J Med. 2012 Nov 8;367(19):1854-60. doi: 10.1056/NEJMsb1205420.

15. Swasthya Slate: http://swasthyaslate.org/usermanual.php

16. Demonstration of the Swasthya Slate Rev 2. Available at: http://www.youtube.com/watch?v=oTe_5IFgc7A

17. Contec Medical Systems Available from: http://www.contecmed.com/main/Default.asp. 2012

18. Loh B, Vuong N, Chan S, Lau C. Automated Mobile pH Reader on a Camera Phone. IAENG Intern. J Computer Science. 2011; 38(3): Advance Online Publication.

19. Gediga, Hamborg & Düntsch (1999). The IsoMetrics Usability Inventory: An operationalisation of ISO 9241-10, Behaviour and Information Technology, 18, 151 - 164.

20. Esquivel A, Sittig DF, Murphy DR, et al. Improving the effectiveness of electronic health record based referral processes. BMC Med Inform Decis Mak. 2012 Sep 13;12:107.

21. Singh H, Sittig DF. A Socio-technical Model to Guide Safe and Effective Health Information Technology Use in India. Indian Journal of Medical Informatics; 6(1); 2012. http://ijmi.org/index.php/ijmi/article/view/189/74

Sittig, D. F., Kahol, K., and Singh H. Sociotechnical Evaluation of the Safety and Effectiveness of Point-of-Care Mobile Computing Devices: A Case Study Conducted in India. (in press MedInfo 2013; Copenhagen, Denmark August 2013). Studies in Health Technology and Informatics, Volume 192: MEDINFO 2013 (in press). DOI10.3233/978-1-61499-289-9-515. Used with permission.

PART IV

CLINICAL DECISION SUPPORT

TEN COMMANDMENTS FOR EFFECTIVE CLINICAL DECISION SUPPORT: MAKING THE PRACTICE OF EVIDENCE-BASED MEDICINE A REALITY

DAVID W BATES, GILAD J KUPERMAN, SAMUEL WANG, TEJAL GANDHI, ANNE KITTLER, LYNN VOLK, CYNTHIA SPURR, RAMIN KHORASANI, MILENKO TANASIJEVIC, and BLACKFORD MIDDLETON

Delivering outstanding medical care requires providing care that is both high-quality and safe. However, while the knowledge base regarding effective medical therapies continues to improve, the practice of medicine continues to lag behind, and errors are distressingly frequent. [1]

Regarding the gaps between evidence and practice, Lomas et al. [2] evaluated a series of published guidelines and found that it took an average of approximately five years for these guidelines to be adopted into routine practice. Moreover, evidence exists that many guidelines—even those that are broadly accepted—are often not followed. [3 4 5 6 7] For example, approximately 50% of eligible patients do not receive beta blockers after myocardial infarction, [8] and a recent study found that only 33% of patients had low-density lipoprotein (LDL) cholesterol levels at or below the National Cholesterol Education Program recommendations. [5] Of course, in many instances, relevant guidelines are not yet available, but even in these instances, practitioners should consider the evidence if they wish to practice evidence-based medicine, and a core part of practicing evidence-based medicine is considering guidelines when they do exist.

Although we strive to provide the best possible care, many studies within our own institution have identified gaps between optimal and actual practice. For example, in a study designed to assess the appropriateness of antiepileptic drug monitoring, only 27% of antiepileptic drug levels had an appropriate indication and, among these, half were drawn at an inappropriate time. [9] Among digoxin levels, only 16% were appropriate in the inpatient setting, and 52% were appropriate in the outpatient setting. [10] Of clinical laboratory tests, 28% were ordered too early after a prior test of the same type to be clinically useful. [11] For evaluation of hypothyroidism or hyperthyroidism, the initial thyroid test performed was not the thyroid-stimulating hormone level in 52% of instances. [12] Only 17% of diabetics who needed eye examinations had them, even after visiting their primary care provider. [13] The Centers for Disease Control and Prevention (CDC) guidelines for vancomycin use were not followed 68% of the time. [14] Safety also is an issue: in one study, we identified 6.5 adverse drug events per 100 admissions, and 28% were preventable [15]; for example, many patients received medications to which they had a known allergy. Clearly, there are many opportunities for improvement.

We believe that decision support delivered using information systems, ideally with the electronic medical record as the platform, will finally provide decision makers with tools making it possible to achieve large gains in performance, narrow gaps between knowledge and practice, and improve safety. [16 17] Recent reviews have suggested that decision support can improve performance, although it has not always been effective. [18 19] These reviews have summarized the evidence that computerized decision support works, in part, based on evidence domain. While this perspective has been very useful and has suggested, for example, that decision support focusing on preventive reminders and drug doses has been more effective than decision support targeting assistance regarding diagnosis, it does not tell one how best to deliver it.

In all the areas discussed above, we have attempted to intervene with decision support to improve care with some successes [20 21] and many partial or complete failures. [22 23 24] For the purposes of this report, we consider decision support to include passive and active referential information as well as reminders, alerts, and guidelines. Many others also have evaluated the impact of decision support, [19 20] and we are not attempting to provide a comprehensive summary of how decision support can improve care but rather to provide our perspective on what worked and what did not. [19] Thus, the goal of this report is to present generic lessons from our experiences that may be useful to others, including informaticians, systems developers, and health care organizations.

9.1 STUDY SITE

Brigham and Women's Hospital (BWH) is a 720-bed tertiary care hospital. The hospital has an integrated hospital information system, accessed via networked desktop personal computers, that provides clinical, administrative, and financial functions. [25 26] A physician order entry application was implemented initially in 1993. [27 28] Physicians enter all patient orders into this application, with the majority being entered in coded form. The information system in general, and the physician order entry system in particular, delivers patient-specific decision support to clinicians in real time. Most active decision support to date has focused on drugs, [29] laboratory testing, [30 22] and radiology procedures. [24] In addition, a wide array of information is available online for physicians to consult, including literature searching, Scientific American Medicine, and the Physician's Desk Reference, among others; these applications are used hundreds of times daily. In the ambulatory practices associated with the hospital, we have developed an electronic medical record, which is the main record used in most practices [31] and which includes an increasing amount of decision support. [32]

We currently are in the process of developing additional applications for the Partners network, which includes BWH and Massachusetts General Hospital, several smaller community hospitals, and Partners Community Healthcare, a network of more than 1,000 physicians across the region. These include a Longitudinal Medical Record, which will serve as a network-wide record across the continuum of care and will include ambulatory order entry, an enterprise master patient index, and a clinical data repository. [31]

9.2   TEN COMMANDMENTS FOR EFFECTIVE CLINICAL DECISION SUPPORT

9.2.1   SPEED IS EVERYTHING

We have found repeatedly, [33] as have others, [34] that the speed of an information system is the parameter that users value most. If the decision support is wonderful, but takes too long to appear, it will be useless. When infrastructure problems slow the speed of an application, user satisfaction declines markedly. Our goal is subsecond "screen flips" (the time it takes to transition from one screen to the next), which appears anecdotally to be the threshold that is important to our users. While this may be a difficult standard to achieve, it should be a primary goal.

Evidence supporting this comes, in part, from user surveys regarding computerized physician order entry. In one such survey, we found that the primary determinant of user satisfaction was speed and that this rated much higher than quality improvement aspects. [35] In fact, users perceived physician order entry primarily as an efficiency technology, [35] even though we found in a formal time–motion study that it took users significantly longer to write orders using the computer than with paper, in part, because many screens were involved. [36] Others have had similar results. [37] Thus, while the hospital administration and clinical leadership's highest priorities are likely to be costs and quality, the top priority of users will be the speed of the information system.

9.2.2   ANTICIPATE NEEDS AND DELIVER IN REAL TIME

It is not enough for the information a provider needs to simply be available someplace in the system—applications must anticipate clinician needs and bring information to clinicians at the time they need it (Fig. 1). All health professionals in the United States face increasing time pressure and can ill afford to spend even more time seeking bits of information. Simply making information accessible electronically, while better than nothing,

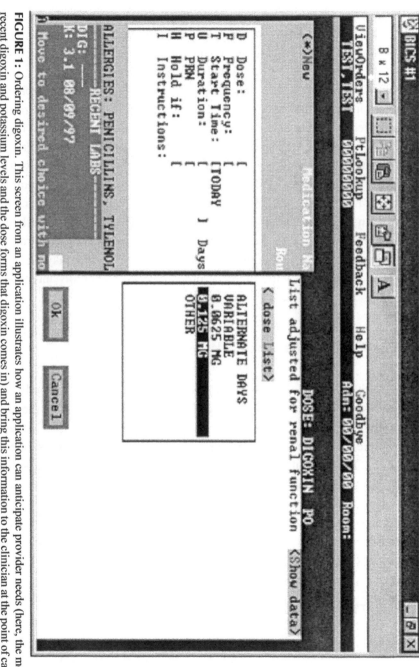

FIGURE 1: Ordering digoxin. This screen from an application illustrates how an application can anticipate provider needs (here, the most recent digoxin and potassium levels and the dose forms that digoxin comes in) and bring this information to the clinician at the point of care.

has little effect. [38] Systems can serve the critical role of gathering and making associations between pieces of information that clinicians might miss because of the sheer volume of data, for example, emphasizing a low-potassium level in a patient receiving digoxin.

Optimal clinical decision support systems should also have the capability to anticipate the subtle "latent needs" of clinicians in addition to more obvious needs. "Latent needs" are needs that are present but have not been consciously realized. Decision support provided through the computer can fill many such latent needs, for example, notifying the clinician to lower a drug dose when a patient's kidney function worsens. [39] Another example of a latent need is a situation that occurs in which one order or piece of information suggests that an action should follow (Fig. 2). [40] Overhage et al. [40] have referred to these orders or information as corollary orders. As did Overhage et al., [40] our group has also found that displaying suggested orders across a wide range of order types substantially increased the likelihood that the desired action will occur. [41]

9.2.3   FIT INTO THE USER'S WORKFLOW

Success with alerts, guidelines, and algorithms depends substantially on integrating suggestions with practice. [38] We have built a number of "stand-alone" guidelines for a variety of conditions, including sleep apnea, for example. However, use counts have been very low, even for excellent guidelines. The vancomycin guideline mentioned above was available for passive consultation, yet was rarely used; only after bringing the guideline to the user on a single screen at the time the clinician was in the process of ordering vancomycin did we see an impact. Understanding clinician workflow, particularly when designing applications for the outpatient setting, is critical.

9.2.4   LITTLE THINGS CAN MAKE A BIG DIFFERENCE

The point here is that usability matters—a lot. Developers must make it easy for a clinician to "do the right thing." In the human factors world, usability testing has had a tremendous impact on improving systems, [42]

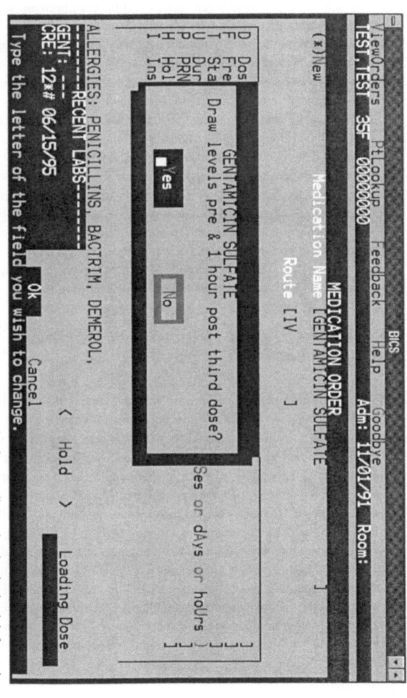

FIGURE 2: Example of a corollary order. Ordering gentamicin sulfate prompts a suggestion for a corollary order: drawing levels before and one hour after the third dose.

and what appear to be nuances can make the difference between success and failure. While it should be obvious that clinical computing systems are no different, usability testing has not necessarily been a routine part of designing them. We have had many experiences in which a minor change in the way screens were designed had a major impact on provider actions. For example, in one application, when the default was set to have clinicians enter the diagnosis as free text rather than from a code list below, a much larger proportion of diagnoses were entered as free text than when we had defaulted to the most likely coded alternative. This, in turn, had down-stream consequences regarding providing decision support, for example, providers did not get reminders about diabetes if diabetes was entered as free text. In a more dramatic example, the Regenstrief group found that displaying computerized reminders suggesting vaccinations for inpatients had no impact when the reminders were easy to ignore, but when the screen flow was altered to make it harder for physicians to ignore the reminder suggestions, they saw a large positive impact. [43]

9.2.5 RECOGNIZE THAT PHYSICIANS WILL STRONGLY RESIST STOPPING

Across a wide array of interventions, we have found that physicians strongly resist suggestions not to carry out an action when we do not offer an alternative, even if the action they are about to carry out is virtually always counterproductive. In a study of decision support regarding abdominal radiography, [24] suggestions that no radiograph be ordered at all were accepted only 5% of the time, even though studies ordered when the alerts were overridden yielded almost no useful findings. Similarly, for tests that were clearly redundant with another test of the same kind performed earlier that day, we found that clinicians overrode reminders a third of the time, even though such results were never useful (Fig. 3). [44]

In counter detailing about drugs, we have found also that if clinicians have strong beliefs about a medication, and either no alternative or an unpalatable alternative is offered, clinicians routinely override suggestions not to order the ketorolac original medication. One example was for intravenous ketorolac, which clinicians believed was more effective than oral nonsteroidals for pain relief, despite little evidence to support this.

Our general approach has been to allow clinicians to exercise their own judgment and override nearly all reminders and to "get past" most guidelines. However, situations arise in which this may not be desirable. For example, we noted several years ago that we were using approximately $600,000 of human growth hormone per year, even though we are not a pediatric hospital. A drug utilization evaluation found that most of this was being used by surgeons in the intensive care unit who believed that giving daily growth hormone to patients with "failure to wean" from the ventilator helped them get off the ventilator more rapidly. However, an examination of the evidence found that there was only one abstract to support this belief. Subsequently, the Pharmacy and Therapeutics Committee formed a group that developed a single-screen, computerized guideline for this medication. Because the medication is never needed urgently and the costs involved were so large ($180 per dose), the guideline stated that one of the indications on the screen had to be present, or the user would have to apply in writing to the chairman of the Pharmacy and Therapeutics Committee (Fig. 4). This had a large impact, and utilization decreased to about one third the former level. However, over time, utilization began again to climb. An evaluation by pharmacy found that users had begun to "game the system" or to state that one of the indications under the guideline was present when, in fact, it was not. However, because of order entry, which requires physicians to log in, it was possible to identify the ordering clinician involved. Targeted discussions with these physicians quickly resulted in utilization returning to previous levels. Thus, in such situations, ongoing monitoring may be required.

9.2.6   CHANGING DIRECTION IS EASIER THAN STOPPING

In many situations, we have found that the computer is an enormously powerful tool for getting physicians to "change direction," and enormous savings can result. Changing physician behavior in this way is especially effective when the issue at hand is one attribute of an order the physician probably does not have strong feelings about, such as the dose, route, or

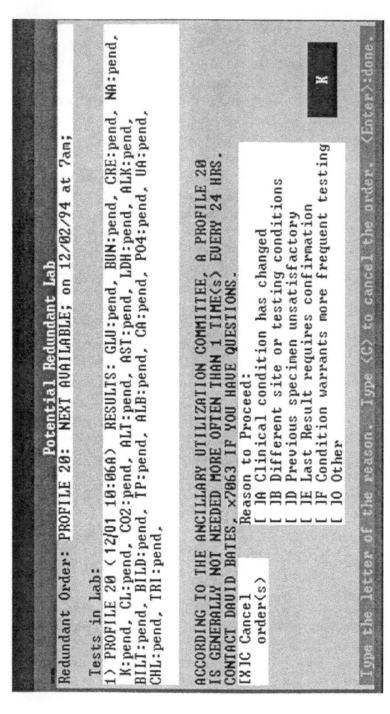

FIGURE 3: Alert for a "redundant" laboratory order. We have found repeatedly that physicians resist stopping; in this instance, alerts for redundant orders often are overridden when there is no alternative plan of action suggested, even when the testing almost never identifies anything useful.

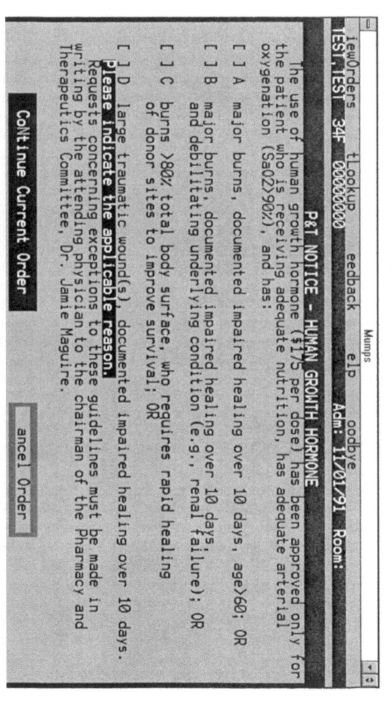

FIGURE 4: Computerized guidelines. These guidelines for the use of human growth hormone were developed to help prevent inappropriate and unnecessary use of this expensive medication. Introducing computerized guidelines to the process of ordering human growth hormone decreased utilization by two thirds.

frequency of a medication or the views in a radiographic study. For example, the Pharmacy and Therapeutics Committee at our institution determined that intravenous ondansetron was as effective if given at a lower dose three times daily rather than the previous routine of four times daily after doing an equivalence study and surveying patients (unpublished data). Simply changing the default dose and frequency on the ordering screen had a dramatic effect on physician behavior. In the four weeks before changing the default frequency, 89.7% of the orders for ondansetron were for four times daily and 5.9% were for three times daily. In the four weeks after changing the default frequency, 13.7% of ondansetron orders were for four times daily, and 75.3% were for three times daily. The cost savings associated with this change were approximately $250,000 in the first year after intervention alone. [41]

Another example of decision support successfully changing physician direction involves abdominal radiograph orders (Fig. 5). For abdominal films, for certain indications, only one view is needed, while for other indications both upright and flat films are needed. [24] In one study, the computer order entry system asked the clinician to provide his or her indication, then suggested the appropriate views if the choice of views did not match the indication. Clinicians accepted these suggestions almost half the time. [24]

9.2.7 SIMPLE INTERVENTIONS WORK BEST

Our experience has been that if you cannot fit a guideline on a single screen, clinicians will not be happy about using it. Writers of paper-based guidelines do not have such constraints and tend to go on at some length. While there is some utility in having the complete backup guideline as reference material, as McDonald and Overhage have pointed out, [45] such guidelines are not usable online without modification, especially during the provision of routine care. An example would be "use aspirin in patients status-post myocardial infarction unless otherwise contraindicated." We have built a number of computerized guidelines, [14 22 24 46] and have repeatedly found this issue to be important. In one study, when clinicians

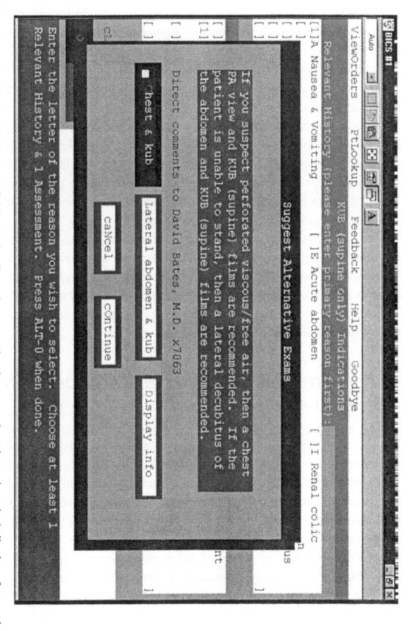

FIGURE 5: Changing direction. In the case of abdominal radiography, suggesting the appropriate views given the indication often results in a change.

ordered several frequently overused rheumatologic tests on inpatients, we developed a Bayesian program that asked clinicians to enter probabilities of disease. [46] However, clinicians needed to provide several pieces of information to get to the key decision support. Eleven percent of intervention orders were cancelled versus less than 1% in the controls. But, we found that in instances in which they cancelled, physicians never got to the decision support piece of the intervention—all the effect appeared to be due to a barrier effect.

Another guideline we evaluated was an adaptation of the CDC guideline for prescribing vancomycin. [14] Getting the guideline to fit on a single screen required substantial condensation and simplification, but we believe this was a key factor in convincing clinicians to use it. In a randomized, controlled trial evaluating the reduction of vancomycin use using computer guidelines, intervention physicians wrote 32% fewer orders than control physicians and had 28% fewer patients for whom a vancomycin order was initiated or renewed. The duration of vancomycin therapy was also 36% lower for patients of the intervention physicians than for patients of the control physicians. [14] Based on a small number of chart reviews, these decreases were clinically appropriate, although a significant amount of inappropriate use persisted.

9.2.8   ASK FOR ADDITIONAL INFORMATION ONLY WHEN YOU REALLY NEED IT

To provide advanced decision support—and especially to implement guidelines—one frequently needs data that are not already in the information system and can be obtained only from the clinician. Examples are the weight of a patient about to be prescribed a nephrotoxic drug and the symptom status of a patient with congestive heart failure. Some situations are perceived as sufficiently risky by clinicians that they will be willing to provide a number of pieces of information, for example, if they are prescribing chemotherapy. However, in many others, the clinician may not want to get a piece of information that is not immediately at hand, such as the weight or whether a young woman could be pregnant. In a trial we performed of guided medication dosing for inpatients with renal insufficiency, [39] we needed to have the patient weight to make suggestions (other variables including age, gender, and creatinine level were all available). Getting consensus that it was acceptable to demand this was in many ways the most difficult part of the project. In approximately one third of patients, no weight was entered at first, although this proportion eventually fell. Overall, our experience has been that the likelihood of success in implementing a computerized guideline is inversely proportional to the number of extra data elements needed. Plans must be made to cover situations in which the provider does not give a piece of information for some reason, and, over time, it makes sense to try to make sure that key pieces of data (such as weight) are collected as part of routine care.

9.2.9   MONITOR IMPACT, GET FEEDBACK, AND RESPOND

If reminders are to be delivered, there should be a reasonable probability that they will be followed, although this probability should likely vary substantially according to the type of reminder. For strongly "action-oriented" suggestions, we try to have clinicians respond positively more than approximately 60% of the time—this is a threshold we reached empirically and somewhat arbitrarily. For other situations, for example when suggesting that a specific type of utilization be avoided, lower thresholds may be reasonable. It is clear that if numerous suggestions are delivered that rarely are useful, clinicians will simply extinguish and miss even very important suggestions. [47] For example, with drug–drug interactions in pharmacies, so many notifications are delivered to pharmacists with similar priority levels that pharmacists have been found to override a third of reminders about a life-threatening interaction. [48] Therefore, we carefully evaluate and prune our knowledge base. For drug–drug interactions, we have downgraded the severity level for many. Achieving the right balance between over-and underalerting is difficult and should be an important topic for further research.

Many of our interventions did not turn out as expected with lower impact for a variety of reasons. We have learned that it is essential to track impact early when supplying decision support by assessing how often suggestions are followed, and then make appropriate midcourse corrections.

For instance, when presenting reminders to use aspirin in patients with coronary artery disease, we found that a major reason for failure to comply was that patients were already receiving warfarin, which we should have anticipated but did not.

9.2.10   MANAGE AND MAINTAIN YOUR KNOWLEDGE-BASED SYSTEMS

Maintaining the knowledge within the system and managing the individual pieces of the system are critical to successful delivery of decision support. We have found it useful to track the frequency of alerts and reminders and user responses and have someone, usually in information systems, evaluate the resulting reports on a regular basis. Thus, if it becomes clear that a drug–drug interaction is suddenly coming up tens of times per day yet is always being overridden, an appropriate corrective action can be taken. The effort required to monitor and address issues in such systems is considerable and is easy to underestimate. It is also critical to keep up with the pace of change of medical knowledge. We have attempted to assign each area of decision support to an individual, and require the individual to assess their assignment periodically to ensure that the knowledge base remains applicable.

9.3   DISCUSSION

The costs of medical care continue to rise, and society is no longer willing to give the medical profession a blank check. An early consequence of rising costs was the increasing penetration of managed care, which has attempted to minimize the provision of unnecessary care, while providing the care that is important. However, even in most managed care situations, many unnecessary things get done, while other effective interventions do not get carried out in part because the number of potentially beneficial things to accomplish is so large that physicians cannot effectively keep track of them all. Information systems represent a critical and underused tool for managing utilization and improving both efficiency and quality. [1]

Especially when combined with an electronic record, decision support is one of the most potent ways to change physician behavior. Some find this approach threatening and fear the loss of physician autonomy. [49] While such fears may not be entirely unfounded, we think the computer can essentially provide a "better cockpit" for clinicians, which can help them avoid errors, be more thorough, and stay closer to the findings of the evidence base. A one-dimensional scale of "degrees of computerization" has been suggested: (1) The computer offers no assistance; humans must do it all. (2) The computer offers a complete set of action alternatives, and (3) narrows the selection down to a few, (4) suggests one, and (5) executes that selection if the human approves, or (6) allows the human a restricted time to veto before automatic execution, or (7) executes automatically, then necessarily informs the human, or (8) informs him or her after execution only if he or she asks, or (9) informs him or her after execution only if it, the computer, decides to. (10) The computer decides everything and acts autonomously, ignoring the human. [50]

Most of medicine in the United States is still at level 1, which we believe is far from optimal. We have found that clinical decision support is most likely to be accepted if it approaches level 5, and while there are comparatively few situations in which this can be achieved, they are very high yield. For instance, there are many "consequent actions," in which one action suggests that another is very likely indicated, for example, ordering aminoglycoside levels after ordering aminoglycosides, and physicians are much more likely to carry out such actions when appropriate suggestions are made. [40] In addition, there are many straightforward situations in which it makes sense to make it as easy as possible for a clinician to carry out an action, for example, ordering a mammogram for a 55-year-old woman. In other instances, level 2 or 3 may be optimal.

Several important, recent trials from England have identified no benefit with computer-based guidelines in chronic diseases in primary care; the studies targeted hypertension, angina, and asthma. [51 52 53] In the most recent of these evaluations, the investigators concluded that key issues were the timing of triggers, ease of use of the system, and helpfulness of the content. [53] These fit with our comments regarding workflow and making messages highly directive. Our own results with chronic diseases and complex guidelines have been largely similar. [38] These results are disappointing because chronic disease management is so important; perhaps the biggest challenge is identifying accurately where the patient is in their care so that helpful suggestions can be made. This remains a vitally important frontier in decision support.

9.4   SURPRISES

A number of features we believed would be valued have either caused major problems, or received relatively little use, or both. Regarding ordering, a major issue was implementation of "free text" ordering—orders that were written simply using free text. While we developed a parser that worked reasonably well, orders written using this mechanism often proved difficult to categorize according to type. As a consequence, relevant decision support was not delivered. Moreover, in these instances, the computer did not know to which ancillary area to send such orders and they thus ended up in a generic pile. However, the clinician had the impression that his or her order had been communicated. A related feature with similar problems was personal order sets. Because of the way the application was designed, such order sets ended up bypassing most decision support. To our surprise, neither free text orders nor personal order sets were used frequently or were highly valued. [35] As a result, we no longer allow either free text orders or personal order sets, although divisions and departments can develop order sets.

Another tool that we thought would be highly valued was links to referential information supporting the decision support. Although this has been used to date less often than we would have hoped, users do rate it as important to them, and part of the reason these get relatively little use may be that the information we have displayed has, as of yet, been quite limited. We currently are building a tool to allow real-time links to Web-based evidence, which should be much more comprehensive and may be more highly valued.

Another surprise came in delivering reminders about redundant tests. [22] We found that these reminders were effective when delivered, but that the overall impact of the decision support was much lower than expected, because the system was often bypassed by test orders going directly to the laboratory, and because tests ordered using order sets were not put through these screens.

9.5 LIMITATIONS AND CONCLUSIONS

Our findings are limited in that many of our experiences to date come from a single, large, tertiary care institution and one large integrated delivery system, so that issues in other types of institutions may vary. Further, a major part of our user group represents residents in training, although many attending physicians use the system on a regular basis.

We conclude that decision support provided using information systems represents a powerful tool for improving clinical care and patient outcomes, and we are hopeful that these thoughts will be useful to others building such systems. Moving toward more evidence-based practice has the potential to improve quality and safety while simultaneously reducing costs. We believe that implementation of computerized decision support through electronic medical records will be the key to actually accomplishing this. However, much remains to be learned about how to best influence physician behavior using decision support—especially around implementing complex guidelines—and this is likely to become an increasingly important area of research as we struggle to provide higher-quality care at lower cost.

REFERENCES

1. Institute of Medicine. Crossing the Quality Chasm: A New Health System for the 21st Century. Washington, DC: National Academy Press, 2001.
2. Lomas J, Sisk JE, Stocking B. From evidence to practice in the United States, the United Kingdom, and Canada. Milbank Q 1993;71:405–10.
3. Schectman JM, Elinsky EG, Bartman BA. Primary care clinician compliance with cholesterol treatment guidelines. J Gen Intern Med 1991;6:121–5.
4. Troein M, Gardell B, Selander S, Rastam L. Guidelines and reported practice for the treatment of hypertension and hypercholesterolaemia. J Intern Med 1997;242:173–8.
5. Marcelino JJ, Feingold KR. Inadequate treatment with HMG-CoA reductase inhibitors by health care providers. Am J Med 1996;100:605–10.
6. Cabana MD, Rand CS, Powe NR, et al. Why don't physicians follow clinical practice guidelines? A framework for improvement. JAMA 1999;282:1458–65.

7. Grimshaw JM, Russell IT. Effect of clinical guidelines on medical practice: a systematic review of rigorous evaluations. Lancet 1993;342:1317–22.
8. Bradford WD, Chen J, Krumholz HM. Under-utilisation of beta-blockers after acute myocardial infarction. Pharmacoeconomic implications. Pharmacoeconomics 1999;15:257–68.
9. Schoenenberger RA, Tanasijevic MJ, Jha A, Bates DW. Appropriateness of antiepileptic drug level monitoring. JAMA 1995;274:1622–6.
10. Canas F, Tanasijevic M, Ma'luf N, Bates DW. Evaluating the appropriateness of digoxin level monitoring. Arch Intern Med 1999;159:363–8.
11. Bates DW, Boyle DL, Rittenberg E, et al. What proportion of common diagnostic tests appear redundant? Am J Med 1998;104:361–8.
12. Solomon CG, Goel PK, Larsen PR, Tanasijevic M, Bates DW. Thyroid function testing in an ambulatory setting: identifying suboptimal patterns of use [abstract]. J Gen Intern Med 1996;11(suppl):88.
13. Karson A, Kuperman G, Horsky J, Fairchild DG, Fiskio J, Bates DW. Patient-specific computerized outpatient reminders to improve physician compliance with clinical guidelines. J Gen Intern Med 2000;15(suppl 1):126.
14. Shojania KG, Yokoe D, Platt R, Fiskio J, Ma'luf N, Bates DW. Reducing vancomycin utilization using a computerized guideline: results of a randomized control trial. J Am Med Inform Assoc 1998;5:554–62.
15. Bates DW, Cullen D, Laird N, et al. Incidence of adverse drug events and potential adverse drug events: implications for prevention. JAMA 1995;274:29–34.
16. Bates DW, Cohen M, Leape LL, Overhage JM, Shabot MM, Sheridan T. Reducing the frequency of errors in medicine using information technology. J Am Med Inform Assoc 2001;8:299–308.
17. Middleton B, Renner K, Leavitt M. Ambulatory practice clinical information management: problems and prospects. Healthc Inf Manag 1997;11(4):97–112.
18. Hunt DL, Haynes RB, Hanna SE, Smith K. Effects of computer-based clinical decision support systems on physician performance and patient outcomes: a systematic review. JAMA 1998;280:1339–46.
19. Johnston ME, Langton KB, Haynes RB, Mathieu A. Effects of computer-based clinical decision support systems on clinician performance and patient outcome. A critical appraisal of research. Ann Intern Med 1994;120:135–42.
20. Bates DW, Kuperman G, Teich JM. Computerized physician order entry and quality of care. Qual Manag Healthc 1994;2(4):18–27.
21. Bates DW, Teich J, Lee J, et al. The impact of computerized physician order entry on medication error prevention. J Am Med Inform Assoc 1999;6:313–21.
22. Bates DW, Kuperman G, Rittenberg E, et al. A randomized trial of a computer-based intervention to reduce utilization of redundant laboratory tests. Am J Med 1999;196:144–59.
23. Solomon DH, Shmerling RH, Schur P, Lew R, Bates DW. A computer-based intervention to reduce unnecessary serologic testing. J Rheumatol 1999;26:2578–84.
24. Harpole LH, Khorasani R, Fiskio J, Kuperman GJ, Bates DW. Automated evidence-based critiquing of orders for abdominal radiographs: impact on utilization and appropriateness. J Am Med Inform Assoc 1997;4:511–21.

25. Safran C, Slack WV, Bleich HL. Role of computing in patient care in two hospitals. MD Comput 1989;6:141–8.
26. Glaser JP, Beckley RF, Roberts P, Marra JK, Hiltz FL, Hurley J. A very large PC LAN as the basis for a hospital information system. J Med Syst 1991;15:133–7.
27. Teich JM, Hurley JF, Beckley RF, Aranow M. Design of an easy-to-use physician order entry system with support for nursing and ancillary departments. Proc Annu Symp Comput Appl Med Care 1992:99–103.
28. Teich JM, Spurr CD, Flammini SJ, et al. Response to a trial of physician based inpatient order entry. Proc Annu Symp Comput Appl Med Care 1993:316–20.
29. Bates DW, Leape LL, Cullen DJ, et al. Effect of computerized physician order entry and a team intervention on prevention of serious medication errors. JAMA 1998;280:1311–6.
30. Bates DW, Kuperman G, Jha A, et al. Does the computerized display of charges affect inpatient ancillary test utilization? Arch Intern Med 1997;157:2501–8.
31. Teich JM, Sittig DF, Kuperman GJ, Chueh HC, Zielstorff RD, Glaser JP. Components of the optimal ambulatory care computing environment. Medinfo 1998;9:t-7.
32. Spurr CD, Wang SJ, Kuperman GJ, Flammini S, Galperin I, Bates DW. Confirming and delivering the benefits of an ambulatory electronic medical record for an integrated delivery system. TEPR 2001 Conf Proc 2001 (CD-ROM).
33. Lee F, Teich JM, Spurr CD, Bates DW. Implementation of physician order entry: user satisfaction and usage patterns. J Am Med Inform Assoc 1996;3:42–55.
34. McDonald CJ. Protocol-based computer reminders, the quality of care and the non-perfectability of man. N Engl J Med 1976;295:1351–5.
35. Lee F, Teich JM, Spurr CD, Bates DW. Implementation of physician order entry: user satisfaction and self-reported usage patterns. J Am Med Inform Assoc 1996;3:42–55.
36. Shu K, Boyle D, Spurr C, et al. Comparison of time spent writing orders on paper with computerized physician order entry. Medinfo 2001;10(pt 2):2–11.
37. Overhage JM, Perkins S, Tierney WM, McDonald CJ. Controlled trial of direct physician order entry: effects on physicians' time utilization in ambulatory primary care internal medicine practices. J Am Med Inform Assoc 2001;8:361–71.
38. Maviglia SM, Zielstorff RD, Paterno M, Teich JM, Bates DW, Kuperman GJ. Automating complex guidelines for chronic disease: lessons learned. J Am Med Inform Assoc 2003;10:154–65.
39. Chertow GM, Lee J, Kuperman GJ, et al. Guided medication dosing for inpatients with renal insufficiency. JAMA 2001;286:2839–44.
40. Overhage JM, Tierney WM, Zhou XH, McDonald CJ. A randomized trial of "corollary orders" to prevent errors of omission. J Am Med Inform Assoc 1997;4:364–75.
41. Teich JM, Merchia PR, Schmiz JL, Kuperman GJ, Spurr CD, Bates DW. Effects of computerized physician order entry on prescribing practices. Arch Intern Med 2000;160:2741–7.
42. Norman DA. The Design of Everyday Things. New York: MIT Press, 2000.
43. Dexter PR, Perkins S, Overhage JM, Maharry K, Kohler RB, McDonald CJ. A computerized reminder system to increase the use of preventive care for hospitalized patients. N Engl J Med 2001;345:965–70.
44. Bates DW, Kuperman GJ, Rittenberg E, et al. Reminders for redundant tests: results of a randomized controlled trial. Symp Comp Appl Med Care 1995:935.

45. McDonald CJ, Overhage JM. Guidelines you can follow and trust: an ideal and an example. JAMA 1994;271:872–3.

46. Solomon DH, Shmerling RH, Schur P, Lew R, Bates DW. A computer based intervention to reduce unnecessary serologic testing. J Rheumatol 1999;26:2578–84.

47. Abookire SA, Teich JM, Sandige H, et al. Improving allergy alerting in a computerized physician order entry system. Proc AMIA Symp 2000:2–6.

48. Cavuto NJ, Woosley RL, Sale M. Pharmacies and prevention of potentially fatal drug interactions. JAMA 1996;275:1086–7.

49. Bogner MS (ed). Human Error in Medicine. Hillsdale, NJ: Lawrence Erlbaum Associates, 1994.

50. Bogner MS Sheridan TB, Thompson JM. People versus computers in medicine. In Bogner MS (ed). Human Error in Medicine. Hillsdale, NJ: Lawrence Erlbaum Associates, 1994, pp 141–59.

51. Montgomery AA, Fahey T, Peters TJ, MacIntosh C, Sharp DJ. Evaluation of computer based clinical decision support system and risk chart for management of hypertension in primary care: randomised controlled trial. BMJ 2000;320:686–90.

52. Eccles M, McColl E, Steen N, et al. Effect of computerised evidence based guidelines on management of asthma and angina in adults in primary care: cluster randomised controlled trial. BMJ 2002;325:941.

53. Rousseau N, McColl E, Newton J, Grimshaw J, Eccles M. Practise based, longitudinal, qualitative interview study of computerized evidence based guidelines in primary care. BMJ 2003;326:314–8.

CHAPTER 10

IMPROVING CLINICAL QUALITY INDICATORS THROUGH ELECTRONIC HEALTH RECORDS: IT TAKES MORE THAN JUST A REMINDER

DEAN F. SITTIG, JONATHAN M. TEICH, JEROME A. OSHEROFF, and HARDEEP SINGH

State-of-the-art electronic health record systems with advanced clinical decision support (CDS) capabilities can fundamentally improve quality and reduce costs of health care. [1,2] However, these outcomes have not been universally achieved.[3,4] As the study by Fiks et al [5] in this issue of Pediatrics demonstrates, providing CDS in the form of "alerts" to encourage desired health care activities may not be sufficient to make a substantial impact. [6] Maximizing the potential of CDS for improving quality and safety of care requires attention to several factors, not all of which are related to the computer system.[7]

The goal for the study by Fiks et al was to increase vaccination rates in asthmatic children, so in examining the results one must first consider what caused the low vaccination rate in their population. Several factors could account for the low initial vaccination rates and, hence, could explain the minimal improvements with alerting. Without knowledge about these factors, it may be too much to expect alerts alone to fix the problem. Alerts are helpful when an unusual occurrence must come to a physician's attention or when a necessary process might be overlooked in a busy encounter. When other underlying problems lead to low vaccination rates, such as poor patient acceptance, difference of opinion about vaccinating patients late in the season, or low priority of vaccination when a patient has an acute problem, they must be addressed before the alert can be successful. Indeed, studies of influenza vaccination reminders in adults have had varying results, and in some cases these results were directly attributable to such noncomputable factors. [8,9] It would have been enlightening if the decision support used in this study also captured the reasons for failure of the providers to act on the alert by having them select or enter a reason for nonvaccination. [10]

In addition, one should also consider whether presentation of the vaccination alert as soon as the patient encounter was opened within the electronic health record was the best CDS intervention to achieve the desired objectives, compared with other intervention types such as facesheet displays, order sets, patient education handouts, and end-of-visit forms. In a guide to CDS implementation that we published in 2005, [11] we suggested that different types of CDS presentation, applied at different parts of the visit workflow, can have very different effects depending on what it is that one is trying to encourage the physician to do. Moreover, communication through group academic detailing (used in this study) may not be the best strategy to educate and change the behavior of clinicians regarding the concepts behind clinical alerts. [12,13]

To achieve a specific clinical objective by using a CDS intervention, one must consider whether the communication and acceptance groundwork has been laid to maximize the intervention's impact, and also consider what type of CDS, applied when in the encounter, is likely to have the greatest impact. [14] From the aforementioned CDS guidebooks [11,14] and other published reviews of CDS effectiveness factors, [15,16] we support the following list of questions to consider before the implementation of any real-time, point-of-care CDS intervention designed to interrupt clinicians during their work.

10.1 COMMUNICATION AND ACCEPTANCE:

1. Has the clinical rule or concept that will be promoted by the intervention been well communicated to the medical staff in advance?

2. Does the intervention, if accepted, change the overall plan of care, or is it intended to cause a limited, corrective action (such as preventing an allergic reaction to a drug)?
3. Are the data used to trigger the alert likely to be accurate and reliable, and are they a reliable indicator for the condition you are trying to change?
4. What is the likelihood that the person receiving the alert will actually change his or her patient management as a result of the alert?
5. Is the patient likely to agree that the recommended actions are beneficial?

10.1.1 INTERVENTION TECHNIQUE:

6. Is an alert the right type of intervention for the clinical objective, and is it presented at the right time?
7. Is the intervention presented to the right person?
8. Is the alert presented clearly, and with enough supporting information, so that the clinician feels confident in taking the recommended action immediately?
9. Does the intervention slow down the workflow?
10. Is the overall alert burden excessive ("alert fatigue")? Were the study providers receiving other types of alerts at the same time?
11. Is the clinical information system, including the use of CDS (eg, the alerts), well-liked and supported by clinicians in general?

10.1.2 MONITORING:

12. Is there a way to monitor the response to the alert on an ongoing basis?

Real-time, point-of-care CDS interventions can be highly effective if the right intervention for the desired clinical objective is used, if the recommendation has been accepted clinically by the physician and patient, if the alert is accurate and clearly understood, if it is presented at a point in the encounter at which the physician can confidently take action on it, and if it makes it easy for the physician to take such action without prolonging or confusing the workflow.

Improving clinical quality objectives through CDS, such as increasing influenza vaccination rates, can be substantially improved by using a systems perspective to address aspects of communication, medical acceptance, clinical workflow, choice of computerized display, and ongoing monitoring. Taken together such extensive interventions can lead to better health outcomes for our patients.

REFERENCES

1. Amarasingham R, Plantinga L, Diener-West M, Gaskin DJ, Powe NR. Clinical information technologies and inpatient outcomes: a multiple hospital study. Arch Intern Med.2009;169 (2):108–114
2. Kaushal R, Jha AK, Franz C, et al; Brigham and Women's Hospital CPOE Working Group. Return on investment for a computerized physician order entry system. J Am Med Inform Assoc.2006;13 (3):261–266
3. Linder JA, Ma J, Bates DW, Middleton B, Stafford RS. Electronic health record use and the quality of ambulatory care in the United States. Arch Intern Med.2007;167 (13):1400–1405
4. Congressional Budget Office. Evidence on the costs and benefits of health information technology. Available at: www.cbo.gov/ftpdocs/91xx/doc9168/05-20-HealthIT. pdf. Accessed May 10, 2009
5. Fiks AG, Hunter KF, Localio AR, et al. Impact of electronic health record–based primary care clinical alerts on influenza vaccination for children and adolescents with asthma: a cluster-randomized trial. Pediatrics.2009;124 (3):159–169
6. Singh H, Arora HS, Vij MS, Rao R, Khan MM, Petersen LA. Communication outcomes of critical imaging results in a computerized notification system. J Am Med Inform Assoc.2007;14 (4):459–466
7. Gerard MN, Trick WE, Das K, Charles-Damte M, Murphy GA, Benson IM. Use of clinical decision support to increase influenza vaccination: multi-year evolution of the system. J Am Med Inform Assoc.2008;15 (6):776–779

8. Tape TG, Campbell JR. Computerized medical records and preventive health care: success depends on many factors. Am J Med.1993;94 (6):619– 625

9. Hak E, Hermens RP, Hoes AW, Verheij TJ, Kuyvenhoven MM, van Essen GA. Effectiveness of a co-ordinated nation-wide programme to improve influenza immunisation rates in the Netherlands. Scand J Prim Health Care.2000;18 (4):237– 241

10. Tang PC, LaRosa MP, Newcomb C, Gorden SM. Measuring the effects of reminders for outpatient influenza immunizations at the point of clinical opportunity. J Am Med Inform Assoc.1999;6 (2):115– 121

11. Osheroff JA, Pifer EA, Teich JM, Sittig DF, Jenders RA. Improving Outcomes with Clinical Decision Support: An Implementer's Guide. Chicago, IL: Health Information and Management and Systems Society; 2005

12. McDonald CJ. Protocol-based computer reminders, the quality of care and the nonperfectability of man. N Engl J Med.1976;295 (24):1351– 1355

13. Simon SR, Smith DH, Feldstein AC, et al. Computerized prescribing alerts and group academic detailing to reduce the use of potentially inappropriate medications in older people. J Am Geriatr Soc.2006;54 (6):963– 968

14. Osheroff JA, ed. Improving Medication Use and Outcomes With Clinical Decision Support: A Step-by-Step Guide. Chicago, IL: Health Information and Management Systems Society; 2009

15. Bates DW, Kuperman GJ, Wang S, et al. Ten commandments for effective clinical decision support: making the practice of evidence-based medicine a reality. J Am Med Inform Assoc.2003;10 (6):523– 530

16. Teich JM, Merchia PR, Schmiz JL, Kuperman GJ, Spurr CD, Bates DW. Effects of computerized physician order entry on prescribing practices. Arch Intern Med.2000;160 (18):2741– 2747

CHAPTER 11

RECOMMENDED PRACTICES FOR COMPUTERIZED CLINICAL DECISION SUPPORT AND KNOWLEDGE MANAGEMENT IN COMMUNITY SETTINGS: A QUALITATIVE STUDY

JOAN S. ASH, DEAN F. SITTIG, KENNETH P. GUAPPONE,
RICHARD H. DYKSTRA, JOSHUA RICHARDSON,
ADAM WRIGHT, JAMES CARPENTER, CARMIT MCMULLEN,
MICHAEL SHAPIRO, ARWEN BUNCE
and BLACKFORD MIDDLETON

11.1 BACKGROUND

11.1.1 INTRODUCTION

There is substantial evidence that computerized provider order entry (CPOE) with clinical decision support (CDS) can enhance health care quality and efficiency [1-5]. We define CDS broadly to include "passive and active referential information as well as computer-based order sets, reminders, alerts, and condition or patient-specific data displays that are accessible at the point of care [[6], p. 524]." Interest in CPOE with CDS is intensifying among clinicians and hospitals in the U.S. as federally funded financial incentives are enacted [7]. At present, only 10 to 20 percent of hospitals have CPOE [8,9], the large majority of which are academic hospitals with teaching programs or hospitals with large numbers of employed physicians, such as Veterans Affairs or Kaiser Permanente hospitals [9]. Although 86% of the 5815 hospitals in the U.S. are community hospitals [10], only 6.9% of them report having even a basic CPOE system [9]. In ambulatory settings, 17% of physicians report that they use clinical information systems, and only 4% of those physicians use systems that include CPOE and CDS [11]. The numbers, however, are rapidly rising.

Until 2006, little research about CDS had been conducted in community hospitals; nearly all had been in academic hospitals [12]. A current series of systematic reviews about the impact of CDS includes more studies from ambulatory and small hospital settings, providing evidence that the impact of CDS on patient outcomes is inconsistent, but its impact on process improvement is stronger [13-16]. A recent report notes that health information technology (HIT) is woefully inadequate in providing cognitive decision support to clinicians, other than that in patient notes and results [17]. Even worse, CPOE can actually produce numerous types of unintended adverse consequences [18], especially related to clinical workflow [19,20].

Because many problems with CDS are associated with behavioral, organizational, and cognitive issues [21,22] in addition to technical issues, the Provider Order Entry Team (POET) based at Oregon Health & Science University in Portland, Oregon conducted two multi-site ethnographic studies and convened an expert panel to focus on these issues. The first study was in community hospitals and the second in ambulatory clinics throughout the US. Their purpose was high level and broad: to identify recommended practices for CDS implementation and knowledge management. We define recommended practices to include procedures and practices actually in use at study sites (themselves exemplars) that both subjects and an external panel of experts deem worthy of consideration by other organizations. Although our main focus for this study was CDS for providers with ordering authority, we also interviewed and observed clinicians in other roles.

11.1.2   THEORY AND FRAMEWORK FOR THE STUDY

To guide this study, we selected a systems-based theoretical framework for understanding the complexity of an organizational system such as a hospital or clinic: the Multiple Perspectives model. We have successfully adopted this approach in the past [23] to study CPOE stakeholders and describe their perspectives using qualitative methods.

The generic Multiple Perspectives model has much to offer, but to use it to structure how we approach the complexities of CDS, it needed further enhancement. The model, originally described by Linstone [24], is useful for approaching any kind of system, but it is incumbent on the model user to carefully identify the "system" (i.e., in a general systems theory sense and not as an information system). Our challenge was to break CDS into subsystems or chunks that could be explored and explained. We did this by 1) breaking the larger system (CDS) into logical components to cope with its complexity while recognizing the dynamic and nonlinear relationships among components, and 2) by using Linstone's Multiple Perspectives model [24] as a framework for studying the system. The CDS system within the dotted oval in Figure 1 contains four components we selected because they represent the major categories of issues we have identified through our grounded theory approach when analyzing field data about unintended consequences and CDS [25]. The components are user, governance, technology, and content issues. These four components overlap at times and they are all surrounded by a permeable barrier, the dotted oval, which represents the unclear boundary between the organization within which the CDS system resides and its surrounding environment. Linstone's Multiple Perspectives approach [24], (perspectives are indicated by the "wings" in Figure 1), provides a framework for how we should view the CDS "system." We need to recognize the technical, organizational, and personal aspects of what is being studied. For the technical perspective, there is only one view because it is ostensibly objective and represents one "inquiring system" [24, p. 63]. By organizational, he means the policies and procedures of the organization, as well as organizational vision, goals, politics, and culture, and there will be more than one view. By personal, he means the individual thoughts and behaviors of key players, who also hold multiple views. We used these views, or lenses through which we studied the system, to guide our subject selection, data gathering, and analysis. When we collected data from clinicians, administrators, and others, we attempted to have them see through the technical, organizational, and personal lenses as much as possible. In addition, as the researchers gathered data, they also attempted to view the CDS system through these three lenses. Finally, we selected experts for development of recommendations based upon this model. This model is a particularly appropriate framework

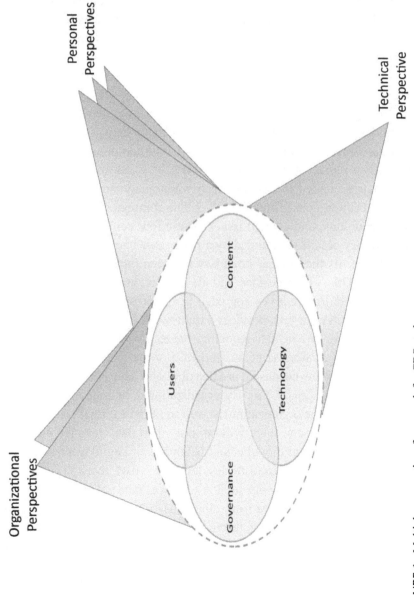

FIGURE 1: Multiple perspectives framework for CDS study.

for qualitative work because the complexity and interrelatedness of perspectives mandate a flexible yet rigorous methodology.

11.2 METHODS

A thorough description of our adaptation of the Rapid Assessment Process has been published elsewhere [26]; we will briefly review it here.

11.2.1 SELECTION OF SITES

Since our goal was to identify recommended practices, we purposively selected sites with reputations for using clinical systems, including CPOE and CDS, well. We sought broad representativeness: we selected organizations with a variety of organizational structures, types of information systems and duration of use. Table 1 outlines attributes of our study sites. The hospitals were community hospitals that used two different commercial systems, one in use for over 30 years and the other for two years. Our definition of community hospitals includes non-teaching hospitals at which private physicians treat most patients. The ambulatory sites, all members of the Clinical Decision Support Consortium (CDSC) [27], used two different commercial systems and three locally-developed systems. As members of the CDSC, they were pre-selected for excellence by the CDSC Steering Committee, but they varied in maturity of information system use, type of system, and organizational structure. Many of these CDSC organizations include both academic and community components, but we deliberately sought out the latter.

The two community hospitals were Providence Portland Medical Center in Portland, OR, which is 1) an urban community hospital, 2) part of a larger 26-hospital system, and 3) was using a commercial system (McKesson, San Francisco, CA), and El Camino Hospital in Mountain View, CA, which is 1) an independent suburban, community hospital with the longest history of CPOE use in the world, and 2) also uses a commercial system (at that time Eclipsys, Atlanta, GA, now Allscripts). Ambulatory sites included Partners HealthCare System in the Boston, MA area. Partners' clinics primarily use the locally developed LMR (Longitudinal Medical Record) system, but a number of their affiliated clinics use commercial systems (GE Healthcare, Fairfield, CT). We studied two groups of clinics in Indianapolis, IN. Clinics affiliated with Wishard Memorial Hospital, a county hospital in Indianapolis, use the locally developed Regenstrief Medical Record System. The Roudebush Veterans Affairs Hospital, also in Indianapolis, uses the VA's nationally developed CPRS system. We also visited many clinics that are members of the Mid-Valley Independent Practice Association (MVIPA) in the Salem, OR area, which uses a commercial system (NextGen, Horsham, PA). Finally, we selected the Robert Wood Johnson (RWJ) Medical Group clinics in New Brunswick, NJ, which also use a commercial system (GE Healthcare, Fairfield, CT). We received human subjects approval from each investigator's home organization (Oregon Health & Science University, the University of Texas at Houston, Kaiser Permanente Northwest, and Brigham and Women's Hospital) and from each study site that has an Institutional Review Board (Brigham and Women's Hospital for Partners HealthCare, Providence Portland Medical Center, El Camino Hospital, the Regenstrief Institute for Wishard, Roudebush Veterans Health Administration, and the Robert Wood Johnson Medical Group), for a total of nine approvals.

11.2.2   SELECTION OF SUBJECTS

To gain multiple perspectives [24], we sought subjects who were experts in CDS content and technology and knowledgeable about CDS governance. We interviewed individuals at each site who had developed CDS, those who managed the CDS and its implementation, those who provided training and support, and users of the system. We gained additional perspectives through use of an interview field survey at the hospital sites. With the help of our sponsor and suggestions from early subjects being shadowed, we selected other users to shadow who were representative of a wide variety of clinicians, deliberately seeking out sceptics as well as regular users and champions. We continued observations and interviews until reaching saturation, the point when we were seeing and hearing the same thing repeatedly.

TABLE 1: Attributes of study sites

	Providence Portland Medical Center	El Camino Hospital	Partners HealthCare	Wishard Memorial Hospital Clinics	Roudebush Veterans Health Administration	Mid-Valley IPA	RWJ Medical Group
Location	Portland, OR	Mountain View, CA	Boston, MA	Indianapolis, IN	Indianapolis, IN	Salem, OR	New Brunswick, NJ
Type of setting	Community hospital	Community hospital	Academic and community outpatient	Academic and county clinics	VA outpatient clinics	Community outpatient	Academic outpatient
Type of system	Commercial	Commercial	Locally developed and commercial	Locally developed	Nationally developed	Commercial	Commercial
Date of visit	Dec-07	Feb-08	Jun-08	Sep-08	Sep-08	Dec-08	Feb-09

11.2.3 DATA COLLECTION METHODS

Researchers in the field of international health have developed expeditious methods for assessing complex site-based situations. Called the Rapid Assessment Process (RAP) [28-30], the approach uses structured assessment instruments, expert interviews, field surveys, and intensive site visits by multidisciplinary research teams. RAP is a multifaceted approach that minimizes the need for extensive fieldwork, and it has been proven to be effective [30]. RAP depends on triangulation, which is the use of multiple methods, a multidisciplinary research team, and a variety of types of settings and subjects, to gain a high level of trustworthiness in data collection and analysis.

We adapted RAP for our purposes. Before each site visit, we asked a local on-site expert to complete a "site profile," a checklist of types of CDS and questions about CDS management [31]. When possible, we also participated in an internet-based demonstration of each system so we could become familiar with local jargon and system capabilities.

Based on this information, we developed interview questions using the language of the site [26]. Topics covered during interviews were backgrounds and roles of interviewees, the culture and history of CDS, barriers and facilitators, knowledge management, governance, and the clinician view of CDS. Formal interviews were semi-structured, recorded, and transcribed. Field notes of observations were guided by the foci identified for the Multiple Perspectives Framework. Field surveys were designed to capture some quantitative data. They included short structured questions for clinicians we were unable to shadow.

Our multidisciplinary team includes clinicians, doctoral level informatics researchers with different backgrounds, and medical anthropologists. One of the most important benefits of ethnography is that ethnographers enter a culture and remain open to learning about it, thus gaining an insider view. In fact, the insiders become the teachers and the researchers become students [32]. For this particular study, the medical ethnographer on the team guided the informaticians through the RAP methodology in such a way that we became well aware of assumptions we held by virtue of our training and expertise. This attention to reflexivity was especially important during observational periods, when we had to be extremely diligent to learn about the user view and not impose our informaticians' view on activities.

After all data were analyzed and themes identified and described in writing, we convened a panel of 17 experts in May of 2010 at a retreat site outside of Portland, OR to review these results and suggest recommendations. The experts represented community hospitals, CDS content vendors and electronic health record vendors, and widely published national CDS researchers. For each theme, these experts discussed practices they would suggest for community hospitals. The format was similar to that used in a prior POET project to produce recommendations for CPOE implementation [33].

11.2.4   DATA ANALYSIS

In order to conduct seven site visits over two years and provide timely feedback to each site, as well as solicit comments from subjects as a form of "member checking" [34, pp. 308-9], we needed to analyze the data quickly. We did this by developing general themes during frequent debriefing sessions and using a template method [34] for roughly coding the data. For each site feedback report we identified organization-specific challenges and possible solutions. Once the site reports were completed, we began using a more traditional grounded theory approach that was both inductive and interpretive. Transcripts of the expert conference were analyzed using the template method [34].

11.3   RESULTS

11.3.1   INTRODUCTION

We interviewed 82 subjects representing clinical, technical, and administrative disciplines. Table 2 indicates the number and roles of those interviewed and observed. We observed 105 clinicians for a total of 194 person-hours and conducted observations in most areas of the hospitals. We visited and observed clinicians working in 41 different clinics. Data analysis, which took place during 90 team meetings, revealed ten general themes.

TABLE 2: Details about interviews and observations at each site

	Provi-dence Portland	El Camino	Partners Health-Care	Wishard	Roude-bush, VA	Mid-Valley IPA	RWJ	Total 7 Sites
Interviews and field surveys								
Roles of Subjects								
Admin-Man-agerial	5	5	2	1	3	1	3	20
Bridger-Clinical*	8	3	4	6	6	3	1	31
Clinical User	13	12	6	4	0	3	-	38
Technical	1	2	2	1	2	3	5	16
Site Total	27	22	14	12	11	10	9	105
Observations								
Hours Ob-serving	36	26	37	20	25	33	17	194
Individuals Observed	10	12	17	16	17	27	6	105
Numbers of Clinics	N/A	N/A	9	6	5	9	12	41

Bridgers are generally nurses or pharmacists who bridge the gap between the clinical and technology worlds

The Multiple Perspectives model was used to help select our subjects, frame our questions and observations, and remain cognizant of relation-ships and dependencies among our four components of CDS: users, con-tent, technology, and governance. It forced us as researchers to use dif-ferent lenses and to gather data from users as they viewed components through the three different lenses: the technical, organizational, and personal, which also overlap and blend at times. Although the themes and patterns arose directly from our data, each is more closely aligned with one system component than others, so the four ovals depicting the CDS components within the dotted oval in the Figure 1 model will serve as an organizing scheme for the following discussion. In addition, because several of the themes that arose directly from the data did not fit into one of the four components of the CDS "system" outlined in the framework, we conducted further analysis which has resulted in our proposing a modification to the framework and a new theoretical construct.

11.3.2 CDS FIELDWORK THEMES

11.3.2.1 COMPONENT ONE: USERS AS A COMPONENT OF THE CDS "SYSTEM"

The end users of CDS are those whose workflow is most affected by it. Users are constantly adjusting their work because of the system and the systems are ideally constantly changing to better facilitate users' work.

THEME 1: WORKFLOW

We were consistently told that any system should fit the workflow of its users as closely as possible. The locally developed systems were designed to fit into the work done at a particular site, but since users differ in their work habits, even these systems needed some customization to match individual workflows. Concomitantly, users must generally adapt their workflows to better fit the system. Those using commercial systems are continuously individualizing or customizing aspects of the system to better fit their ways of doing things, or adapting to the system's requirements. There are limits to what buyers of commercial systems are allowed to customize, however, which is often why workflow must be adapted.

Reengineering the workflow

The sites using commercial systems had all conducted workflow analyses in each clinic prior to implementation. The sites with locally developed systems seem to be in a perpetual state of workflow engineering. A researcher wrote in fieldnotes: "I speak to the workflow fellow who calls himself an EMR Workflow Engineer. He observes how the staff uses the computer system and helps them to trouble shoot workflow problems. His team observes the lean manufacturing/production philosophy. He uses time/motion studies and asks the practice about what needs they have." At one site we were told "So now what we're doing is we're sort of going back to all these sites and saying okay, we're going to start from scratch with you. We'll go over all of your workflows and all the ways that you document and make your decisions and we'll show you how to do this in the EMR now."

In-line applications and CDS that fit the workflow

By in-line applications we mean computer-enabled help that seamlessly fits the workflow, that does not interrupt the clinician, and that is nearly invisible. Applications are in-line if they provide needed information at the appropriate time in the encounter. Templates are an excellent example of an in-line application providing decision support. These were especially useful in the ambulatory setting when clinicians used the system during the patient encounter. One researcher's fieldnotes said: "She uses the point and click charting templates to complete her review of systems [and] history and physical very quickly." Another noted: "[The provider] uses templates and occasionally brings notes forward. I asked him whether he did this because it made it faster or because it helped him remember. He said mainly because it made it faster, occasionally for remembering." Some users were critical of the documentation generated by use of the templates, so they entered free text into the template instead of or in addition to filling in the fields. Some clinicians would not use a computer in the exam room because they thought it would hamper physician-patient interactions. Some, however, were observed to be remarkably facile, brought the patient into the encounter skilfully, and enjoyed using the templates. Often, these were the clinicians who had taken the time to modify templates to their liking.

Most clinicians who had e-prescribing available praised its ability to help them. One researcher said in fieldnotes: "If he prescribes a med, he does it in the room on the computer. It [then] prints out [so he can] hand it to the patient or to fax, or may fax directly. The app is populated by a list of pharmacies. The patient's usual choice is there as the default value."

Variability of workflow

We were told that the prime reason why workflow analysis is needed prior to implementation or on an ongoing basis is that each physician has developed his or her own way of doing things. One interviewee said: "People practice in very different ways. Some physicians look at the screen once before they see the patients, and then they don't really touch the computer [again] until they have to write prescriptions. So, the opportunities to interact with the computer and receive decision support can be limited for those practitioners." Others carry laptops or tablet computers with them at all times and have multiple opportunities to receive CDS.

Location of the encounter

We observed that CDS usefulness depends a great deal on where the physician opts to use the computer. Clinicians who use templates during the patient encounter receive timely, helpful, welcome, seamless decision support: "Her process is to use her laptop in the exam room, filling out the smart form [template] for her note. She further edits the smart form in her office." On the other hand, clinicians who waited to use the templates, often until after the patient had left, missed an opportunity to be reminded of important issues.

Temporal issues

Timing of the CDS presentation, especially alerts, is important to users. We heard complaints about alerts firing at the wrong time, both too early in the encounter and too late. Clinicians wanted them at "the point in time during the encounter where it's really going to be most helpful and most actionable." Time pressures had an impact as well. None of the outpatient sites we studied had many alerts aimed at physicians. We were told: "They're overwhelmed, they're too busy, they have too many demands on their time." An informatician noted about alerts: "We thought that it was a much bigger downside to frustrating people by constantly interrupting their workflow than missing the alerts." One site turned them all off and a representative told us: "Now they need to turn the alerts back on, condition by condition. They plan on customizing the alerts before they turn them back on; having the task force review the logic before they turn them back on; turning them on clinic by clinic."

11.3.2.2   COMPONENT TWO: CONTENT AS A COMPONENT OF THE CDS "SYSTEM"

Content issues include development or purchase and management of CDS.

THEME 2: KNOWLEDGE MANAGEMENT

By knowledge management, we mean the entire process of developing and translating pieces of knowledge so that they are available in the system. Knowledge management also includes acquiring, tracking, evaluating, and maintaining knowledge, just as libraries gather, catalog, and maintain library collections.

Knowledge creation

The sites we studied that had locally developed systems also had locally developed CDS, which, because of the way it was developed over many years by innovative individuals, is hard to track. However, they are making progress in developing ways to monitor their CDS. Individuals at these sites continue to develop new CDS, which now tends to be more carefully managed. Close ties with the pharmacy and therapeutics committees and quality assurance staff members yield ideas about "new drugs as they are introduced as possible candidates for CDS." Although our study sites that used commercial systems did not develop CDS de novo, they followed many of the same processes when customizing content they obtained from others, including content vendors. All of our sites with commercial systems had informaticians in leadership roles and CDS analysts who could modify CDS content.

Content library management

We use this term because we see an analogy between traditional library functions such as acquisitions, cataloging, maintenance, provision of access, and "weeding" of materials and the functions that appear to be needed for CDS content management. The acquisition phase includes either development or modification of CDS, described above. Once an organization acquires a certain amount of CDS, it starts to lose track of what it has, so an inventory is wise if it has not been conducted from the beginning. Following the inventory, a means of cataloging, or indexing, is needed so that analysts can search to find out what exists. Model sites conduct cyclical reviews for curation and maintenance and have mechanisms for scanning the environment to keep up to date about new evidence. Organizations with commercial systems can take advantage of software offered by vendors to help manage this process. Unlike libraries, holders of CDS do not often share their locally developed or modified CDS. We asked interviewees about their willingness to share CDS. The reasons for not sharing included lack of a technical ability to do so and a hesitation to share without remuneration what they had spent time developing. There are also legal issues that inhibit sharing. On the other hand, there was interest in sharing among sites that have a particular vendor-based system and also when an organization wants new CDS. Organizations would like to be on the receiving end but not the giving end of the exchange.

11.3.2.3 COMPONENT THREE: TECHNOLOGY AS A COMPONENT OF THE CDS "SYSTEM"

Several of our themes relate to this component: data as a foundation for CDS; user computer interaction; and measurement and metrics.

THEME 3: DATA AS A FOUNDATION FOR CDS

Many types of CDS require that data about individual patients reside in the system. For example, before a reminder that a mammogram should be scheduled can be generated, the system needs to know the age and gender of the patient, when her last mammogram was performed, whether they have a mammogram already scheduled, and finally, if they are status post bilateral mastectomy or in a hospice program. We were told that if decision support is to be highly sensitive and patient-specific, then accurate, complete, structured information about the patient must already exist in the system.

Having enough information about the patient

None of our study sites has truly complete data about its patients because patients receive care from many different organizations. Even VA patients sometimes get care outside of the VA system. Some data, such as those in medication lists, are especially hard to keep accurate and up to date. Other data must come from sources such as laboratories and agreements as well as technical interoperability are needed if these data are to be shared. For example, one interviewee noted: "The patient we were looking at had an LDL reminder but the patient had actually had the LDL done. The reminder didn't work correctly since he didn't have lab results in the EMR (so it thought the test hadn't been done when it had been)." We often heard remarks such as: "We're working on getting university radiology, a radiology site to send us their results electronically, because right now they come over as paper and we have to scan them." Clinicians uniformly desire having all the right information, but not too much information, at the point of care.

Quality

Often our subjects worried about the accuracy of data that had to be entered manually. One said "Even my own partner doesn't really, you know, capture or do the data. I mean a lot of it is just getting the work done at that moment in time." A nurse confided that "at times the nurses will simply cut and paste medication profile information from [the system] into the medication reconciliation document without properly verifying all of the medications on the list."

Sharing Data

Data are often stored in separate silos, with laboratory and radiology information in separate systems that cannot share information with an EMR. The extent of the ability to share data within and across sites varies a good deal. One site, which included a group of outpatient clinics, shares nothing but demographic data between clinics. The VA shares nationally, Partners sites share some information such as allergy information, and the Wishard clinics using the Regenstrief system are part of a statewide network sharing some patient-specific clinical information.

Varied uses for these data

Administrators and informaticians told us they value data availability not only as a basis for patient specific CDS but also for quality measures reported after the fact. One informant said "It is frustrating that we have not been able to get any quality indicators out" because data were not being entered by all clinicians. Another use is for research purposes, and both accurate and complete data are needed. Others would like population-based data.

THEME 4: USER COMPUTER INTERACTION

We think of user computer interaction as ease of use of the system, including the equipment, the screen layout, the number of clicks needed to accomplish a task, the cognitive energy needed to figure out what to do next, and the speed of use. There are two major sub-themes that emerged: customization, which can take place on many different levels, and usefulness.

Customization

All of the systems we studied could be customized and these successful sites all devoted considerable staff time to this endeavor. Even sites with locally developed systems were constantly providing further customization: "We sat down with the [EMR] team and they had to change the user interface of how pediatricians would order medications, because now we're doing it through weight based dosing vs. flat dosing." An analyst at a site with an EMR that provides templates noted: "We can edit the forms and customize them for the practice. We have to build custom-like orders, we have to build for the practice, medications, problems, custom lists for each practice and when they log into the system, it automatically defaults to their custom list." Analysts also make changes to simplify use of the system. As one analyst noted: "I look at it and say no, this will never fly. Ten clicks to get here, forget it, we've got to simplify this."

Usefulness

During observations, we found that presentation of the CDS was of utmost importance. Where CDS was "in-line" with workflow, we often observed that simple presentation decisions could be extremely powerful. For example, the use of color draws attention to data without changing workflow: "It flags it in red, so it's a visual cue to the physicians that it's a little bit outside of the range and if you're ordering something with a narrow therapeutic index, you need to be aware." Actionability was likewise critical. If reminders are "actionable," meaning that the clinician can respond to the reminder without needing to access another part of the system, usually with one click, they minimize impact on workflow and tend to be used. At one site, most decision support is provided this way, and the positive outcome is that reminders tend to be voluntarily viewed and acted on. In addition, structured data are collected and reports generated about responses to reminders. Reliability is very much valued by clinicians. We were told that CDS cannot be useful if clinicians avoid the system because it is not available at times. Finally, correctness and applicability to the patient are important. There are times when the system simply is not correct. One clinician noted: "When you order inhalers, it often rejects the dose that it suggested you use!"

THEME 5: MEASUREMENT AND METRICS

We were told that patient-specific, accurate, and complete information that already exists in the system is needed to measure both the effect of clinical decision support and the use of it. Also, metrics need to be established so that the impact of the EMR can be measured over time. For example, it is useful to know how often alerts are being overridden and why.

Administrative needs; quality reporting

With increasing pressure to be accountable for quality, the sites we studied either already take advantage of measures that can be extracted from the system based on CDS interventions, or they are planning to conduct ongoing measurement once the system is fully implemented across all clinics. We were told at several sites that provide performance feedback to clinicians that such feedback is welcomed. One site with a "dashboard" provides direct feedback to clinicians. An interviewee noted: "So, it's at the clinician level, sort of their performance on key indicators compared to their peers and compared to some external benchmarks." Some sites provide incentives for meeting performance goals: "we are reporting on things that ultimately become these accountability metrics. . . people are either going to get bonuses if they do certain things and if they don't, they don't." At another site we were told: "most physicians will use the reminders because they get report cards on their completion rates. . . they are attended to as opposed to other systems in other organizations where there's not this tracking reporting type system. If you go down into the clinics you'll see graphs that compare clinics to one another as a form of competition."

Monitoring and control of CDS

Some of the study sites monitor how effective some CDS is: "How usable is our decision support such that for example we are now putting in routine efforts to track override rates." They might also monitor the effort put into maintaining CDS: "we are now better able track the timeliness and the labor required to meet those maintenance obligations." Sites that do not monitor CDS at present are planning to do it soon.

11.2.3.4   COMPONENT FOUR: GOVERNANCE AS A COMPONENT OF THE CDS "SYSTEM"

All of our study sites had formal governance structures for managing CDS.

THEME 6: GOVERNANCE

Governance includes formal and informal mechanisms for making decisions about the system and about CDS in particular; four subthemes emerged from our data.

Environmental factors/Motivation

We were told in interviews that while the ultimate motivator for implementation of CDS is the desire to improve patient care, there are other intermediary factors pressing for it. These include increasing attention to rewarding patient safety and healthcare quality by accrediting bodies, payors, and professional societies. As one quality assurance director noted: "We moved to the EMR because we felt it would standardize or help quality and would standardize our, some of our practice." Another motivator is competition in the health care sector. As one interviewee stated: "I think the underlying drive, perhaps not surprisingly, it's the recognition that we need to distinguish ourselves as an organization from amongst the competitors in terms of safety and quality."

Setting priorities and resource management

We were told that one of the most difficult aspects of CDS governance is the setting of priorities. With outside pressures to meet certain measures and internal pressures to decrease costs or improve specific local outcomes, organizations must decide where to put their energy. One of our sites has a committee that developed a list: "A top ten list of what we thought should be standardized across the enterprise." Each site has a somewhat different approach to setting priorities, but all have multidisciplinary committees that provide oversight and make ultimate decisions.

Governance structure

We found three aspects of governance structure related to CDS, which our study sites consider crucial: committees, process, and feedback to the governance system. Committees play a vital role in governance. The more mature CDS sites have several layers of committees, with higher-level decisions made by higher-level committees. These are generally multidisciplinary, with a mix of clinicians, administrators, and technology representatives. One was described by an interviewee: "It's called the EMR IT Advisory Group. The physicians, some of the IT staff, some of the clinical staff, and the analysts." All tend to gather task forces of clinical experts when needed. Each site has a process for discovering new evidence or environmental changes that impact CDS. One example of this is a process for learning about changes made by the Pharmacy and Therapeutics Committee. Finally, mechanisms for feedback to the governance system are imperative. Each site also has a process for reviewing requests from users. At one site, "the clinical content committee reviews requests that come up from the user base and they are funnelled to and from the [information system] management team about decision support."

Relationships with vendors

The sites with commercial systems must depend a great deal on decisions about CDS that are made by their EMR vendors. Therefore, they must be in close contact with the vendor. We heard at one of these sites: "We sort of have a very tight knit connection with [our vendor]. So, I think everyone sort of collaborates with them and cross-communicates with them on practically everything. We really can't do very much on our own here without [the vendor]." The EMR vendors generally purchase content for CDS from content vendors. Sites with locally developed EMRs often purchase directly from content vendors, especially for medication information.

Proposed New Construct, Translational Interaction

Several themes emerged from our analysis of the data that did not easily fit into the framework originally proposed, which included components for content, users, governance, and technology. Instead, the additional themes all included aspects of "translation," which we define as communicating meaning through language.

THEME 7: TRANSLATION FOR COLLABORATION

For groups to collaborate effectively, they must understand the cultures of the different involved groups. Culture implies a shared system of meaning and language. The different groups for which collaboration is necessary include: the developers and analysts, IT staff, clinic staff, the vendors, clinicians, and administration.

Collaboration for development

At sites that build new CDS, the development process involves a development analyst who facilitates discussions among clinical specialists, knowledge engineers, and programmers. A researcher explained in fieldnotes: "She is a 'development analyst' and the team leader for similar analysts. They write specs, test, and modify and they serve as liaisons between the users and IT. There are other analysts who are implementation and support analysts." The development analysts and knowledge engineers exist at the interface of the clinical and information technology worlds and are familiar with the vocabularies of both.

Translation for vendor collaboration

At the sites with commercial systems, analysts modify CDS content provided by vendors and to do so, they must often work with members of the vendor's staff. As one analyst stated it: "A lot of her job and a lot of my job is working with [the vendor] to make sure things are running correctly." Often, those within the purchasing organization feel that they are not sufficiently supported by vendors, although it is usually incumbent on them to purchase services in order to receive them.

Translation between users and IT

Both analysts and training and support staff translate or explain the clinical culture to information technology staff. One analyst noted: "Our local IT people said 'oh, that can't be done. . . then I realized it wasn't that it couldn't be done. The IT people we were working with didn't understand what the clinicians were asking to get done. I realized then that there needs to be some kind of an intermediary who understands the IT world and the clinical side."

Collaboration among clinical organizations

The cultures of outpatient clinics which house physicians in private practice and the cultures of the hospitals to which those physicians refer patients are different enough that information systems are impacted. The business models are different, of course, and some vendors do not have products for both or will not sell to both except under certain circumstances. In addition, there is sometimes competition for patients if the hospital performs outpatient procedures. We were told that collaboration between the organizations that purchase content and EMRs and the vendors is essential.

THEME 8: THE MEANING OF CDS

We asked each interviewee how he or she would define CDS, primarily because we wanted insight into different perspectives. We quickly learned that CDS generally means something quite different to the informatics experts than it does to the clinical users. It is important to note that meaning goes beyond definition: it is making sense of a phenomenon. Much of what we learned about these mental models our subjects hold came from observations and informal comments. Their view surprised us: often they did not know what "clinical decision support" is, so we had to explore the idea by asking how the computer helps them make clinical decisions. The users see CDS as an opportunity for the system to help them get through their day. They focus on the help and assistance the EMR can offer. Experts usually describe CDS in terms of sophisticated alerts or reminders. Interestingly, CDS implementers at each site seem to have a unique philosophy that guides their CDS efforts, a shared mental model or organizational meaning. We divide this theme into two sub-themes: the multiple meanings of CDS and different informatics philosophies of CDS.

Multiple meanings of CDS

Clinical decision support means different things to different disciplines and to individuals within those disciplines. One of our sites has a position called "Coordinator of Clinical Decision Support" which deals exclusively with administrative data in the form of reports about clinicians' actions and not at all with how clinicians make clinical decisions. We heard similar definitions echoed by quality assurance staff. When asked for a definition, informaticians usually offered a very broad definition such as "presenting information to somebody in a way that's going to help them to make decisions or take actions." However, those individuals often went on to describe alerts and reminders, most likely because these forms of CDS are most interesting to them. On the other hand, most of the practicing clinicians we observed thought of CDS as anything that could help them finish their work in a timely manner. Any information in either the clinical information system or the office practice system that assists the clinician's workflow constitutes CDS in their view. Some clinicians described talking with or e-mailing other clinicians or even reading another clinician's notes as decision support. They make little distinction between clinical information and other types of information such as demographic or scheduling information. To them, all of this information helps them take care of their patients.

Informatics philosophy of CDS

Experts at several of our sites expressed philosophies that guided their organization's development of CDS. One of the study sites held a philosophy "we're not trying to tell the physicians what to do, we're trying to give them the information." Informants at another site used the terms "guardrails" and "helping the clinician to do the right thing." One informatics professional noted: "I've seen a lot of decision support done as forcing people down this path or that path, always has been the carrot or the stick. . . what is the grade of the ground? You can get that mule pulling that cart, are you whipping them, are you enticing them, but the truth is that if you just make it easier to go down one path. . . To me that's the ideal decision support is when the person doesn't even realize that it is happening." Elsewhere we heard "giving vaccinations when patients were in the hospital and the most effective way to do it was to give it to nursing and make it part of their protocol; and take it out of the decision tree of the doctor. Sometimes the best decision support is not to give them the decision." Administrators at one site clearly saw CDS as an "enabler of standardization."

THEME 9: ROLES OF SPECIAL, ESSENTIAL PEOPLE FOR CDS

In prior studies, we have identified and described typical "special essential people" roles for CPOE implementation and maintenance [35]. These roles include administrative leaders, clinical leaders, champions, opinion leaders, and bridgers of different types who span the gap between the clinical world and the technology world and generally provide support and training. This study confirmed that these roles are critical for effective CDS as well. However, this study also identified several new and emerging roles directly related to CDS, which will become increasingly important. We arrived at this list through analysis of statements our informants made during interviews and through field observations.

Essential people as previously defined

We found the same types of essential people at these sites that we described after visiting five organizations for a prior study about CPOE success factors [35]: champions, who are clinicians in the forefront of information technology; opinion leaders, who are clinicians well respected for their clinical expertise who are spokespeople for systems; administrative leaders, who are not clinicians, but who hold a vision of what CIS can do; clinical leaders, who are clinicians by background but hold administrative positions; and "bridgers," who are usually clinically trained but who have enough IT expertise so they can train and support users or serve as analysts who develop or modify systems. These designations are not mutually exclusive, since clinical champions may also be administrators, for example. In addition to these roles, we discovered in this CDS study a number of variations of the roles we previously identified. For example, two sites that have commercial systems have on-site analysts who actually work for the vendor and not for the hospital or practice. This arrangement has both advantages and disadvantages and seems to work best when the analysts have experience working for the organization they serve. One analyst of this type described how difficult it had been for outsiders hired as analysts because "They had to get used to the flow. . . they had to get used to that because this is a completely different environment for them. So it took them a while to kind of figure that out, whereas I already knew, that so that was an advantage for me."

Newly found essential roles for CDS

These include knowledge engineers, subject matter experts, outpatient clinic champions, pharmacy informaticians, and ambulatory clinic chief medical information officers.

Knowledge engineers and analysts

The sites we studied that have non-commercial systems were unique in that they each have knowledge engineers who are clinicians, usually physicians, who have developed and evaluated decision support through grant funding. These knowledge engineers help to develop the content for CDS and are skilled facilitators who seek to gain consensus from clinicians. They translate human readable content into a form that the system can use, so they are technically as well as clinically astute. Their role was well described by one informant: "We do have people who are practicing clinicians who are helping create the rules. You definitely need someone who knows the technical side of the equation." Analysts are generally clinically trained as well and they perform many of the same tasks of knowledge engineers, often modifying content available through commercial systems.

Clinical CDS Subject Matter Experts (SMEs)

Each organization has a cadre of clinicians who assist with development or modification of decision support. Organizations seem to have difficulty motivating SMEs as time goes on. By SME motivation, we mean that once these individuals are identified and they are taking their SME roles seriously, they need to be nurtured and continuously updated and motivated to continue being SMEs. These people are clinicians who are interested in information technology and the potential of computerized CDS. When systems are new, they seem naturally motivated by the challenge of implementation. However, as CDS is continuously rolled out, these SMEs grow weary. Some of the sites compensate these experts: "I know how challenging it is for clinicians to take time to address these important issues. That has been compensated and I think that's another whole, you know, another whole dimension."

Outpatient clinic champions, often non-clinical

In office practice settings, there is usually someone who serves as office champion. This go-to person is sometimes one of the clinicians who has an aptitude for computer systems, but more often it is one of the office administrative staff members who devotes part time to working with the system. Having such a point person who is both knowledgeable and personable seems to be important for success.

Pharmacists who are Pharmacy and Therapeutics (P and T) Committee connectors

Hospitals have Pharmacy and Therapeutics committees, which oversee medication use. Pharmacists who bridge the gap between these P and T committees and CDS developers are uniquely capable of assisting with medication related CDS development and maintenance. They play a critical role in communicating between the committee and the developers so that the developers are well informed about P and T priorities.

Ambulatory clinic CMIOs

Each of the two freestanding clinic organizations we studied hired physicians with informatics training to fill the role of a chief medical information or information systems officer. Each used a commercial system, so these individuals played a key role in expressing the clinic's needs to the vendor, in facilitating the work of the CDS analysts, and in communicating with users.

THEME 10: COMMUNICATION, TRAINING AND SUPPORT

Communication, training, and support are critical success factors for any clinical information system, but there are unique issues when the focus is

CDS. This theme includes communication and training about new CDS and CDS modifications as well as ongoing support efforts.

Communication about CDS takes many forms, and staff members at our study sites feel it is exceedingly difficult. Like training, communication is hard to do when busy clinicians are the target audience. One informatician said: "there are always new features that come up and I think we still completely suck at letting people know about new features." Types of communication include e-mail, on site meetings and presentations, "lunch and learns," use of feedback buttons, and personal contacts with CDS analysts or super users. Communication between clinicians and patients, we found, can be enhanced through CDS, both through the use of reminders about health maintenance schedules and other forms of communication. For example, one informatician noted: "We actually make it very easy [for clinicians] to write patients a letter describing their test results in a patient-friendly format."

Training, primarily conducted one-on-one at the sites we studied, needs to be ongoing, especially as more decision support is added, and organizations find it exceedingly difficult. It is hard to separate training from communication and support or to differentiate it from education or efforts to motivate clinicians. As one physician developer noted: "asking them [providers] to do something with decision support, it's just, you know, to really make that behavior change requires lining up more than the reminder. You've got to line up education and incentives and a whole bunch of things and generally we don't do that for too many [providers]."

Initial training needs to show the user how a particular CDS type might fit that user's individual workflow. One trainer noted: "We have to understand what the physician is going to be doing. Are they going to be dictating, are they going to be typing their notes?. . . So, really trying to gear the training around workflow." Ongoing training is especially necessary as new CDS is added. However, organizations were somewhat apologetic about their inability to do this well. We found that users rarely felt their knowledge about changes to CDS was up to date. One physician said "A lot of it you learn by trial and error," and a researcher's fieldnotes noted someone "had developed some work-arounds that seemed valuable, but that required him to do many inefficient actions within [the system]."

By support, we mean providing help to users at the time of need. Support related to CDS involves continuous feedback to and from users, generally by phone to a help desk or through e-mail. One clinician's quote is characteristic of what we heard at all of our study sites: "whenever we e-mail them [IT support] or have a problem with them or feel like things should come up differently or pop up differently or whatever, I mean, they're great."

11.3   DISCUSSION

11.3.1   THE THEMES

Many of our results, including the importance of workflow integration, well designed user interfaces, ongoing knowledge management and intentional interaction among stakeholders, confirm statements made by others based on their experience and expert opinion [6,36-41]. While much of what we have described may seem familiar, one characteristic of good qualitative research is the ability of those studied to see themselves, and their world, reflected in the results. In grounding the findings in carefully collected data from seven varied sites, this research validates and strengthens previous work. It also extends the findings to community hospitals and ambulatory clinics, sites which are historically under-represented. In addition, we offer actionable recommendations based on our findings, thus furthering the ability of hospitals and clinics to increase the quality, safety and efficiency benefits from CPOE with CDS. The process for identifying recommended practices was as follows. First, interviewees were asked about them. Second, observers recorded noteworthy practices in fieldnotes. Third, debriefings and team analysis meetings identified them for the reports. Recipients of the site reports were asked for feedback as a form of member checking. Finally, descriptions of recommended practices were presented to the panel of experts during a two-day conference and discussed at length. Those recommendations are offered below.

11.3.2 RECOMMENDATIONS ABOUT USERS AS A COMPONENT OF THE CDS "SYSTEM"

11.3.2.1 THEME 1 WORKFLOW

Organizations should pay attention to workflow assessment prior to any intervention. There are good examples of CDS types that fit the workflow of users, with order sets and templates among the best. Even the smallest clinics we visited were using these with success once some customization had been done. These are good places to start, and any organization with an EMR can do it. Higher level, interruptive CDS types like alerts need careful screening and they should be a goal, carefully planned with clinician involvement. We recommend that organizations with EMRs move forward with simple CDS no matter what their size. Order sets, checklists and templates can be considered "low hanging fruit" and they suit the purposes of all stakeholder groups by providing standardization and gathering structured data that can serve multiple purposes. Some of this low hanging fruit is available from vendors, but, as others have noted in the past, organizations must plan on customizing it so that it fits local practice and workflows [20,42].

11.3.3 RECOMMENDATIONS ABOUT CONTENT AS A COMPONENT OF THE CDS "SYSTEM"

11.3.3.1 THEME 2 KNOWLEDGE MANAGEMENT

Organizations should plan early and establish procedures for the maintenance of CDS. Knowledge used in CDS changes rapidly, so organizations should have the resources to purchase and to keep knowledge bases up to date. Some organizations avail themselves of services offered by content vendors to help them to manage their CDS. At a national level, if there is greater utilization of Continuity of Care Document (CCD) standards, making it easier for external applications to individual patient data as part of the clinical workflow, "clinical content development organizations will begin to make available actionable, real-time, clinical decision support interventions on a widespread scale. [[43], p. 616]"

11.3.4   RECOMMENDATIONS ABOUT TECHNOLOGY AS A COMPONENT OF THE CDS "SYSTEM"

11.3.4.1   THEME 3 DATA AS A FOUNDATION FOR CDS

Organizations should take all possible steps to assure acquisition of high quality data. Clinicians should be educated about why good structured data are needed and why data integrity is so important [44]. At the national level, standards for health information exchange are evolving, and they should be supported. Standard triggers, which cause certain decision rules to be invoked, need to be defined. Finally, standards for input data need to be defined. Of course, use of standard vocabularies is needed so that CDS can be both robust and shared across implementations.

11.3.4.2   THEME 4 USER COMPUTER INTERACTION

As CDS is developed, it should be tested on real users prior to implementation. Mechanisms need to be in place for receiving user feedback and acting on it [40]. The in-line CDS described here is most usable in that it does not interrupt workflow. If CDS must interrupt workflow, it should be designed so that it is actionable. In other words, the user should be offered choices that can be selected immediately, without navigating to another part of the system.

11.3.4.3   THEME 5 MEASUREMENT AND METRICS

Measurement and refinement of CDS content is critical for CDS interventions to be effective. Organizations should design metrics as content is developed or purchased, and they should be diligent about implementing the measures. Once measurements are available, reports should be communicated and the CDS interventions should be refined as needed. Decision makers need to plan what will be measured as early as possible, and each stakeholder group should be included in the decision-making. Clinicians themselves will be interested in measures of their own clinical patterns, implementers will be interested in how well the CDS is working, and administrators and quality assurance staff will desire measures of safety such as those required by accrediting bodies.

11.3.5   RECOMMENDATIONS ABOUT GOVERNANCE AS A COMPONENT OF THE CDS "SYSTEM"

11.3.5.1   THEME 6 GOVERNANCE

CDS is a powerful tool for influencing clinician behavior. It is important to have an effective governance process in place to keep clinical leadership, end users, and IT aligned. Existing committees like a Pharmacy and Therapeutics or quality committee may be able to serve this purpose, but in many cases, they will need to be modified or new committees will have to be developed, especially as the content grows and becomes more complex. Clinicians must be involved and, to motivate continued involvement, a suitable reward system is needed.

11.3.5.2   A NEW THEORETICAL CONSTRUCT: TRANSLATIONAL INTERACTION

We crafted our questions and foci for observations around the four components of users, governance, technology, and content, so it was not surprising when the themes of workflow, governance, usability, measures and metrics, data as a foundation for CDS, and knowledge management were identified as themes. However, four themes spontaneously and surprisingly arose from the data: translation for collaboration, the meaning of CDS, new roles for essential people, and communication, training, and support. When we realized that they all had in common the notion that meaningful exchanges between actors with diverse worldviews are difficult but critical at the points of overlap that exist among our original four components, we sought further insight about the commonalities of these four themes.

The medical anthropologists on the team were familiar with the work of Michael Agar, which seems especially applicable here. He describes Rich Points, which occur at the point of interaction between actors with different understandings of a situation and lead to "moments of incomprehension and unmet expectations [45]." According to Agar, Rich Points like these require a translation between the different ways of understanding, or worldviews, in order to explain the meaning of the situation. Translation is especially difficult because it goes beyond words and vocabulary and includes cultural meaning. For example, "system" to a physician might mean the physiological system but to an information technology staff member it usually means hardware and software. In fact, Agar has coined the term "languaculture" to emphasize that language and culture shape one another. Informaticians, for example, often bridge both worlds and can explain the cultural and language differences between them. We adopted the term "translation" from Agar because the languages of the clinicians and the information technology workers are different and the languages need to be mutually understood by individuals involved in CDS. "Language is not a prison," according to Agar, however: "it is a room you are comfortable in--you can move out of it but it is uncomfortable [[46], p. 68]." Successful negotiation of these Rich Points leads to shared understanding and expectations, which in turn enables communication and action. Our team noted that translation alone, with its focus on language and culture, fails to take into account this process, which includes moving among worlds. For example, a physician may collaborate with others working to modify a CDS module by virtue of his clinical expertise, but he may hold a meaning of CDS as "alerts and reminders" by virtue of informatics training. That same person might fill the role of a new kind of essential person as a knowledge engineer, and may spend part of his time training other physicians as their peer. In other words, there is active movement between and among the components, so we are calling this aspect Interaction. The entire process of building this shared system of meaning and language (or, integrating multiple systems of meaning and language) across disciplines and worldviews we call Translational Interaction.

It seems to us that the intersections of users, governance, content, and technology give rise to the four new themes, which all describe elements of translation among the original components. This leads to a theory that the four new translational themes need a great deal of attention if CDS is to live up to its promise. They provide Rich Points for research, for workforce development, and for policy. Figure 2 provides our new model, which includes an oval, symbolizing Translational Interaction, which hovers over the intersections of the four elements. It hovers because it should not obscure the intersections and instead should call attention to them. Insight about each Translational Interaction theme and recommendations follow.

11.3.5.3   THEME 7 TRANSLATION FOR COLLABORATION

Different stakeholder groups need to share their understandings of CDS. Stakeholders who primarily view CDS as a vehicle for promoting standardization, quality, and safety need to understand that clinicians see it differently and vice versa. This sharing can be done during the processes of decision making about new modules, and of development or modification. Knowledge engineers, even if they are clinicians, should observe and work with users to learn the local workflows and language. Since vendors are collaborators in the CDS process, their perspectives must be understood by organizations.

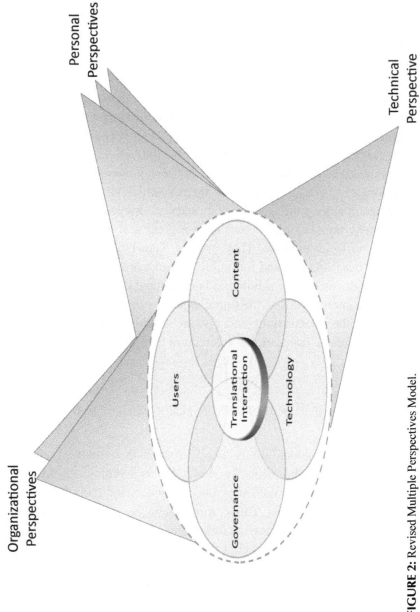

FIGURE 2: Revised Multiple Perspectives Model.

11.3.5.4   THEME 8 THE MEANING OF CDS

Because the end users of clinical information systems hold different mental models about CDS from developers, implementers, and organizational decision makers, they cannot always be "on the same page" as these other groups that are responsible for CDS. If users believe the best CDS is that which increases their efficiency and others view CDS as cognitive assistance that sometimes must decrease users' efficiency, there is a large problem. Users are not getting what they need and want and the other groups have difficulty convincing the clinicians that CDS is useful. We urge all stakeholder groups to view CDS broadly. Using our general definition of CDS as "passive and active referential information as well as reminders, alerts, and guidelines [6, p. 524]," we saw excellent uses of CDS in the field, including use of actionable templates in exam rooms in the ambulatory setting. This is a kind of CDS which fits the clinician's mental model as positive, which is being provided by vendors, and which is successful. Our recommendation is that the user view should be considered before CDS is implemented or even developed and that clinicians should be closely involved in any implementation that could possibly decrease efficiency. Also, research is needed to identify different mental models and strategies must be developed for helping to reach a point where a shared mental model exists.

11.3.5.5   THEME 9 ROLES OF SPECIAL, ESSENTIAL PEOPLE

The new, emerging roles that center around CDS represent changes in the structure of the health information technology and informatics workforce. Some of the knowledge engineers, pharmacy informaticians, and clinic champions have had no formal informatics training, so we predict that training programs addressing their needs will be needed in the future. Organizations must understand from the beginning that even when they purchase a commercial system, customization will be necessary and knowledge engineers/analysts will be critical. These organizations need to formalize these roles and plan to either create or hire individuals to fill them. By create, we mean provide professional development for them. Finally, individuals with the talent to bridge the gap between the clinical and IT worlds need to consider careers playing these essential roles.

11.3.5.6   THEME 10 COMMUNICATION, TRAINING, AND SUPPORT

These are never ending processes as they relate to CDS and they need considerable ongoing resources. Users need to know about current CDS and to be aware of upcoming CDS. Implementers should make sure users are involved from the beginning of the CDS design process, and their feedback should be solicited and taken seriously.

Theory and framework

The Multiple Perspectives Framework served to guide us in subject selection and development of questions for interviews and foci for observations, and continuously reminded us of the complex nature of information systems within health care environments. The new construct we have added to the framework, that of Translational Interaction, could be useful for future applied informatics research efforts.

11.4   LIMITATIONS

The results of this study, while not generalizable in a quantitative sense, should be transferable to similar contexts. Each recommended practice should be assessed at the local level; sites may need to modify practices depending on their maturity, organizational structure, resources, and information system. The methods were designed to be efficient; results could be different if prolonged periods of time were spent in the field. We did not study sites without EHRs, so our sites are not representative of the majority of hospitals and clinics in the U.S. Because we were funded to only study outpatient sites that belong to the CDS Consortium, and because several of these have locally developed systems with sophisticated CDS, they are not typical of most clinics. On the other hand, these sites provided excellent examples of existing recommended practices.

11.5   CONCLUSIONS

In the US, efforts to encourage widespread use of clinical information systems by hospitals and health care providers are likely to succeed only if these systems meet the needs of the major stakeholders. Optimal use and acceptance of clinical decision support is necessary for meaningful use and desired outcomes. For this reason, it is imperative that policy makers, health care administrators, and clinicians reach a mutual shared understanding of CDS and agreement on its goals. A broad view of CDS could include quality and safety aims as well as user workflow assistance, for example. Such aggressive movement will only be possible if the next generation of informatics manpower is available, however. The essential people who will customize, implement, manage and support CDS efforts are key to national efforts and meaningful use of health information technology.

REFERENCES

1.   Hunt DL, Haynes RB, Hanna SE, Smith K: Effects of computer-based clinical decision support systems on physician performance and patient outcomes: a systematic review. JAMA 1998, 280(15):1339-46.
2.   Devine EB, Hansen RN, Wilson-Norton JL, Lawless NM, Fisk AW, Blough DK, Martin DP, Sullivan SD: The impact of computerized provider order entry on medication errors in a multispecialty group practice. J Am Med Inform Assoc 2010, 17:78-84.
3.   Kawamoto K, Houlihan CA, Balas EA, Lobach DF: Improving clinical practice using clinical decision support systems: a systematic review of trials to identify features critical to success. BMJ 330(7494):765.
4.   Garg AX, Adhikari NK, McDonald H, Rosas-Arellano MP, Devereaux PJ, Beyene J, Sam J, Haynes RB: Effects of computerized clinical decision support systems on practitioner performance and patient outcomes: a systematic review. JAMA 2005, 293(10):1223-38.
5.   Kaushal R, Jha AK, Franz C, Glaser J, Shetty KD, Jaggi T, Middleton B, Kuperman GJ, Khorasani R, Tanasijevic M, Bates DW: Return on investment for a computerized physician order entry system. J Am Med Inform Assoc 2006, 13(3):261-6.
6.   Bates DW, Kuperman GJ, Wang S, Ghandi T, Kittler A, Volk L, Spurr C, Khorasani R, Tanasijevic M, Middleton B: Ten commandments for effective clinical decision support: making the practice of evidence-based medicine a reality. J Am Med Inform Assoc 2003, 10(6):523-30.

7. Blumenthal D: Stimulating the adoption of health information technology. N Engl J Med 2009, 360(15):1477-1479.

8. Ash JS, Gorman PN, Seshadri V, Hersh WR: Computerized physician order entry in U.S. hospitals: results of a 2002 survey. J Am Med Inform Assoc 2004, 11(2):95-9.

9. Jha AK, DesRoches CD, Campbell EG, Donelan K, Rao SR, Ferris TG, Shields A, Rosenbaum S, Blumenthal D: Use of electronic health records in U.S. hospitals. N Engl J Med 2009, 360(16):1628-38. American Hospital Association [http://www.aha.org/research/rc/stat-studies/fast-facts.shtml]

10. DesRoches CM, Campbell EG, Rao SR, Donelan K, Ferris TG, Jha A, Kaushal R, Levy DE, Rosenbaum S, Shields A, Blumenthal D: Electronic health records in ambulatory care--a national survey of physicians. N Engl J Med 2008, 359(1):50-60.

11. Chaudhry B, Wang J, Wu S, Maglione M, Mojica W, Roth E, Morton SC, Shekelle PG: Systematic review: impact of health information technology on quality, efficiency, and costs of medical care. Ann Int Med 2006, 144(10):742-52.

12. Souza NM, Sebaldt RJ, Mackay JA, Prorok JC, Weise-Kelly L, Navarro T, Wilczynski NL, Haynes RB: Computerized clinical decision support for primary preventive care: A decision-maker-researcher partnership systematic review of effects on process of care and patient outcomes. Implem Sci 2011, 6:87.

13. Hemens BJ, Holbrook A, Tonkin M, Mackay JA, Weise-Kelly L, Navarro T, Wilczynski NL, Haynes RB: Computerized clinical decision support for drug prescribing and management: A decision-maker-researcher partnership systematic review. Implem Sci 2011, 6:89.

14. Sohota N, Lloyd R, Ramakrishna A, Mackay JA, Prorok Jc, Weise-Kelly L, Navarro T, Wilczynski NL, Haynes RB: Computerized clinical decision support systems for acute care management: A decision-maker-researcher partnership systematic review of effects on process of care and patient outcomes. Implem Sci 2011, 6:91.

15. Roshanov PS, Misra S, Gerstein H, Garg AX, Sebaldt RJ, Mackay JA, Weise-Kelly L, Navarro T, Wilczynski NL, Haynes RB: Computerized clinical decision support systems for chronic disease management: A decision-maker-researcher partnership systematic review. Implem Sci 2011, 6:92.

16. Stead WW, Linn HS: Computational technology for effective health care: immediate steps and strategic directions. Washington, D.C.: The National Academies Press; 2009.

17. Campbell E, Sittig DF, Ash JS, Guappone K, Dykstra R: Types of unintended consequences related to computerized provider order entry. J Am Med Inform Assoc 2006, 13(5):547-556.

18. Campbell E, Guappone KP, Sittig DF, Dykstra RH, Ash JS: Computerized provider order entry adoption: implications for clinical workflow. J Gen Int Med 2009, 24(1):21-6.

19. Karsh B-T: Clinical practice improvement and redesign: how change in workflow can be supported by clinical decision support. AHRQ Publication No. 09-0054-EF. Rockville, MD, Agency for Healthcare Research and Quality; 2009.

20. Berner ES: Clinical decision support systems: state of the art. AHRQ Publication No. 09-0060-EF. Rockville, MD: Agency for Healthcare Research and Quality; 2009.

21. Moxey A, Robertson J, Newby D, Hains I, Williamson M, Pearson S: Computerized clinical decision support for prescribing: provision does not guarantee uptake. J Am Med Inform Assoc 2010, 17:25-33.

22. Ash JS, Gorman PN, Lavelle M, Lyman J: Multiple perspectives on physician order entry. AMIA Proc 2000, 26-30.

23. Linstone HA: Decision making for technology executives: using multiple perspectives to improve performance. Boston, MA, Artech House; 1999.

24. Ash JS, Sittig DF, Poon EG, Guappone K, Campbell E, Dykstra RH: The extent and important of unintended consequences related to computerized provider order entry. J Am Med Inform Assoc 2007, 14(4):415-23.

25. McMullen CK, Ash JS, Sittig DF, Bunce A, Guappone K, Dykstra R, Carpenter J, Richardson J, Wright A: Rapid assessment of clinical information systems in the healthcare setting: An efficient method for time-pressed evaluation. Meth Inform Med 2011, 50(4):299-307.

26. Middleton B: The Clinical Decision Support Consortium. Stud Health Technol Inform 2009, 150:26-30.

27. Beebe J: Rapid assessment process: an introduction. Walnut Creek, CA, AltaMira Press; 2001.

28. Handwerker WP: Quick ethnography. Walnut Creek, CA, AltaMira Press; 2001.

29. Trotter RT, Needle RH, Goosby E, Bates C, Singer M: A methodological model for rapid assessment, response, and evaluation: the RARE program in public health. Field Methods 2001, 13:137-59.

30. Sittig DF, Wright A, Simonaitis L, Carpenter JD, Allen GO, Doebbeling BN, Sirajuddin AM, Ash JS, Middleton B: The state of the art in clinical knowledge management: an inventory of tools and techniques. Int J Med Inform 2010, 79:44-57.

31. Spradley JP: Participant observation. New York, NY, Holt, Rinehart and Winston; 1980.

32. Ash JS, Stavri PZ, Kuperman GJ: A consensus statement on considerations for a successful CPOE implementation. Journal of the American Medical Informatics Association 2003, 10(3):229-234.

33. Crabtree BF, Miller WL (Eds): Doing qualitative research. 2nd edition. Thousand Oaks, CA, Sage; 1999.

34. Ash JS, Stavri PZ, Dykstra R, Fournier L: Implementing computerized physician order entry: the importance of special people. Int J Med Inform 2003, 69:235-250.

35. Miller RA, Waitman LR, Chen S, Rosenbloom ST: The anatomy of decision support during inpatient care provider order entry (CPOE): empirical observations from a decade of CPOE experiences at Vanderbilt. J Biomed Inform 2006, 38(6):469-85.

36. Lorenzi NM, Novak LL, Weiss JB, Gadd CS, Unertl KM: Crossing the implementation chasm: a proposal for bold action. J Am Med Inform Assoc 2008, 15(3):290-6.

37. Metzger J, MacDonald K: Clinical decision support for independent physician practice. California Healthcare Foundation; 2002. Available at http:/ / www.chcf.org/ publications/ 2002/ 10/ clinical-decision-supportfor-the-i ndependent-physician-practice Accessed October 15, 2011

38. Osheroff JA, Pifer EA, Teich JM, Sittig DF, Jenders RA: Improving outcomes with clinical decision support: an implementer's guide. Chicago, IL, HIMSS; 2005.

39. Saleem JJ, Patterson ES, Militello L, Render ML, Orshansky G, Asch SM: Exploring barriers and facilitators to the use of computerized clinical reminders. J Am Med Inform Assoc 2005, 12(4):438-47.

40. Tamblyn R, Huang A, Taylor L, Kawasumi y, Bartlett G, Grad R, Jacques A, Dawes M, Abrahamowicz M, Perreault R, Winslade N, Poissant L, Pinsonneault A: A randomized trial of the effectiveness of on-demand versus computer-triggered drug decision support in primary care. J Am Med Inform Assoc 2008, 15(4):430-8.

41. Ash JS, Sittig DF, Wright A, McMullen C, Shapiro M, Bunce A, Middleton B: Clinical decision support in small community practice settings: a case study. Journal of the American Medical Informatics Association 2011, 18(6):879-882.

42. Berner ES, Kasiraman RK, Yu F, Ray MN: Data quality in the outpatient setting: impact on clinical decision support systems. AMIA Proc 2005, 41-5.

43. Wright A, Goldberg H, Hongsmeier T, Middleton B: A description and functional anatomy of ruled-base decision support content at a large integrated delivery network. J Am Med Inform Assoc 2007, 14(4):489-96.

44. Agar M: Culture: can you take it anywhere? Int J Qual Meth 2006., 5(2): See http://www.ualberta.ca/~iiqm/backissues/5_2/pdf/agar.pdf webcite Accessed December 28, 2009

45. Agar M: Language shock: understanding the culture of conversation. New York, N.Y., William Morrow; 1995.

Ash, J. .S, Sittig, D. F., Guappone, K. P. , Dykstra, R. H., Richardson, J., Wright, A., Carpenter, J., McMullen, C., Shapiro, M., Bunce, A., and Middleton, B. Recommended Practices for Computerized Clinical Decision Support and Knowledge Management in Community Settings: A Qualitative Study. BMC Medical Informatics and Decision Making 2012, 12:6 doi:10.1186/1472-6947-12-6. Re-used as per the Creative Commons Attribution License.

CHAPTER 12

GOVERNANCE FOR CLINICAL DECISION SUPPORT: CASE STUDIES AND RECOMMENDED PRACTICES FROM LEADING INSTITUTIONS

ADAM WRIGHT, DEAN F. SITTIG, JOAN S. ASH,
DAVID W. BATES, JOSHUA FEBLOWITZ, GREG FRASER,
SAVERIO M. MAVIGLIA, CARMIT MCMULLEN,
W. PAUL NICHOL, JUSTINE E. PANG, JACK STARMER,
and BLACKFORD MIDDLETON

12.1 INTRODUCTION AND BACKGROUND

Clinical decision support (CDS) represents a critical tool for improving the quality and safety of healthcare. CDS has been defined in many ways, but at its core, it is any computer-based system that presents information in a manner that helps clinicians, patients, or other interested parties make optimal clinical decisions. For the purposes of this paper, we will limit our attention to real-time, point-of-care, computer-based CDS systems, such as drug–drug interaction alerting, health maintenance reminders, condition-specific order sets, and clinical documentation tools. A substantial body of evidence suggests that, when well-designed and effectively implemented, CDS can have positive effects for healthcare quality, patient safety, and the provision of cost-effective care. [1 2]

Although the benefits of decision support are numerous, only a small number of sites in the USA have achieved significant success with it. [3] A variety of challenges limit the wide adoption of CDS, but a critical one is the difficulty of developing and maintaining the required knowledge bases of clinical content. [4 5] Effective CDS often requires extremely large knowledge bases of clinical facts (eg, drug-interaction tables). This content must be engineered (or purchased) and must also be kept current as clinical knowledge, guidelines, and best practices evolve. [6] The knowledge bases that are developed must reflect both universal best practices and local practices and needs. Knowledge management is an iterative process that involves both the creation of new content and the continuous review and revision of existing content.

To develop these clinical knowledge bases and ultimately work toward "meaningful use" of CDS, organizations must implement and operate governance processes for their clinical knowledge. [5 7] These governance processes take many forms. Some organizations use existing clinical committees to develop and screen decision-support content (such as a Pharmacy and Therapeutics Committee) or appoint a single person to review and approve content (such as the Chief Medical Informatics Officer), while others develop new committee structures along with intranet-based content creation, review, and approval systems. Governance can vary widely depending on the type and size of the organization. For example, large organizations, such as academic medical centers and government-run hospitals, can potentially develop and implement CDS internally, while smaller organizations, such as group practices and community hospitals, may need to rely on a partnership with a commercial vendor.

Careful consideration of governance issues when developing and implementing CDS can be as important as the quality of the decision support itself. In the absence of effective governance practices, implementation of CDS may fail, despite the purchase or development of a sophisticated system. A notable example of this issue is the decision-support system at Cedars-Sinai Medical Center that had to be shut down because of usability issues. [8] Employing better governance practices throughout the design and implementation phases, such as increased end-user involvement, can potentially stave off these types of problems.

Although governance and other organization factors have been noted as an essential aspect of high-quality CDS [9 10] and requisite data warehousing and management, [11] limited research exists about optimal and real-world CDS governance practices. Outside of the healthcare industry, a variety of models have been proposed to describe knowledge management and IT governance practices.[12–14] These models emphasize the need for continuous knowledge management, the value of studying real-world governance best practices and the importance of well-planned implementation. Researchers also note the substantial investment required to implement IT and knowledge management systems and the uncertainty associated with these investments, further underscoring the need for effective governance. [12 15] In order to establish effective governance practices and realize the potential of IT and knowledge management systems, a broad understanding of the institutional pressures organizations face and real-world assessment of these institutional pressures is both valuable and necessary. [16]

Any organization embarking on a new initiative to develop decision support (or simply expanding an existing mandate) faces the choice of how to design its governance structures and the underlying technology to support these efforts. In this paper, we show how five diverse healthcare organizations developed their governance structures and discuss some of the tools they are using to support these activities. We examine each organization's governance, content management, and technical approaches. After presenting the approaches, we synthesize the lessons learned and develop a set of recommended practices in the three areas. For the purposes of this paper, we refer to "governance practices" as any formal leadership structure, governing bodies, and institutional policies related to the development and implementation of clinical information systems. In general, "governance" refers to the process by which an institution decides on what content will be implemented and how this will occur. In contrast, "content management" refers to the organizational structures and clinical information systems used to view, manage, and update clinical content on an ongoing basis following implementation. Content management allows for continuous tracking of existing CDS systems and allows institutions to generate reports for committee review. In this paper, we analyze both of these interrelated issues at each of the participating sites.

12.2 METHODS

This work is part of a larger initiative called the Clinical Decision Support Consortium. [17] The Consortium is focused on sharing CDS content and is pursuing several related aims, including the creation of knowledge representation standards, [18] development of CDS services, and execution of a number of demonstrations of Consortium decision-support content at sites across the country. One of the foremost aims of the Consortium, however, is the study of decision-support best practices including governance practices. [19]

Members of the Clinical Decision Support Consortium research team conducted three site visits and five comprehensive surveys (the three original sites plus two validation sites) at institutions across the country to learn about their CDS capabilities and governance practices with the goal of distilling a set of recommended governance and content management practices based on observations and interviews during field research. Our sampling strategy for these visits was purposive; we selected five exemplary institutions with a history of successful CDS research and utilization.

The team used the Rapid Assessment Process for all fieldwork. [20] At each site visit, a team of four to seven researchers (physicians, nurses, pharmacists, and informaticians) traveled to the site and conducted interviews with decision-support developers and information system leaders, as well as observations of clinical end users. Interviews were tape-recorded, and detailed field notes were captured for each observation. Each day at midday and in the evening, the team debriefed and modified the approach as needed. During these meetings, the research team reviewed field notes, discussed their observations and worked to identify themes and recurring patterns. After returning from the site visit, audio recordings were transcribed, and field notes were typed. The research team, lead by trained ethnographers, identified themes in the data using a grounded theory approach. NVivo 8 qualitative data-analysis software (QSR International, Victoria, Australia) was used to facilitate the process. Field notes and transcripts of interviews were read into NVivo, and then recurring concepts and themes were identified by the team members using the software. The data collected during site visits covered the entire breadth of CDS, including issues such as user interface and technical considerations. For this analysis, only data coded under the themes of content management and governance were reviewed in detail.

After conducting the initial analysis in NVivo, and identifying several hundred concepts across several thousand lines of notes and transcripts, the team used a card-sorting technique to develop an initial set of governance and content-management practices we had observed in the field and then distilled these practices into a summary set of themes. We then developed questions based on these themes and sent written questionnaires to a purposive sample of five sites: three from our initial site visits and two new sites to validate and extend our initial findings. We also asked each site to fill out an inventory of decision-support content at their site based on the six key categories of CDS developed by Osheroff et al. [21]

The five organizations studied are Partners HealthCare System in Boston, Massachusetts; the Mid-Valley Independent Physicians Association (MVIPA) in Salem, Oregon; Vanderbilt Medical Group, in Nashville, Tennessee; Veterans Health Administration (VA), a national healthcare delivery organization headquartered in Washington, DC; and the University of Texas Physicians' Practice Plan, in Houston, Texas. Site visits were conducted at Partners HealthCare, MVIPA and the VA Health System in Indianapolis.

Based on these case studies, we develop a theoretical framework for studying decision-support governance and present a set of recommended practices that other institutions might consider as they develop their own governance approaches. Because formal governance models for decision support are relatively new, no interventional (or even wide-scale observational) evidence exists for the effect of various CDS governance practices, and there is no particular regulation relevant to such practices. Thus, for the purpose of this paper, we refer to "recommended practices" as practices which the sites identified as critical to their success and which appear to have face validity. We believe that this is the best proxy for consensus available, given the relative novelty of inquiry in the area of CDS governance.

12.3 RESULTS

12.3.1 OVERVIEW OF ORGANIZATIONS

These five organizations encompass a variety of academic and community hospitals, and comparatively small and large ambulatory practices. They use both commercially available and in-house-developed clinical information

TABLE 1: Overview of the organizations' characteristics

	Mid-Valley Independent Physicians Association*	University of Texas Physicians' Practice Plan	Vanderbilt Medical Group	Partners HealthCare*	Veteran's Health Administration*
Location	Salem, OR	Houston, TX	Nashville, TN	Boston, MA	National
Characteristics of setting	Community outpatient	Academic, outpatient	Academic	Academic	Government
Volume of care	Over 500 practitioners at 262 practices; more than 40 000 patients	More than 1200 practitioners at 88 clinics in 80 medical specialties and subspecialties	More than 1400 practitioners in 96 practice groups; 1.2 million clinic visits yearly; 52 000 inpatient admissions yearly	More than 7000 practitioners; 2.0 million ambulatory visits yearly; 200 000 inpatient admissions yearly	More than 17 000 practitioners in 1300 sites of care; 5.5 million patients; 62.3 million outpatient visits yearly; 590 000 admissions and 5 million inpatient bed days of care yearly
Clinical information systems	Uses NextGen Healthcare Information Systems EHR; supported by Mid-Valley Independent Physicians Association	75% of all clinicians have used Allscripts EMR system, live since 2004; no paper charts (all paper information scanned in)	Internally developed EHR, StarChart, and internally developed care provider order entry, WizOrder	Integrated internally developed outpatient EHR, the Longitudinal Medical Record; patient access to online health record application	Computerized Patient Record System developed by VA available in all areas
Decision support characteristics	Built-in clinical decision support tools (eg, drug–drug interaction, health maintenance reminders, order sets); tailored clinical content for 14 specialties; patient care plan dashboard; prescribing module	Medication related CDS content (eg, drug–drug, drug allergy) purchased from Allscripts (little to no modifications); UpToDate access; Surescripts for prescriptions; lab results received electronically from Quest; order sets	Computerized provider order entry (over 1000 order sets and advisors); clinical reminders; barcode medication administration	Clinical alerts; order sets; comprehensive chronic disease-management systems for diabetes and coronary disease; outpatient results management application	Supports numerous types of CDS, such as clinical reminders, order checks, order menus, and record flags; chronic disease-management systems including patient registries; bar code medication administration; patient web portal with wellness reminders

Site visit conducted

systems. They also include for-profit, not-for-profit, and government-provided healthcare as well as the full gamut of medical and surgical clinical specialties. Their key characteristics are shown in table 1. We visited Partners, MVIPA, and the VA Health System in Indianapolis, Indiana. The University of Texas and Vanderbilt were used as our validation sites and were characterized through written questions and interviews.

In addition to the broad demographic characteristics in table 1, we found that each site had at least one example of each of the six decision-support types in the Osheroff taxonomy, suggesting that each site had sufficient breadth of content to necessitate some level of decision-support governance.

Despite having similar breadth of CDS, the sites varied dramatically in the depth of decision support they had. For example, the number of different condition-specific order sets ranged from less than 50 to more than 800, and the number of unique clinical alerts ranged from less than 50 to more than 7000. This pattern of differing "depths" of CDS implementation accounts in large part for the differences in the structure, complexity, and size of the clinical governance infrastructure that each organization has developed.

12.3.2   GOVERNANCE APPROACHES

All five sites in our analysis had at least some degree of decision-support governance, although the form and pattern of governance models differed greatly. Table 2 describes the approaches, including CDS-related staff, committees, governance process, tailoring of content, levels of governance, and tools for soliciting and managing user feedback. The five organizations are listed left to right across the top according to size, starting with the two smaller strictly ambulatory sites that use commercial systems. They are followed by the two academic health centers with locally developed inpatient as well as outpatient systems. The national VA health network, in the final column, is the largest and includes inpatient, outpatient, long term, and home-based care. Table 2 compares governance styles and structures across each of the five case studies.

TABLE 2: Governance approaches at each of the five sites

	Mid-Valley Independent Physicians Association*	University of Texas	Vanderbilt	Partners*	Veterans Health Administration*
CDS-related staff	A medical director of information systems and 13 informatics staff members help support the system	Most content is purchased, so CDS-focused staff is minimal	Large academic informatics staff, including physicians, nurses, pharmacists, and informaticians	Physicians, pharmacists, nurses, informaticians, analysts, and software developers	National and local software developers, clinical subject-matter experts, and local clinical application coordinators
Committees	EHR Communications and Policy Committee comprising key Mid-Valley Independent Physicians Association staff and representatives from the Mid-Valley Independent Physicians Association board of directors helps guide ongoing CDS operations and development of new content. A Physician Advisory Committee discusses and prioritizes development activities.	Content governed by the Chief Information Officer and an 'Allscripts Review Board' composed of key clinical and administrative leaders from the practice, including six practicing physician representatives	Decentralized organization-wide committees for example, Patient Safety and Clinical Practice Committees. System-specific committees: Horizon Expert Documentation advisory board (nurse charting) and user groups (Horizon Expert Orders, StarPanel). Also pharmacy and condition specific groups for example, Medication Use and Safety Improvement, Patient Falls and Vascular Access Committees. Committees are not overseen by central authority and may not interact with one another.	Centralized organization, different teams concentrate on different clinical domains. For example, an enterprise-wide medication-related content group consists of pharmacists and physicians working in collaboration with engineers and broader clinical groups, such as an adult primary care expert panel, a diabetes panel, and a host of ad hoc clinical work groups. Committees/content groups regulated and coordinated by central authority.	At the local level (ie, individual VA site), clinical councils or boards, pharmacy and therapeutics committees, quality management committees, primary care committees, and/or clinical informatics committees. Nationally, a National Clinical Reminders Committee.

TABLE 2: *cont.*

	Mid-Valley Independent Physicians Association*	University of Texas	Vanderbilt	Partners*	Veterans Health Administration*
Process	Almost all content comes from EMR vendor. New development (eg, additional drug–drug interaction rules) is primarily based on requests made by member physicians. The user community includes subject matter experts (SMEs), who are polled or convened as necessary.	Content purchased from commercial vendor. Day-to-day CDS operations are run by a small team that is responsible for managing all servers, desktop support, and issues escalated to the Allscripts review board.	Relatively decentralized. Content is typically requested by end users or experts most familiar with that subset of available tools and developed in collaboration with informatics experts by that group, or centrally.	Full-time clinically trained subject matter experts (SMEs) work in small teams with knowledge engineers to develop and implement CDS, using a three-stage life cycle process of knowledge creation, knowledge deployment, and periodic review	Performance measures established nationally based on quality goals and utilization review, corresponding reminders are developed either locally or nationally. Local, regional, and national committees have input into the content developed.
Customization	Practices are permitted to develop their own content if desired, and NextGen system allows sufficient customization so specific templates, rules, and actions can be filtered to a specific practice without affecting others	Generally not permitted	Local customization is allowed within the constraints of the agreed upon standard practice (eg, a screening practice might vary by clinical unit, but all patients must still be screened)	Partners consists of a large number of hospital and outpatient sites, and, although they support local customization of content where necessary (eg, to adapt to differences in hospital formularies), common enterprise-wide content is preferred.	Governance for performance measures and drug–drug and drug-allergy checks at national level. Previously, sites developed local clinical reminders; national reminders are preferred. Order menus/sets, templates, and consult requests done at facility level.
CIS usage required	Use of CDSS encouraged	Use of CDSS encouraged, no paper chart	Use of CDSS encouraged	Mandated usage	Mandated Usage

TABLE 2: *cont.*

	Mid-Valley Independent Physicians Association*	University of Texas	Vanderbilt	Partners*	Veterans Health Administration*
Review/monitoring	Regular review of EMR performance with reports issued	Monthly reports issued to clinics by vendor regarding EMR performance	Regular review of usage statistics and research project evaluations	Regular review of usage statistics when available and research project evaluations	Measure outcomes against national measures. Regular review of EMR performance with reports issued.
User feedback	Direct interaction between end users and the medical director and support staff through user-group meetings	Informal user feedback, surveys and help-desk issue tracking	Email, regular contact by content owners with the clinical teams, clinical user group meetings, and regularly scheduled review of content and usage statistics with the clinical teams	Applications have built-in features to enable users to provide granular feedback in response to CDS interventions. Users are invited to participate in user groups and the content development process depending on interest/expertise.	Users interact primarily with local clinical application coordinators to provide feedback
References			31-33	34, 35	36, 37

* Site visit conducted

Variation in governance strategies was observed across the five sites. CDS-related staff ranged from a small staff responsible for overseeing a vendor system to large academic informatics departments that included numerous clinicians, informaticians, and software developers. Most sites employed the use of committees to govern development, implementation, and maintenance of CDS systems, although committee structure and overall organization varied. In some cases, content was purchased from an outside vendor, and in others it was developed by in-house staff based on institutional needs. Sites also varied in the degree to which they allowed tailoring of CDS content in individual practices or hospital services. Some form of regular review was common across all sites studied, although mechanisms of user feedback varied significantly in form and frequency.

One particularly notable finding was that governance approaches differed substantially between institutions relying on vendor-based clinical information systems and those with "home-grown" internal clinical information systems (CIS). These differences were largely related to each type of institution's involvement in CDS development, implementation and management. Organizations that rely on vendor-based CDS require governance structures largely limited to collaboration with vendors and ongoing day-to-day operational management. In contrast, organizations with internally developed systems are responsible for the entire process of development, implementation, and ongoing management and assessment. These fundamental differences result in diverging governance practices, which are summarized in table 3.

12.3.3 OVERVIEW OF CONTENT-MANAGEMENT APPROACHES

Our research findings clearly revealed that sites needed coordinated ways to manage their decision-support content, particularly as the amount and complexity of the content grew.

At Partners, a great deal of the CDS content was developed as part of research projects, and balancing research and operational decision-support projects has been challenging, as research content must be maintained (or decommissioned) after the research project ends. Over the last 5 years, with the maturation of the knowledge management group's processes, content is increasingly re-evaluated on a periodic basis, which includes analysis of usage data, such as acceptance and override rates for alerts. [22 23] The most robust review mechanisms are in place for formulary drug information (dose and frequency lists), drug–drug interaction rules, [24] age- and renal-based drug dosing guidance rules, [25] and health maintenance reminders. For these assets, Partners conducts regularly scheduled reviews of content, at differing frequencies. In addition, on-demand reviews are prompted by user feedback and external events gleaned from regular scans of health-information sources, such as FDA and pharmaceutical company announcements and the medical research literature.

TABLE 3: Comparison of governance practices at sites with internal CIS (clinical information systems) development and vendor-based CIS

Governance	Internally developed CIS	Vendor-based CIS
Clinical decision-support-related staff	Require large staff with specialized clinical knowledge	Fewer staff members who support system and collaborate with vendor
Committees	More, specialized committees	Fewer (possibly one) centralized committee(s)
Process	Content developed by committee, employing subject matter experts and knowledge engineers	All or almost all content comes from content vendor; system operations may be run locally
Customization	Permitted, although standardization may be preferred	Limited or not permitted
Central governance	Content managed through organization-wide committees with distinct specializations	Content managed centrally by vendor
CIS usage required	Use of clinical decision-support system more likely to be mandated	Use of clinical decision-support system more likely to be encouraged
Review/monitoring	Regular usage monitoring and research evaluation	Regular reports from vendors
User feedback	Variety of tools employed	Variety of tools employed

Vanderbilt has several mechanisms to assess ongoing proper functioning of clinical content. Surveillance data are collected on order set usage, responses to decision-support pop-up alerts, and other CDS items to adjust the support to the desired outcome. Vanderbilt conducts regular reviews of content and then updates the content as clinical evidence surfaces that would necessitate a change. Vanderbilt prioritizes changes based on quality, safety, clinical volumes, and cost/benefit.

In contrast to the other academic institutions, the University of Texas, Houston Physicians' Practice Plan relies heavily on Allscripts' content, and updates are tied to the Allscripts' release schedule. The Practice Plan conducts surveys of clinical users and creates monthly reports that provide all clinics with a breakdown of the utilization of all aspects of the EHR (electronic health record) (eg, percentage of prescriptions written electronically).

CDS capabilities at the VA are constantly being updated and revised to reflect internal research activities, review of performance measures, input from regulatory groups, networking with academic affiliates, changing emphasis of national program and patient priorities, and involvement in national professional societies and working groups. Evidence-based guidelines from nationally recognized authorities are also reviewed regularly for inclusion. Additionally, the VA national pharmacy program is pursuing integration of a commercially available database for drug–drug/allergy interactions, which would be maintained and periodically updated. Evaluation of the effectiveness of the CDS is indirect and based on the measurement of outcomes it was designed to impact.

Finally, at MVIPA, the primary method of evaluating the effectiveness of CDS is ongoing field testing. Content is updated periodically through the NextGen release cycle and is first tested by MVIPA staff. Design changes that affect clinical content are reviewed by the medical director of information systems. The director also monitors regulatory requirements and prioritizes updates according to their effective dates and their impact.

12.3.4   COMPARISON OF CONTENT-MANAGEMENT APPROACHES

The content-management practices of the organizations differed significantly based on the nature of the organizations. Academic medical centers reported that much of their content was, at least initially, developed by researchers as a part of research projects. Identifying and maintaining this content, particularly after research projects concluded, appeared to be challenging. Sites also reported developing content based on user requests, regulatory and quality reporting requirements, and other organizational priorities.

All sites reported some form of ongoing content review, but the frequency and regularity of these reviews varied. Some organizations carried out an annual review, while other organizations reviewed content based on user feedback or as new evidence became available. Sites which relied more heavily on vendor content were more likely to report periodic updates or refreshes, often tied to vendor release schedules.

Sites also mentioned and underscored the importance of field-testing content and listening and responding to user feedback. These feedback mechanisms ranged from passive receipt of reports to active feedback tools embedded in the EHR and periodic site visits and assessments. Some sites also reported monitoring usage of content in order to prioritize the most highly used content.

In addition to direct CDS-related evaluation, some sites (particularly the VA) reported a strong focus on associated quality measures. The VA also emphasizes standard practice and common data elements within and across their system of care, and is in the process of standardizing such practices when there is evidence or experience to support such efforts. Other sites, including Partners, reported less standardization.

12.4   DISCUSSION

Based on our data collection and analysis, we identified a set of recommended practices for CDS governance and content management. These strategies are designed for organizations developing or expanding CDS efforts at their sites. Based on the sites we studied, these practices seem to be effective general approaches to CDS governance. As evidenced in the case studies, however, decision support is an intensely local phenomenon,26 and as such, sites may need to tailor or selectively adopt these practices to develop solutions that work for them.

12.4.1 RECOMMENDED PRACTICES FOR GOVERNANCE

Delivering excellent CDS requires addressing many governance issues. Among these are defining who will determine if, when, and in what order new decision support will be added; developing a process for assessing the impact of new decision support on information systems' response time and reliability; building tools to enable tracking of what decision support is in place; developing an approach for testing decision support in silico; defining approaches for dealing with rules that interact; developing solid processes for getting feedback from users and letting them know what changes have been made in the underlying systems; and building tools for automated monitoring of decision support. These recommended CDS governance practices are summarized below.

12.4.1.1 PRIORITIZE THE ORDER OF DEVELOPMENT FOR NEW CDS AND DELEGATE CONTENT DEVELOPMENT TO SPECIALIZED WORKING GROUPS

One of the most important issues is developing a sound approach for determining what new decision support will be added and establishing a timeline for development and implementation. A high-level group should prioritize new and ongoing work (eg, blood transfusion-related CDS versus CDS around medications in the neonatal intensive care unit) while specific content work groups develop the prioritized content. Ideally, knowledge-management work groups should consist of local experts in each clinical content area. This process may be carried out internally or delegated to a vendor.

12.4.1.2   CONSIDER THE POTENTIAL IMPACT OF NEW CDS ON EXISTING CLINICAL INFORMATION SYSTEMS (SUCH AS THE EHR APPLICATION OR COMPUTERIZED PROVIDER ORDER ENTRY SYSTEM)

With all new CDS content or functionality it is vitally important to consider the potential impact on all related systems upon implementation. Organizations need a sound process in place for assessing any potential impact on their larger clinical information system ecosystem (ie, EHR, computerized provider order entry, laboratory results system). For example, what are the effects of a new intervention on usability, response time and reliability of the surrounding information system? Each organization is unique in institutional structure and culture, and thus assessments must be performed de novo for each institution, regardless of whether a new CDS is internally developed or purchased from a vendor. Careful evaluation is necessary to avoid potentially problems with related and interacting CIS.

12.4.1.3   DEVELOP TOOLS TO MONITOR CDS INVENTORY, FACILITATE UPDATES, AND ENSURE CONTINUITY

Robust tools must be built to monitor and maintain existing decision support. These tools facilitate tracking of when changes were made, when updating is due, and who is responsible for these activities within an organization. Having one person who can review all content (eg, a chief informatics officer) is very helpful, but when the amount of content increases, this may not be possible. Furthermore, planning for inevitable leadership transitions is essential in order to ensure continuity and maintain up-to-date content. The volume of clinical content and rule logic contained in these systems makes these tools necessary for ensuring the system is up to date and functioning properly, and for guiding future development and implementation.

12.4.1.4   IMPLEMENT PROCEDURES FOR ASSESSING THE IMPACT OF CHANGES AND ADDITIONS TO CDS SYSTEM ON THE SYSTEM'S OWN FUNCTIONALITY

Within any existing CDS system, it is crucial to test decision support before it "goes live" to reduce the likelihood that it will create problems with the existing decision support, or slow down the live system. [27] A related issue is that many rules interact, and as more rules are added, interactions become more frequent, one example being rules relating to reducing cholesterol levels in patients with diabetes and coronary disease. [28] To the extent possible, conflicts and interactions should be addressed in the background so that users are not confronted with redundant or inconsistent warnings. Committees may be required to interact to resolve conflicts fairly and transparently. Specific CDS system testing and rule interaction resolution (related to the stability of the CDS system itself) should be carried out in addition to testing of the impact of CDS systems on all clinical information systems (as outlined in recommendation 2).

12.4.1.5   PROVIDE MULTIPLE ROBUST CHANNELS FOR USER FEEDBACK AND THE DISSEMINATION OF SYSTEMS-RELATED INFORMATION TO END USERS

Building processes that make it possible for users to deliver feedback about the decision support is critical to user acceptance. When a significant issue or problem is identified, it is also crucial to have a process for responding to user suggestions and making appropriate changes. Some organizations such as Vanderbilt have gone so far as to deliver routine, individual reports back to providers after such feedback has been addressed. All organizations will need approaches for notifying providers of important changes in decision support (eg, new alerts, changes to the interface).

12.4.1.6   DEVELOP TOOLS FOR ONGOING MONITORING OF CDS INTERVENTIONS (EG, RULE FIRINGS, USER RESPONSE)

Approaches that enable automated monitoring of systems will be increasingly important, so that one can determine how often rules are firing and how users are responding to them. [29] Flags should be set to enable the counting of rule firing, and approaches are needed to track user responses, including when users cancel or "escape" following a warning. Often, a seemingly minor change can have a major impact on how many warnings are being delivered, and even on overall system performance. In addition to ongoing monitoring of CDS inventory (as outlined in Recommendation 3), monitoring of CDS interventions is necessary for properly assessing the impact of CDS on clinician behavior and patient care. The combination of these tools provides continuous system feedback that can guide changes and additions to the CDS system.

12.4.2   RECOMMENDED PRACTICES FOR CONTENT MANAGEMENT

The development and implementation of effective CDS also depend on sound content-management strategies. The large knowledge bases required for robust CDS necessitate frequent and thorough management in order to keep clinical content up to date. Based on our comparison of the five case studies, we define four recommended practices for content management.

12.4.2.1   DELINEATE THE KNOWLEDGE-MANAGEMENT LIFE CYCLE

The knowledge-management life cycle is an iterative and cyclical process for maintaining the large knowledge bases that CDS requires. The life cycle typically extends from recognition of a clinical need to maintenance and periodic review with modification, retirement, or replacement of the intervention as needed. Every site had at least some component of a knowledge-management life cycle (even if only the creation part);

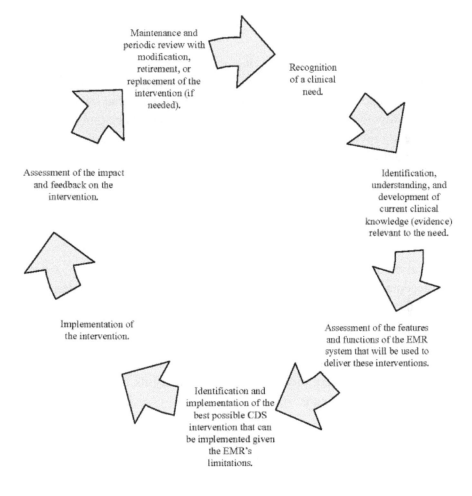

FIGURE 1: Knowledge-management life cycle. CDS, clinical decision support; EMR, electronic medical record

however, we found seven commonly occurring life-cycle phases, shown in figure 1.

12.4.2.2   DEVELOP TOOLS TO FACILITATE CONTENT MANAGEMENT

Several of the sites reported having special-purpose software tools for managing content throughout this knowledge management life cycle. The availability and use of these tools, when well designed, can improve efficiency, allow for asynchronous communication, and ensure that content is periodically reviewed and kept up to date.30 Such tools can also enhance the auditability of content, as decisions can be traced.

12.4.2.3   ENABLE ONGOING MEASUREMENT OF ACCEPTANCE AND EFFECTIVENESS OF CDS INTERVENTIONS

Several of the studied sites had robust measurement programs, where the acceptance and effectiveness of their content are measured after roll-out and on an ongoing basis. Measurement allows content developers to assess the impact of their content and to identify opportunities for improvement. Common metrics included firing rate, acceptance rate, analysis of override reasons, and measurement of the decision support's effects on intermediate processes, and ultimately its effects on patient safety and quality of care.

12.4.2.4   IMPLEMENT USER-FEEDBACK TOOLS THAT ENCOURAGE FREQUENT END-USER INPUT

All of the sites provided some capability for user feedback, ranging from feedback buttons embedded in the EHR application to email, helpdesk query tracking, and clinical representation on committees. Listening and responding to feedback is an important tool for product improvement. It also has the added advantage of fostering a sense of ownership of the product by end users when they feel that their input is valued.

12.4.3 CONSIDERATIONS FOR SMALLER SITES

The governance and content-management strategies we identified are most applicable for large sites with mature and robust CDS. However, small sites that are earlier in the process of developing CDS also face similar governance challenges. The primary differences are that, in general, most small sites have a limited ability to develop and monitor CDS and, as a result, tend to purchase their decision support from commercial content suppliers, rather than developing the content themselves, and tend to rely on general-purpose software tools and built-in EHR functions. In a small practice environment, some tasks, such as monitoring inventory and user feedback, may be simpler to accomplish. Overall, small sites must confront the same issues but with the added challenge of limited financial resources and personnel.

12.4.4 LIMITATIONS AND FUTURE WORK

The purpose of this project was to develop an initial framework for thinking about governance for CDS and to identify a set of recommended practices based on our work. However, this approach has several important limitations, which correlate with opportunities for future work. First, we presented data on a total of five exemplary sites which are purposefully non-representative of typical practice—we believe that this approach maximized what we could learn, but it also limits the generalizability of our data. Further exploration of more sites (especially sites with more typical CDS environments) would contribute to a more well-rounded understanding of CDS governance practices, as widely applied. In addition, it may also be worthwhile to expand our assessment of CDS governance practices to include the role of professional organizations, national regulatory bodies, and clinical content vendors. The governance issues discussed in this paper are not limited to commercial EHR vendors and healthcare institutions, and in the future, we hope to investigate the role of these additional key plays in CDS development and implementation. Finally, the sites studied included only US institutions, which further limits the generalizability of our findings—future study of an internationally representative collection of sites is also likely to be fruitful.

In addition, although we employed a well-established method of qualitative data collection (RAP), complementary future quantitative research could shed further light on CDS governance practices and enhance generalizability. We identified recommended practices based on consensus and expert opinion, and as a result, some effective practices may have been missed. Ideally, these practices would be studied further through a combination of observational or even experimental studies in order to more rigorously quantify the methods for and value of governance. Because of the present relative paucity of sites with advanced (or even formal) governance structures, it may yet be premature to perform such a study, but once there exists a sufficient set of institutions with reasonably robust governance practices, we believe that such a study would add great value to the literature.

Finally, we were not able to characterize the cost of CDS governance, or to study the financial implications of different governance approaches. It would be valuable to assess the comparative cost of different approaches to CDS governance across multiple institutions. However, given the small number of sites with extensive experience in CDS governance and the difficulty in determining costs of large and multifaceted governance structures, such an analysis was not possible at this time but would be a useful future research endeavor.

12.5 CONCLUSIONS

We have synthesized five case studies and identified a set of recommended practices for governance and content management. The five sites we studied were quite diverse; however, they had also learned many overlapping and complementary lessons about governance for CDS. Although the needs of every implementer of decision support are different, we believe that many of these recommended practices may be nearly universal and that all implementers of decision support should consider employing them.

REFERENCES

1. Garg AX, Adhikari NK, McDonald H, et al. Effects of computerized clinical decision support systems on practitioner performance and patient outcomes: a systematic review. JAMA 2005;293:1223–38.
2. Kawamoto K, Houlihan CA, Balas EA, et al. Improving clinical practice using clinical decision support systems: a systematic review of trials to identify features critical to success. BMJ 2005;330:765.
3. Chaudhry B, Wang J, Wu S, et al. Systematic review: impact of health information technology on quality, efficiency, and costs of medical care. Ann Intern Med 2006;144:742–52.
4. Sittig DF, Wright A, Osheroff JA, et al. Grand challenges in clinical decision support. J Biomed Inform 2008;41:387–92.
5. Wright A, Bates DW, Middleton B, et al. Creating and sharing clinical decision support content with Web 2.0: Issues and examples. J Biomed Inform 2009;42:334–46.
6. Sittig DF, Wright A, Simonaitis L, et al. The state of the art in clinical knowledge management: an inventory of tools and techniques. Int J Med Inform 2009;79:44–57.
7. Bates DW, Kuperman GJ, Wang S, et al. Ten commandments for effective clinical decision support: making the practice of evidence-based medicine a reality. J Am Med Inform Assoc 2003;10:523–30.
8. Morrissey J. Harmonic divergence. Cedars-Sinai joins others in holding off on CPOE. Mod Healthc 2004;34:16.
9. Teich JM, Osheroff JA, Pifer EA, et al., CDS Expert Review Panel. Clinical decision support in electronic prescribing: recommendations and an action plan: report of the joint clinical decision support workgroup. J Am Med Inform Assoc 2005;12:365–76.
10. Osheroff JA, Pifer EA, Teich JM, et al. Outcomes with Clinical Decision Support: An Implementer's Guide. Chicago, IL: Health Information Management Systems Society, 2005.
11. Watson HJ, Fuller C, Ariyachandra T. Data warehouse governance: best practices at Blue Cross and Blue Shield of North Carolina. Decision Support Systems 2004;38:435–50.
12. Burstein F, McKay J, Zyngier S. Knowledge management governance: a multifaceted approach to organizational decision and innovation support. Proceedings of the IFIP Conference on Decision Support Systems. Prato, Italy; 2004.
13. Onions PEW, de Langen R. Knowledge Management Governance. Budapest, Hungary: 7th European Conference on Knowledge Management (ECKM 2006), Cornivus University, 2006.
14. Grant G, Brown A, Uruthirapathy A, et al. An Extended Model of IT Governance: A Conceptual Proposal. Americas Conference on Information Systems. Keystone, Colorado; 2007.

15. Nunes MB, Annansingh F, Eaglestone B, et al. Knowledge management issues in knowledge-intensive SMEs. J Doc 2006;62:101–19.
16. Jacobson DD. Revisiting IT Governance in the Light of Institutional Theory. 42nd Hawaii International Conference on Systems Science. Hawaii: Waikoloa, Big Island, 2009.
17. Middleton B. The clinical decision support consortium. Stud Health Technol Inform 2009;150:26–30.
18. Boxwala A, Rocha B, Maviglia S, et al. Multilayered Knowledge Representation as a Means to Disseminating Knowledge for Use in Clinical Decision-Support Systems. Orlando, FL: Spring AMIA Proc, 2009.
19. Ash J, Sittig DF, Dykstra R, et al. Identifying best practices for clinical decision support and knowledge management in the field. Stud Health Technol Inform 2010;160:806–10.
20. McMullen C, Ash J, Sittig D, et al. Rapid assessment of clinical information systems in the healthcare setting: an efficient method for time-pressed evaluation. Methods Inf Med 2010;50(2).
21. Osheroff J, Pifer E, Teich J, et al. Improving Outcomes with Clinical Decision Support: An Implementer's Guide. Chicago, IL: HIMSS, 2005.
22. Shah NR, Seger AC, Seger DL, et al. Improving acceptance of computerized prescribing alerts in ambulatory care. J Am Med Inform Assoc 2006;13:5–11.
23. Abookire SA, Teich JM, Sandige H, et al. Improving allergy alerting in a computerized physician order entry system. Proc AMIA Symp 2000:2–6.
24. Paterno MD, Maviglia SM, Gorman PN, et al. Tiering drug–drug interaction alerts by severity increases compliance rates. J Am Med Inform Assoc 2009;16:40–6.
25. Palchuk MB, Seger DL, Alexeyev A, et al. Implementing renal impairment and geriatric decision support in ambulatory e-prescribing. AMIA Annu Symp Proc 2005:1071.
26. Miller RA. Computer-assisted diagnostic decision support: history, challenges, and possible paths forward. Adv Health Sci Educ Theory Pract 2009;(14 Suppl 1):89–106.
27. Campbell EM, Sittig DF, Guappone KP, et al. Overdependence on technology: an unintended adverse consequence of computerized provider order entry. AMIA Annu Symp Proc 2007:94–8.
28. Ganda OP. Refining lipoprotein assessment in diabetes: apolipoprotein B makes sense. Endocr Pract 2009;15:370–6.
29. Sittig DF, Campbell E, Guappone K, et al. Recommendations for monitoring and evaluation of in-patient computer-based provider order entry systems: results of a Delphi survey. AMIA Annu Symp Proc 2007:671–5.
30. Sittig DF, Wright A, Simonaitis L, et al. The state of the art in clinical knowledge management: an inventory of tools and techniques. Int J Med Inform 2010;79(1):44–57.
31. Miller RA, Waitman LR, Chen S, et al. The anatomy of decision support during inpatient care provider order entry (CPOE): empirical observations from a decade of CPOE experience at Vanderbilt. J Biomed Inform 2005;38:469–85.

32. Geissbuhler A, Miller RA. Distributing knowledge maintenance for clinical decision-support systems: the 'knowledge library' model. Proc AMIA Symp 1999:770–4.
33. Chiu KW, Miller RA. Developing an advisor predicting inpatient hypokalemia: a negative study. AMIA Annu Symp Proc 2007:910.
34. Goldman DS, Colecchi J, Hongsermeier TM, et al. Knowledge management and content integration: a collaborative approach. AMIA Annu Symp Proc 2008:953.
35. Kuperman GJ, Marston E, Paterno M, et al. Creating an enterprise-wide allergy repository at Partners HealthCare System. AMIA Annu Symp Proc 2003:376–80.
36. Fung CH, Tsai JS, Lulejian A, et al. An evaluation of the Veterans Health Administration's clinical reminders system: a national survey of generalists. J Gen Intern Med 2008;23:392–8.
37. Asch SM, McGlynn EA, Hogan MM, et al. Comparison of quality of care for patients in the Veterans Health Administration and patients in the Veterans Health Administration and patients in a national sample. Ann Intern Med 2004;141:938–45.

CHAPTER 13

USE OF ORDER SETS IN INPATIENT COMPUTERIZED PROVIDER ORDER ENTRY SYSTEMS: A COMPARATIVE ANALYSIS OF USAGE PATTERNS AT SEVEN SITES

ADAM WRIGHT, JOSHUA C. FEBLOWITZ,, JUSTINE E. PANG,
JAMES D. CARPENTER, MICHAEL A. KRALL,
BLACKFORD MIDDLETON, and DEAN F. SITTIG

13.1 INTRODUCTION AND BACKGROUND

Computerized provider order entry (CPOE) with embedded clinical decision support (CDS) has been shown to improve the quality and efficiency of patient care, reduce errors and increase adherence to evidence-based care guidelines [1], [2], [3], [4] and [5]. Many CPOE systems allow for the use of order sets, collections of clinically related orders grouped together for convenience and efficiency. Order sets may be designed for a wide variety of clinical scenarios including any type of hospital admission (e.g. cardiology admission), condition (e.g. myocardial infarction), symptom (e.g. chest pain), procedure (e.g. angiography), or treatment (e.g. chemotherapy). Such tools have existed in paper form for many years – long before the advent of electronic medical records or CPOE – and continue to be used today [6], [7] and [8]. However, CPOE allows order sets to be deployed more widely and consistently across the hospital setting. For the purpose of this paper, we consider an "order set" to be a collection of orders designed around a specific clinical purpose and intended to be used together. This differs from an "order pick list" which lists related orders

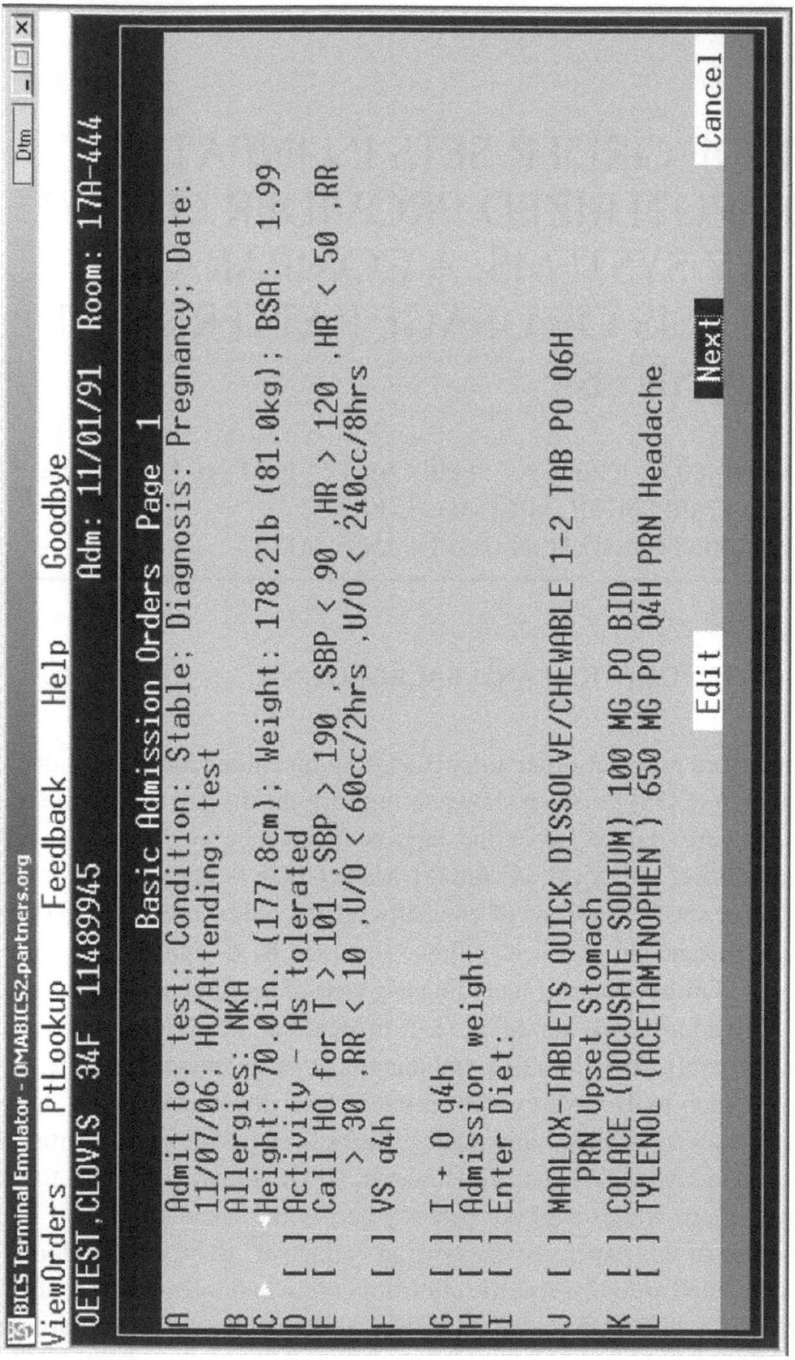

BICS Terminal Emulator - OMABICS2.partners.org   [Dtm] [_][□][X]

ViewOrders   PtLookup   Feedback   Help   Goodbye

OETEST,CLOVIS   34F   11489945   Adm: 11/01/91   Room: 17A-444

                    Basic Admission Orders   Page 1

A   Admit to: test; Condition: Stable; Diagnosis: Pregnancy; Date:
     11/07/06; HO/Attending: test
B   Allergies: NKA
C   Height: 70.0in. (177.8cm); Weight: 178.2lb (81.0kg); BSA: 1.99
D [ ] Activity - As tolerated
E [ ] Call HO for T > 101 ,SBP > 190 ,SBP < 90 ,HR > 120 ,HR < 50 ,RR
         > 30 ,RR < 10 ,U/O < 60cc/2hrs ,U/O < 240cc/8hrs
F [ ] VS q4h

G [ ] I + 0 q4h
H [ ] Admission weight
I [ ] Enter Diet:

J [ ] MAALOX-TABLETS QUICK DISSOLVE/CHEWABLE 1-2 TAB PO Q6H
         PRN Upset Stomach
K [ ] COLACE (DOCUSATE SODIUM) 100 MG PO BID
L [ ] TYLENOL (ACETAMINOPHEN) 650 MG PO Q4H PRN Headache

                      Edit   Next   Cancel

FIGURE 1: Sample order set from BICS (Brigham Integrated Computing System).

that are not designed to be used as a unified group (e.g. a list of antibiotics). A sample electronic admissions order set used at Brigham & Women's Hospital is shown in Fig. 1.

The use of order sets has been shown to improve the quality and efficiency of care and increase adherence to evidence-based guidelines [8], [9], [10], [11], [12] and [13]. They accomplish these aims by influencing provider behavior at the point of order entry. Order sets serve a function similar to a checklist, ensuring critical steps are not missed during a given care process. Rather than entering desired orders from memory, providers are presented with a list of orders relevant to the particular clinical scenario.

In addition to preventing steps in a clinical process from being overlooked, order sets also provide tacit decision support based on their content. For example, the use of an "acute myocardial infarction" order set has been shown to increase the probability that a beta blocker is administered (as well as other evidence-based treatments such as aspirin, ACE inhibitors, heparin therapy, tenecteplase and eptifibatide) [7]. In an electronic format, such an order set might also (1) ensure that the most effective beta blocker is used (by listing the preferred standard-of-care as the only option, the default selected choice, or first on the list of choices), (2) enable documentation of a contraindication to beta blocker therapy if no beta blocker is chosen and (3) enable more widespread tracking and measurement of the delivery of evidence-based case.

Despite evidence suggesting that order sets may be of value for improving patient care, only limited research exists on order set usage patterns and much current research is focused on narrow clinical applications (such as the implementation of a single order set for a specific condition). Payne et al. [14] were among the first to conduct a broad investigation of "order configuration entities" that might improve CPOE efficiency and increase provider acceptance of CPOE, including: order dialogs (guided ordering), quick orders (preconfigured orders), order menus (a organizational hierarchy of orders), and order sets (collections of related orders). They found that, although time-consuming and resource-intensive to produce, such entities were valuable tools for accomplishing these goals. In addition, they found that the majority of usage was skewed toward a subset of all implemented content. The investigation was limited to a single site (Veterans Affairs Puget Sound Health Care System, Seattle & Tacoma, WA) and thus our goal in this project was to expand and update these results by examining order set usage across multiple clinical sites.

Given that the development of orders sets is both time- and resource-intensive [14] and [15], an improved understanding of order set usage patterns could be of value for both vendors and institutions attempting to develop and implement these tools. Although some automated methods of generating order sets have been proposed [16] and [17], order sets are generally designed and implemented using manual processes, with content determined by local governance committees. Researchers and standards developers are also currently exploring ways to share order set content across sites [18] and [19]. Through automation and content sharing, it may be possible to make the order set a more efficient, cost-effective and widely used tool.

In order to generate useful order set content, a better understanding of order set usage patterns and identification of "high-value" order sets is needed. Expanding on previous research [20], we developed a basic order set classification scheme to describe the different types currently in use and analyzed order set usage across a purposive sample of seven sites with CPOE. The goal of this project was to identify specific order set usage patterns that could aid clinical sites and vendors in prioritizing development of high-value order sets.

13.2 METHODS

13.2.1 SAMPLE

We selected a diverse purposive sample of ten clinical sites with computerized order sets and requested information on each site's order set usage in the inpatient setting for a period of 1 year. This sample was designed to include a geographically diverse mix of small and large, community and academic medical centers with a range of CPOE systems (both self-developed and commercially developed systems with a mix of vendors), case heterogeneity and patient volume (measured by case-mix index, which represents the average diagnosis related group relative weight for a hospital). Seven sites agreed to participate in the project, two did not have usage data available and one declined to participate due to time constraints. Site characteristics are presented in Section 3. Data on staffing, case mix index, discharges, and patient days were based on information provided by American Hospital Directory (28).

13.2.2   DATASET

Order set usage data (for 1914 total order sets) was obtained from the seven sites. Use of an order set was defined as opening and submitting the order set. It did not matter whether the user activated a single item from an order set or every order in a single set – each counted as one use of an order set. Participating sites were asked to provide anonymized logs of inpatient system-wide order set usage for a full year (including time, date and order set name for each instance of use). Information on unused order sets (order sets with zero uses during the study period) was available at only four sites and thus "zero-use" order sets were excluded from analysis. One site was able to provide only 6 months of data due to the system's data storage capabilities. Given that order set usage for this site was largely consistent across the two quarters provided, we doubled the order set use counts in the analysis phase to compensate for the shorter data collection period. All other sites provided a full year of order set data. Start and end dates varied across sites.

13.2.3   CLASSIFICATION OF ORDER SETS

Due to granularity and naming mismatches across sites, it was not possible to conduct a cross-site comparison based on order set name alone. In addition, given the wide variation in order set content and large data set, we believed it would be extremely challenging – and not necessarily fruitful – to analyze order set content directly across sites. Thus, we developed an order set classification scheme in order to (1) provide a method of comparing order set usage across sites with varying naming conventions and order set granularity and (2) create unifying basic categories for a large database of order sets with potentially variable content.

Following qualitative assessment of the collected order set usage data, the following five categories were developed based on order set type as determined by the name of each order set (and, when needed, review of the order set content in a small number of cases):

- ADT (admissions/discharge/transfer): Groups of orders related to admission to any hospital service (including general admissions orders), discharge from the hospital or transfer internally or externally. These types of order sets are further divided into subcategories: admission, discharge or transfer.
- Perioperative (pre-operative/post-operative/unspecified): Collections of orders related to preparation for surgery or care following surgery (not necessarily specific to a certain procedure) and any surgery-related order sets with a purpose not otherwise specified. These types of order sets are divided into subcategories: pre-operative, post-operative or unspecified (not-otherwise-specified based on order set name).
- Condition-specific: Order sets pertaining to a specific diagnosis (e.g. myocardial infarction) or symptom (e.g. abdominal pain). For each condition-specific order set, the related condition was recorded.
- Task-oriented: Order sets related to a specific diagnostic (e.g. chest X-ray) or therapeutic procedure (e.g. transfusion) or to administration of a particular medication (e.g. insulin) or other treatment. For each task-specific order set, the related task was recorded.
- Service-specific: Order sets related to a specific hospital service (e.g. ICU). For each service-specific order set, the related service was recorded.

In addition, two other categories were identified on the basis of each order set's function and origin:

- Convenience: Order sets that catalog laboratory tests, medications or clinical consult orders organized for ordering convenience, but not for any particular clinical purpose. For example, some sites used order sets like "AM Labs" or "Common STAT Labs" that allow common orders to be placed quickly. Unlike regular order sets, users are generally expected to pick only a single or small number of orders from a convenience set, and the convenience set lacks an associated clinical purpose – only some sites had convenience sets, and they were frequently used as workarounds when other mechanisms of organizing orders (e.g. order menus) were not available. As previously mentioned, we do not consider convenience sets to be "true" order sets but define these here for completeness.

• Personal: Order sets created or modified for use by an individual or group of practitioners rather than institution-wide committees.

The categories listed above are not mutually exclusive (e.g., a cardiology admission order set would be both "ADT" and "service-specific"). All order sets surveyed fall into at least one category, with many falling into multiple categories. In order to maintain consistency, rules for classification of recurring types of order sets were devised on an ongoing basis and are shown in Appendix A. When an order set was classified into one of the first five categories, specific details (e.g. the condition, task or service) were also recorded.

In order to further compare usage patterns across sites, we also developed an attribute called "order set signature" which combines multiple order set classifications into a single descriptive term. For example, using this strategy, all order sets classified as "ADT (admit)" and "Service-specific (medicine)" can be grouped across sites into the signature "Admit to Medicine." We utilized this attribute to group related order sets across sites and create a list of top signatures.

13.2.4   DATA ANALYSIS

Once our list of order set types was finalized, classification of order sets was carried out by study staff (JF). Consensus checks were conducted with the primary author (AW) for a random subset of the order sets, high-use order sets and all those with potentially ambiguous categorization. Additional information was requested from study sites on an as-needed basis when an order set name was ambiguous. All data analysis was carried out in Microsoft Excel and SAS 9.2, including calculation of order set counts and category-specific usage statistics.

13.3 RESULTS

13.3.1 SITES

Order set usage data was collected from a diverse sample of sites with CPOE. The characteristics of each of the participating sites, including CPOE system, CPOE install year, order set vendor, location, hospital type, teaching hospital status, number of staffed beds (median: 395, average: 431), case mix index (median: 1.61, average: 1.59), discharges per year (median: 18,384, average: 25,021) and patient-days per year (median: 102,421, average: 129,791), are shown in Table 1. Participating sites included a geographically diverse mix of small and large, academic and community hospitals. Five sites had commercial CPOE systems, while two sites had internally developed systems.

13.3.2 ORDER SET TYPES AND USAGE

Our data set consisted of 1914 order sets. These order sets were used a total of 676,142 times in a 1 year period. Table 1 shows the number of order sets and total order set uses by category for each of the seven sites. Order sets from each site were classified into non-mutually exclusive categories as described above. The total by category and average uses per order set are shown on the right-hand side of Table 1. By count, task- (n = 1100) and service-specific (n = 956) order sets were the most common, while personal (n = 79) order sets were least common. Service-specific order sets contributed the most (53.3%) to overall usage, while personal order sets contributed the least (0.2%). ADT order sets had the highest uses per set (812.5) while personal order sets had the lowest (13.7).

Additional order set usage data is presented in Table 2a, Table 2b, Table 2c, Table 2d and Table 2e. For ADT (Table 2a) and perioperative (Table 2b) order sets, total number, total uses, average uses per set and number of sites with each order set type are shown for each subcategory. Admission order sets were the predominant ADT order set subtype by both count and usage. Post-operative sets were the most common perioperative order set subtype by both count and usage.

TABLE 1: Order set usage by category.

Order set category	BWH	Faulkner	KPNW	MGH	KT	NSMC	PPMC	Total		
	Order sets (total uses)	Order sets (total uses)	Order sets (total uses)	Order sets (total uses)	Order sets (total uses)	Order sets (total uses)	Order sets (total uses)	Order sets	Uses	Uses/set
ADT	29 (20,339)	8 (1354)	48 (18,154)	58 (109,450)	48 (6351)	20 (19,256)	19 (11,982)	230 (12.0%)	186,885 (27.6%)	812.5
Perioperative	26 (1170)	15 (290)	148 (32,982)	155 (117,551)	30 (6010)	23 (4180)	10 (781)	407 (21.3%)	163,565 (24.2%)	401.9
Condition	24 (4130)	1 (134)	211 (34,653)	82 (34,544)	191 (7792)	17 (2472)	55 (11,352)	581 (30.5%)	95,077 (14.1%)	163.6
Task	45 (4765)	24 (934)	298 (50,454)	179 (70,850)	98 (4850)	76 (14,392)	380 (66,078)	1100 (57.5%)	212,323 (31.4%)	193
Service	20 (3308)	7 (631)	410 (89,032)	281 (212,458)	144 (18,399)	58 (23,544)	36 (13,255)	956 (49.9%)	360,627 (53.3%)	377.2
Convenience	2 (11)	2 (1283)	43 (19,888)	8 (4124)	40 (4976)	42 (11,210)	335 (157,399)	472 (24.7%)	198,891 (29.4%)	421.4
Personal	2 (8)	3 (33)	53 (377)	12 (156)	0 (0)	0 (0)	9 (510)	79 (4.1%)	1084 (0.2%)	13.7

WH, Brigham and Women's Hospital; KPNW, Kaiser Sunnyside Medical Center; MGH, Massachusetts General Hospital; KT, Memorial Hermann Katy Hospital; NSMC, North Shore Medical Center Union Hospital; PPMC, Providence Portland Medical Center

WH, Brigham and Women's Hospital; KPNW, Kaiser Sunnyside Medical Center; MGH, Massachusetts General Hospital; KT, Memorial Hermann Katy Hospital; NSMC, North Shore Medical Center Union Hospital; PPMC, Providence Portland Medical Center

TABLE 2A: Order set number and usage: ADT.

Top order sets	Count	Uses	Uses per set	Sites with order set type
Admit	209 (90.8%)	181, 166 (96.9%)	871	7
Discharge	14 (6.1%)	5140 (2.8%)	367.1	2
Transfer	6 (2.6%)	521 (0.3%)	86.8	4
Other	1 (0.4%)	55 (<0.1%)	55	1

TABLE 2B: Order set number and usage: perioperative

Top order sets	Count	Uses	Uses per set	Sites with Order set type
Pre-operative	90 (22.1%)	23, 502 (14.3%)	261.1	6
Post-operative	262 (64.4%)	119, 222 (72.9%)	455	7
Unspecified	55 (13.5%)	20, 841 (12.7%)	378.9	7

TABLE 2C: Order set number and usage: condition (top ten).

Top order sets by usage	Uses	Uses/ set	# Sites with order set type	Top order sets by % of total usage	Average % of overall usage	Uses/ set	# Sites with order set type
Peripartum/labor	31,247 (32.9%)	600.9	5	Peripartum/labor	4.80%	600.9	5
Chest Pain/ACS/MI	1,035 (11.6%)	356	6	Chest Pain/ACS/MI	1.80%	356	6
Diabetesb	6724 (7.1%)	3362	2	Abdominal/Flank Pain/GI Complaint	1.30%	643.7	3
Abdominal/Flank Pain/GI Complaint	6437 (6.8%)	643.7	3	Diabetesb	0.80%	3362	2
DVT, VTE and/or PE	5392 (5.7%)	173.9	6	Cardiac Complaint	0.70%	514.5	1
Hypoglycemiab	3192 (3.4%)	1064	3	Stroke/TIA	0.60%	70.9	6
Stroke/TIA	2270 (2.4%)	70.9	6	DVT, VTE and/or PE	0.50%	173.9	6
Burn/Smoke Inhalation	1985 (2.1%)	248.1	3	Pneumonia	0.40%	48.3	6

TABLE 2C: *Cont.*

Top order sets by usage	Uses	Uses/ set	# Sites with order set type	Top order sets by % of total usage	Average % of overall usage	Uses/ set	# Sites with order set type
Pneumonia	1882 (2.0%)	48.3	6	Respiratory Complaint (RDS, Distress, Virus)	0.30%	190.5	4
AAAb	1862 (2.0%)	465.5	2	Neurological Complaintb	0.30%	487	1

TABLE 2D: Order set number and usage: task (top ten).

Top order sets by usage	Uses	Uses/ set	# Sites with order set type	Top order sets by % of total usage	Average % of overall usage	Uses/ set	# Sites with order set type
Insulin	17,568 (8.3%)	532.4	6	Insulin	2.10%	532.4	6
Angiography/angioplasty	15,401 (7.2%)	394.9	4	Angiography/angioplasty	2.00%	394.9	4
Arthroplasty	8322 (3.9%)	489.5	6	Epidural/intrathecal	1.70%	347.4	5
Epidural/intrathecal	7295 (3.4%)	347.4	5	Detoxb	1.50%	126	2
Electrolyte replacement	6877 (3.2%)	343.9	5	Patient-controlled analgesia	1.30%	425	5
Patient-controlled analgesia	5100 (2.4%)	425	5	Arthroplasty	0.90%	489.5	6
Blood transfusion	5014 (2.4%)	557.1	5	Albuterol and Ipratropiumb	0.90%	49	1
Heparin	4153 (2.0%)	207.7	4	Circumcisionb	0.70%	374.7	3
Craniotomyb	4116 (1.9%)	823.2	3	Heparin	0.60%	207.7	4
Thoracic Surgery	3915 (1.8%)	1957.5	2	Total Parenteral Nutritionb	0.60%	155.8	4

TABLE 2E: Order set number and usage: task (top ten).

Top order sets by usage	Uses	Uses/ set	# Sites with order set type	Top order sets by % of total usage	Average % of overall usage	Uses/ set	# Sites with order set type
Emergency/trauma	48,258 (13.4%)	258.1	4	Emergency/ trauma	7.60%	258.1	4
Obstetrics and Gynecology/ Labor and Delivery	36,639 (10.2%)	516	5	Anesthesia	6.20%	649.1	4
Anesthesia	31,807 (8.8%)	649.1	4	Obstetrics and Gynecology/ Labor and Delivery	5.70%	516	5
Orthopedic Surgery	24,148 (6.7%)	575	5	Newborn Nursery	2.50%	836.9	3
Hospitalist	16,960 (4.7%)	1211.4	2	ICU	2.50%	104.8	6
Cardiac Surgery	14,579 (4.0%)	857.6	3	Cardiology	2.40%	581.5	4
Cardiology	14,538 (4.0%)	581.5	4	Medicine	2.40%	1266.4	2
Pediatrics	13,508 (3.7%)	314.1	4	Orthopedic Surgery	2.00%	575	5
Neurosurgery	13,133 (3.6%)	938.1	3	Hospitalist	1.70%	1211.4	2
Gynecological Surgery	9197 (2.6%)	306.6	3	Surgery	1.50%	132.4	4

For condition-specific (Table 2c), task-specific (Table 2d) and service-specific (Table 2e) order sets, the top ten subcategories are shown by number and use as well as the number of sites with each subtype. The top ten conditions, tasks and services by usage accounted for 75.8%, 37.2%, and 63.9% of usage respectively within each category. In addition, 472 convenience order sets and 79 personal order sets were identified, accounting for 29.4% and 0.2% of total usage respectively.

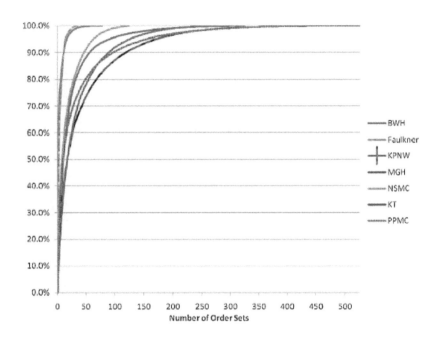

FIGURE 2: Cumulative distribution of order set usage by site.

Out of all 1914 order sets, the top 20% of order sets (383 order sets) by use account for 90.1% of total usage. The cumulative distribution of order set usage by site is shown in Fig. 2. The top ten individual order sets by usage (excluding convenience and personal order sets) are shown by site in Table 3a. In addition, the top 20 "order set signatures" (described in the methods section) are shown in Table 3b.

TABLE 3A: Top ten order sets by site based on total usage.

Rank	BWH	Faulkner	KPNW	MGH	KT	NSMC	PPMC
1	Basic admissions (ADT)	Medicine Admission (ADT, Service)	Diabetes Management (Condition, Task, Service)	Standard Admission (ADT)	Anesthesia Post-Op – PACU (Perioperative, Service)	Medicine Admission (ADT, Service)	Hospitalist Admission (ADT, Service)
2	Patient-controlled analgesia (Task)	Addiction Recovery (Task)	PACU Post-Op (Perioperative, Service)	Anesthesia Same Day Surgical Unit (Perioperative, Service)	OB/GYN Triage (Service)	Cardiology Admission (ADT, Service)	Insulin Correction (Task)
3	Post-Partum (Condition, Service)	Admit to Surgery (ADT, Service)	Standard Admission (ADT)	Labor, Birth and Recovery Admission (ADT, Condition, Service)	Anesthesia Pre-Op (Perioperative, Service)	Albuterol and Ipratropium (Task)	Guidelines for Hypoglycemia (Condition)
4	Post-Cardiac Catheterization/Intervention (Perioperative, Task)	Parenteral Nutrition (Task)	Standard Pre-Op (Perioperative)	Post-Op Cardiac Surgery ICU (Perioperative, Service)	Anesthesia Labor Epidurals (Task, Condition, Service)	Newborn Admission (ADT, Service)	Deep Vein Thrombosis Prophylaxis (Condition)
5	Routine Admit Post-Cardiac Catheterization (ADT, Task)	Rule-Out Myocardial Infarction (Condition)	Patient-controlled analgesia (Task)	Neurology Admission (ADT, Service)	Gastrointestinal Complaint – ED (Condition, Service)	Obstetrics Admission (ADT, Service)	Blood Product Transfusion (Task)
6	Labor Admission Template (ADT, Condition, Service)	Addiction Recovery – Opiates (Task)	Expedited Admission – ED (ADT, Service)	Post-Op Same Day Surgical Unity (Perioperative, Service)	Neonatal Circumcision (Task)	Psych Admission (ADT, Service)	Oxygen Ordering (Task)

TABLE 3A: *Cont.*

Rank	BWH	Faulkner	KPNW	MGH	KT	NSMC	PPMC
7	Admit-Ischemia Pathway (ADT, Condition)	Endoscopy (Task)	Chest Pain â€" ED (Condition, Service)	Orthopedic Surgery Post-Op (Perioperative, Service)	Cardiac Complaint (ED) (ADT, Service)	ICU Admission (ADT, Service)	Universal Respiratory Therapy Protocol (Task)
8	Post-Partum (New) (Condition, Service)	Medicine Admission â€" Psych (ADT, Service)	Blood Transfusion (Task)	Pediatrics Admission (ADT, Service)	Intrathecal/Epidural Narcotics (Anesthesia) (Task, Service)	Post-Partum â€" Vaginal Birth (Condition, Service)	Echocardiogram Orders (Task)
9	Stroke Admission (ADT, Condition)	Hemodialysis (Task)	Abdominal Flank Pain â€" ED (Condition, Service)	Medical ICU Admission (ADT, Service)	Neurological Complaint â€" ED (Condition, Service)	Pediatric Admission (ADT, Service)	Potassium IV Replacement (Task)
10	Insulin Protocol (Task)	ICU Admission (ADT, Service)	Chest Pain â€" Possible Cardiac â€" ED (Condition, Service)	Post-Op â€" General (Perioperative)	GBS Prophylaxis (Condition)	Transitional Care Unit Admission (ADT, Service)	Admission (ADT)
Count by category	ADT = 5Perioperative = 1Condition = 5Task = 4Service = 3	ADT = 4Perioperative = 0Condition = 1Task = 5Service = 4	ADT = 2Perioperative = 2Condition = 4Task = 3Service = 6	ADT = 5Perioperative = 5Condition = 1Task = 1Service = 8	ADT = 0Perioperative = 2Condition = 4Task = 3Service = 7	ADT = 7Perioperative = 0Condition = 1Task = 1Service = 8	ADT = 2Perioperative = 0Condition = 2Task = 5Service = 1

TABLE 3B: Top 20 order set signaturesa overall based by percent of total usage.

Order set signature	Average percent of total usage (%)	# Sites with order set signature
Admit	16.2	7
Post-Operative, Anesthesia Service	3	3
Admit to Medicine Serviceb	2.3	1
Peripartum/Labor, Labor and Delivery/ Obstetrics and Gynecology Servicese	1.8	4
Admit to Cardiology Serviceb	1.7	4
Admit to Labor and Delivery/Obstetrics and Gynecology Servicesa,e	1.6	3
Pre-Operative, Anesthesia	1.5	2
Drug and Alcohol Detox Protocolsb	1.4	1
Abdominal/Flank Pain/GI Complaint, Emergency/Trauma Service	1.3	3
Admit, Peripartum/ Delivery, Labor and Delivery/Obstetrics and Gynecology Servicesb,e	1.3	3
Admit to Psychiatry Serviceb	1.2	4
Admit to Pediatric Serviceb	1	2
Chest Pain/ACS/ MI Evaluation and Managementc	1	5
Patient-controlled analgesia	0.9	3
Epidural/Intrathecal for Peripartum/Labor, Anesthesia Service	0.9	3

TABLE 3B: *Cont.*

Order set signature	Average percent of total usage (%)	# Sites with order set signature
Insulin for Diabetes, Hospitalist Serviceb,d	0.8	1
Insulin (General)d	0.8	4
Admit to ICU	0.8	4
Chest Pain/ACS/MI, Emergency/Trauma Servicec	0.7	3
Admit to Emergency/ Trauma	0.7	3

a For definition of "order set signature," see Section 2.3.
b Based on <5 individual order sets.
c These order sets fell into two related but distinct signatures. The first group includes chest pain evaluation and management order sets designed for hospital-wide use and the second group includes those specific to the emergency/trauma service.
d These order sets fell into two related but distinct signatures. The first group includes insulin order sets designed for diabetes management within the hospitalist service while the second group includes insulin order sets for broader clinical use hospital-wide.
e The granularity and content of OB/GYN order sets varied considerably and fell into three related but distinct signatures. The first group includes peripartum care not related to hospital admission, the second includes admission to L&D and OB/GYN services not related to peripartum conditions, and the third includes admission to the hospital for peripartum conditions.

13.4   DISCUSSION

We have studied the types and utilization of order sets in a small but diverse sample of hospitals in the United States (US), and learned that at all participating sites, order sets were widely used, although the count and total usage statistics varied drastically. We have dramatically expanded results reported in our previous work [20], which included only a high-level analysis of the top order sets at each site, and data on the cumulative distribution of order set usage. The order set classification scheme, complete review of order set database (n = 1914) and the extensive category-specific analysis of usage patterns presented in this manuscript are novel findings not previously described.

Our sample was intentionally diverse covering a range of community hospitals and academic medical centers, with a case-mix index (CMI) ranging from 1.12 (a community hospital) to 2.06 (a large academic medical center), a median of 1.61, and an average of 1.59. The CMI is calculated by adding diagnosis-related group (DRG) weight for the hospital's Medicare patients and dividing by the total number of discharges. Medicare, a national health insurance program in the US administered by the federal government, provides health care to individuals older than 65 or to younger individuals with disabilities; Medicare uses DRGs to determine the payment amount for reimbursement according to a patient's diagnosis, procedures performed while in hospital, and other demographic characteristics. Consequently, the CMI takes into account the complexity of the patient's illness and reflects the diversity of the patients treated in a hospital by averaging the DRGs for all patients treated in one fiscal year. For fiscal year 2010, the median CMI for all hospitals in the United States was 1.38, the average was 1.42, with a range of 0.50–3.77 [21].

We encountered a large range of order set usage per set, usage per discharge and usage per bed across the seven sites. This may be due in part to differences in the CPOE systems and order set catalogs (the complete library of all order sets) at each site. For example, convenience order sets were especially common at Portland Providence Medical Center (PPMC). In PPMC's CPOE system, order sets are the most efficient mechanism for entering orders, and the PPMC staff have created many convenience sets. In fact, the system has two different constructs for order sets: order outlines (which operate in the Java-based CPOE front end) and iForms (HTML documents rendered in an external window) – these two constructs are the predominant mode of entry for the system, and the entry of individual orders through non-order set means is less common. However, at other sites, such as Brigham & Women's Hospital, providers seem to rely on other tools in the CPOE for entering individual orders, so convenience orders are uncommon.

In addition, there were notable differences in the granularity of sites' order set catalogs. For example, Faulkner Hospital had only eight ADT order sets covering major hospital services while Massachusetts General Hospital had 58 ADT sets covering a wide range of services as well as specific patient states and procedures. There were also important differences between the order set usage profiles of each site. At some hospitals, ADT order sets predominated while other hospitals appeared to use order sets primarily for convenience ordering. The difference in granularity may reflect differences in each site's order set approach. For example, although all hospitals had the ability to create order sets without needing customization by their vendor, their approach varied. Some hospitals began with model content provided by their EHR vendor or by a commercial order set vendor, while others started from scratch. Further, some allowed users to create personal order sets (a functionality which is generally being phased out in our study sites), while others required departmental sponsorship for order sets. Unfortunately, there is no objective measure regarding the ease or difficulty in creating order sets therefore, we were not able to evaluate this potential confounding factor across organizations. Consequently, we could not distinguish whether the approach to order set creation and modification varied because of the difficulty of this task or due to other reasons.

Overall, much of the variation observed is likely to be due to differences in the clinical information systems (CIS) implemented at each site, local governance practices regarding the use of CIS and differences between the sites themselves (size, patient volume, available services, etc.). Within and across order set categories, we identified several salient usage patterns which are discussed in depth below.

13.4.1   MAJOR USAGE PATTERNS

13.4.1.1   ADT

The highest usage per set occurred in the ADT category and can be attributed primarily to the use of admissions sets – including generic, service-specific, and condition-specific sets. Usage per ADT set was roughly double the next most frequently used categories. It appears that hospitals get a great amount of utility from these types of order sets, likely because admission is a common occurrence at any large, multi-specialty inpatient facility and requires that many orders be entered at one time. The top order sets by site (Table 3a) and top cross-site order set signatures (Table 3b) also showed a high instance of admissions order sets (including the top order set signature overall, "Admit").

We recommend that, at minimum, a basic admission order set be part of any implementation project. When feasible, additional service-specific admissions sets and condition-specific admission sets should also be developed.

13.4.1.2   PERIOPERATIVE

Post-operative order sets were the most common and most frequently used type of perioperative order set, accounting for approximately 73% of total usage within the category. These order sets were often task-specific or service-specific. Pre-operative order sets were also commonly used, and, in some cases, order sets spanned both the pre-operative and post-operative period. We recommend that sites implement a standard pre-operative and post-operative order set and also develop or purchase additional content based on high-volume services and commonly performed procedures.

13.4.1.3   CONDITION-SPECIFIC

Within the category of condition-specific order sets, we observed that certain common conditions and clinical states dominated overall usage. Peripartum/labor order sets alone accounted for approximately a third of all condition-specific order set usage. The top order sets by site (Table 3a) and top cross-site order set signatures (Table 3b) also showed a high instance of peripartum/labor order sets. Order sets such as those related to cardiac events (Chest Pain/ACS/MI) and thrombotic disease (DVT, VTE and/or PE prophylaxis and treatment) also accounted for a disproportionately large number of uses. Hospitals should prioritize the implementation of order sets related to common conditions and presentations and study their billing and discharge data to determine the highest-value conditions to target.

13.4.1.4   TASK-SPECIFIC

Task-specific order sets were by far the most common type of order set in number (1100 total order sets or 57.5%); however, they were used disproportionately less often, accounting for only 31.4% overall, and a large number of task-specific order sets went essentially unused. Thus, it is important that sites work to identify common or especially important tasks for which the development and implementation of order sets is worthwhile.

Based on usage alone, our findings indicate that task-specific order sets may be valuable for frequent procedures or treatments, especially those applicable across conditions and services such as epidural/intrathecal anesthesia, patient-controlled analgesia, electrolyte replacement and blood transfusion. Order sets for common complex surgical procedures such as arthroplasty, angiography and angioplasty were also often used and appear to be supported by order sets based on usage. Sites should create or purchase procedure- and treatment-oriented order sets based on (1) the degree of standardization of the associated task (a more standardized task lends itself more easily to the use of order sets) and (2) the volume of these tasks performed at that particular site. Sites should also identify and implement important task-specific order sets based on other factors such as cost of care and quality and safety initiatives.

13.4.1.5   SERVICE-SPECIFIC

As was the case with condition- and task-specific order sets, a small number of services accounted for a disproportionately large amount of overall usage. The top three services by usage (emergency/trauma, anesthesia and obstetrics and gynecology) accounted for approximately one third of total usage and the top ten services (out of 68) generated over 61% of usage. While sites should develop order sets for all major services, they should preferentially develop order sets targeted to high-volume services, especially the emergency department, obstetrics and gynecology, and anesthesia as applicable. These top services can also be noted frequently in the top order sets by site (Table 4a) and top cross-site order set signatures (Table 3b).

13.4.1.6   CONVENIENCE

We observed a substantial number of convenience order sets: roughly one quarter of the order sets studied fell into this category. However, the instance of convenience orders varied widely across sites. Usage was also highly skewed toward a small minority of order sets: a mere 7.6% of convenience sets account for 80% of usage. The most highly used convenience sets were generally lab or medication pick lists. As previously mentioned, we do not consider convenience sets to be "true" order sets. Convenience sets are generally more akin to pick-lists and are often a workaround when other mechanisms of grouping orders or facilitating the entry of common orders are unavailable. The demand for and use of convenience order sets should be studied to improve the CPOE system as heavy reliance on convenience sets may indicate gaps or deficiencies in the user interface of the system.

13.4.1.7   PERSONAL

Although many of the sites allowed users to create new order sets or customize existing order sets, personal order sets were uncommon and infrequently used in our study. This indicates that end users are unlikely to generate their own content, probably due to time constraints and lack of system expertise. While it may be valuable in limited instances to have this functionality available, our results suggest that it is not very likely to be utilized. In fact, several of the sites with personal order sets indicated that they were phasing personal order set capability out, and asking users to substitute standard order sets. We recommend that sites should first research whether personal order sets would be useful in their system and if not, concentrate on developing standard order sets that will be more widely used.

13.4.1.8   GENERAL PATTERNS

At each of the studied sites, we observed that a small number of order sets accounted for a large proportion of total order set usage (shown in Fig. 2). A similar phenomenon was observed with specific categories of order sets as well, as described above. For example, 144 distinct conditions and symptoms were identified within the category of condition-specific order sets. Yet, the top ten accounted for 76% percent of condition-specific order set usage. A similar phenomenon was also observed by Payne et al. in their investigation of order configuration entities at VA Puget Sound [14]. They found that usage of "order configuration entities" was concentrated in a small number of orders and that 47% of all content went unused during their six-month evaluation period. We have also shown similar patterns for the distribution of medication, problem and laboratory data in an electronic medical record [22].

These findings suggest that sites should attempt to identify high-value order sets before initiating any development and implementation project. Even at the site at which order set use was least concentrated, 80% of total usage came from less than 70 order sets and 95% of usage came from under 175. This indicates that, if thoughtfully chosen, a catalog of 150–200 order sets may meet the vast majority of a site's order set needs. The top order sets (Table 3a) and top order set signatures (Table 3b) may serve as a valuable starting point for sites wishing to develop or purchase order sets. Data such as service volume, admission and discharge diagnosis frequencies and procedure volume can all be used to inform and tailor the development of a robust order set catalog, and such data is generally available from departmental or institution-wide billing systems, even for institutions that have not implemented CPOE. Substantial time and resources may be wasted if order sets are developed or purchased without preliminary usage research and a strong implementation plan.

While it is beneficial to focus on order sets that are likely to be used frequently, it is also important to note that "high-value" order sets are not limited only to high-volume sets. Although this investigation focuses on usage statistics, sites may also find it useful to create order sets based on other institutional priorities such as reducing the incidence of adverse events or decreasing the cost of care. Sites should be sure to balance the development and implementation of "high-use" order sets with order sets they believe will be critical for other reasons (even if they are less frequently used).

13.4.2   IMPLICATIONS AND FUTURE DIRECTIONS

Our findings clearly show that order sets are a frequently used tool when available as part of CPOE. Given that order sets can be time- and resource-intensive to create, it is important to focus on those high-volume order sets that will be the most used. Our findings indicate that a small proportion of order sets will ultimately be most employed at any given site. Institutions hoping to implement order sets should work to identify high-value order sets based on local needs and focus their attention and resources on this subset.

We hope that sites planning to implement order sets will use these findings to guide the development or purchase of order set content. For those sites that have not yet implemented any order sets, it may be of value to analyze available discharge and billing data to identify areas ripe for the application of order sets. Final selection of order sets to be implemented should be tailored based on local priorities, governance practices [23] and available resources. In addition, we hope that those sites that have already implemented order sets will expand these findings based on their own order set usage data and continue to refine their catalogs.

For smaller sites and those with limited resources for developing order sets, it may be of value to purchase content from an established order set vendor rather than developing content "in-house". Such vendor-generated order sets can serve as a good starting point for a local catalog that can, over time, be customized to suit institutional needs. Vendor-generated order sets may offer an alternative to local development although both can require substantial investments of time and resources.

Another potentially valuable approach to encouraging order set use is to facilitate sharing of validated content. Our data suggests that there are order set types that many sites have in common. As such, it may be possible to develop high-value order sets that can be shared widely and then tailored to local needs. HL7 is developing a standard for representing order sets [18], and, if adopted, this approach may enable wider sharing of content. In fact, many EHR vendors already have electronic libraries where customers can share order set content [24] and [25]; however, until the HL7 standard work is completed and the standard is adopted, interoperability of order set content across vendors is not possible; additional obstacles to content sharing include security concerns and economic loss to competitors [25], which may especially hinder vendors from creating sharing capabilities. Nonetheless, we believe it would be both technically feasible and highly valuable to create, through multi-site collaboration, a freely available "starter kit" of high-value order sets that could then be tailored to institutional needs and expanded based on local priorities.

Finally, sites looking to implement new order sets need to realize that post-implementation maintenance is crucial as a large corpus of order sets need periodic review. In order to restrict unintended adverse consequences of order sets, systems need content update and information review (26). As important as multidisciplinary collaboration may be during planning stages of new order sets (27), the same cooperation is needed during the maintenance stages. However, if periodic order set review is difficult for a specific site, it may choose not to develop as many start-up order sets.

13.4.3   LIMITATIONS

We examined a purposive sample that included only seven hospitals using CPOE. Our sample was designed to be diverse, but it is not random and is not necessarily representative of hospitals in the United States. In particular, our findings may not be generalizable to sites not represented in our sample (e.g. specialty, VA or children's hospitals), though many of the themes and analysis techniques we identify are likely to hold.

Considerable differences in order set naming convention and granularity made it challenging to directly compare order sets across sites. However, we believe that the order set classification scheme described above serves as a useful means of unifying order set data across sites. The designed classification scheme is an original approach that has not been employed before. Furthermore, because only one member of the study team classified the order sets, we were not able to calculate a kappa coefficient.

In addition, given the size of our database and the data sites were able to provide, analysis of the specific content of each order set and the usage patterns of individual providers was beyond the scope of this investigation. Differences in order set content and provider order set usage warrant further study, as the extent of homogeneity or heterogeneity of content is likely to influence the extent to which such content can be shared and individual provider behavior may be relevant to understanding variable order set usage across and within sites. Finally, we were unable to obtain complete information on order sets with zero uses from all sites, so such sets were excluded from our analysis. However, studying such sets could be useful for discerning patterns of order sets that are infrequently used.

13.5 CONCLUSION

We observed important patterns in order set usage across multiple sites as well as meaningful variations between sites. A small number of order sets accounted for the large majority of overall order set usage. Vendors and institutional order set developers should focus on high-value order set types in order to optimize the resources devoted to development and implementation and maximize the value of this important tool.

REFERENCES

1. D.W. Bates, L.L. Leape, D.J. Cullen et al.Effect of computerized physician order entry and a team intervention on prevention of serious medication errors JAMA, 280 (15) (1998), pp. 1311–1316
2. F. van Rosse, B. Maat, C.M. Rademaker, A.J. van Vught, A.C. Egberts, C.W. Bollen The effect of computerized physician order entry on medication prescription errors and clinical outcome in pediatric and intensive care: a systematic review Pediatrics, 123 (April (4)) (2009), pp. 1184–1190
3. M.T. Holdsworth, R.E. Fichtl, D.W. Raisch et al. Impact of computerized prescriber order entry on the incidence of adverse drug events in pediatric inpatients Pediatrics, 120 (November (5)) (2007), pp. 1058–1066
4. R. Kaushal, A.K. Jha, C. Franz et al. Return on investment for a computerized physician order entry system J. Am. Med. Inform. Assoc., 13 (May–June (3)) (2006), pp. 261–266

5.   E. Ammenwerth, P. Schnell-Inderst, C. Machan, U. Siebert The effect of electronic prescribing on medication errors and adverse drug events: a systematic review J. Am. Med. Inform. Assoc., 15 (September–October (5)) (2008), pp. 585–600

6.   J. Chan, K.G. Shojania, A.C. Easty, E.E. Etchells Does user-centred design affect the efficiency, usability and safety of CPOE order sets? J. Am. Med. Inform. Assoc., 18 (May (3)) (2011), pp. 276–281

7.   C.J. Santolin, L.S. Boyer Change of care for patients with acute myocardial infarctions through algorithm and standardized physician order sets Crit. Pathways Cardiol., 3 (June (2)) (2004), pp. 79–82

8.   S.T. Micek, N. Roubinian, T. Heuring et al. Before–after study of a standardized hospital order set for the management of septic shock Crit. Care Med., 34 (November (11)) (2006), pp. 2707–2713

9.   D.J. Ballard, G. Ogola, N.S. Fleming, et al., The Impact of Standardized Order Sets on Quality and Financial Outcomes, Culture and Redesign, vol. 2, 2008. Available from: http://www.ahrq.gov/downloads/pub/advances2/vol2/Advances-Ballard_12.pdf (cited 31.03.11).

10.   A.S. McAlearney, D. Chisolm, S. Veneris, D. Rich, K. Kelleher Utilization of evidence-based computerized order sets in pediatrics Int. J. Med. Inform., 75 (July (7)) (2006), pp. 501–512

11.   A. Ozdas, T. Speroff, L.R. Waitman, J. Ozbolt, J. Butler, R.A. Miller Integrating "best of care" protocols into clinicians' workflow via care provider order entry: impact on quality-of-care indicators for acute myocardial infarction J. Am. Med. Inform. Assoc., 13 (March–April (2)) (2006), pp. 188–196

12.   S. Fishbane, M.S. Niederman, C. Daly et al. The impact of standardized order sets and intensive clinical case management on outcomes in community-acquired pneumonia Arch. Inter. Med., 167 (August (15)) (2007), pp. 1664–1669

13.   N.S. Fleming, G. Ogola, D.J. Ballard Implementing a standardized order set for community-acquired pneumonia: impact on mortality and cost Joint Comm. J. Qual. Patient Saf./Joint Comm. Resour., 35 (August (8)) (2009), pp. 414–421

14.   T.H. Payne, P.J. Hoey, P. Nichol, C. Lovis Preparation and use of preconstructed orders, order sets, and order menus in a computerized provider order entry system J. Am. Med. Inform. Assoc., 10 (July–August (4)) (2003), pp. 322–329

15.   J. Meleskie, D. Eby Adaptation and implementation of standardized order sets in a network of multi-hospital corporations in rural Ontario Healthcare Quart. (Toronto, Ont.), 12 (1) (2009), pp. 78–83

16.   A.S. Rothschild, H.P. Lehmann Information retrieval performance of probabilistically generated, problem-specific computerized provider order entry picklists: a pilot study J. Am. Med. Inform. Assoc., 12 (May–June (3)) (2005), pp. 322–330

17.   A. Wright, D.F. Sittig Automated development of order sets and corollary orders by data mining in an ambulatory computerized physician order entry system AMIA Annual Symposium Proceedings/AMIA Symposium (2006), pp. 819–823

18.   J.C. McClay, J.R. Campbell, C. Parker, K. Hrabak, S.W. Tu, R. Abarbanel Structuring order sets for interoperable distribution AMIA Annual Symposium Proceedings/AMIA Symposium (2006), pp. 549–553

19. B. Middleton The clinical decision support consortium Stud. Health Technol. Inform., 150 (2009), pp. 26–30

20. A. Wright, D.F. Sittig, J.D. Carpenter, M.A. Krall, J.E. Pang, B. Middleton Order sets in computerized physician order entry systems: an analysis of seven sites AMIA Annual Symposium Proceedings/AMIA Symposium (2010), pp. 892–896

21. Services CfMM, FY 2010 Final Rule Home Page, 2011. Available from: https://www.cms.gov/acuteinpatientpps/10fr/itemdetail.asp?itemid=CMS1227442 (cited 06.01.11).

22. A. Wright, D.W. Bates Distribution of problems, medications and lab results in electronic health records: the Pareto principle at work Appl. Clin. Inform., 1 (1) (2010), pp. 32–37

23. A. Wright, D.F. Sittig, J.S. Ash et al. Governance for clinical decision support: case studies and recommended practices from leading institutions J. Am. Med. Inform. Assoc., 18 (March (2)) (2011), pp. 187–194

24. A. Wright, D.W. Bates, B. Middleton et al. Creating and sharing clinical decision support content with Web 2.0: issues and examples J. Biomed. Inform., 42 (April (2)) (2009), pp. 334–346

25. I-Form Library. Available from: http://www.iformlibrary.com/ (cited 16.04.11).

PART V

REFERRALS

CHAPTER 14

IMPROVING THE EFFECTIVENESS OF ELECTRONIC HEALTH RECORD-BASED REFERRAL PROCESSES

ADOL ESQUIVEL, DEAN F. SITTIG, DANIEL R. MURPHY, and HARDEEP SINGH

14.1 INTRODUCTION

Outpatient referrals, defined as processes that include a transfer of responsibility for some aspect of patient's care from a referring provider to a secondary service or provider, [1] are an important but challenging aspect of primary care practice. Successful coordination of referrals hinges upon effective and timely communication to facilitate information sharing and transfer of patient care responsibilities between outpatient providers [2-10]. However, referral communication related to both provider-provider and provider-patient interactions [3,11-14] is prone to breakdown [2,14-22]. The growing use of referral care [23] suggests the need for improving reliability and efficiency of the referral process to create a greater impact on health care quality.

In accordance with the 2009 Health Information Technology for Economic and Clinical Health Act (HITECH) and its Meaningful Use goals for effective use of electronic health records (EHRs), healthcare institutions are increasingly adopting technology to support patient care. By 2015, hospitals are expected to demonstrate, among other things, the capability to exchange key clinical information among providers of care and other patient-authorized entities electronically [24]. This increasing adoption of health information technology holds promise for improving referral communication in health care [25-28]. However, early adopters of these technologies, mostly large integrated systems, have encountered novel communication challenges and unintended consequences that are important to understand in order to reduce future care delays [18,29-35].

Many referrals between primary care providers (PCPs) and specialists do not take place within the same practice or institution; and in general, providers don't have access to the same EHR. However, efforts to address communication challenges using EHRs will be essential given the emphasis on coordination of care and exchange of relevant clinical information by the Patient Protection and Affordable Care Act of 2010 [36]. Recent reform initiatives call for healthcare institutions to become Accountable Care Organizations (ACOs) [37] and demonstrate the use of evidence-based medicine and the application of evolving technologies to support a strong foundation for coordinated primary care. They also create an expectation of continuous process improvement based on measurement of clinical quality and outcomes [38]. EHR-based referrals thus would be an essential component of patient care through ACOs. Even when supported by technology, referral communication between PCPs and specialists is often unsatisfactory [39]. This might be partially due to lack of attention on how communication technology fits with the social environment in which it is implemented [40,41]. Addressing these key challenges in making electronic referral communication effective [11,12,42] requires a multifaceted "socio-technical" approach [43].

Although efforts have been made to improve and standardize overall EHR usability, [44,45] there are presently no standards that specifically address the design or use of electronic systems in outpatient referral communication, and best practices in this area are limited [6,19,39,46-48]. In fact, no available turn-key EHR system can fully support the complexities of most referral processes. Furthermore, referral processes are highly variable across health care settings, and EHRs that support referrals are often heavily customized to reflect unique organizational requirements [19,49,50]. Although complete standardization of referral practices is neither possible nor desirable, several aspects of referral communication are amenable to strategies to reduce the risk of unintended consequences and delays in patient care.

This article describes ten recommendations that represent potential best practices to design, develop, implement, improve, and monitor electronic outpatient referral communication. Recommendations are grounded in a socio-technical model for health information technology [43]. This model uses 8 interrelated dimensions to identify challenges related to developing, implementing, and using information technology within health care (hardware & software, clinical content, human-computer interface, people, workflow & communication, organizational features, external rules and regulations, and measurement & monitoring). The recommendations are also based on current literature, sound clinical practice, our previous work, and a systems-based approach to understanding and implementing health information technology solutions. We also categorized recommendations according to the dimensions of the socio-technical model with which they are most closely related (Table 1). Some recommendations have an established evidence-base and others are based on our experiences or perspectives, but most are not widely adopted by institutions and/or current EHRs. Thus, we believe these recommendations are relevant to all system designers, practicing clinicians, and other stakeholders considering the use of EHRs to support referral communication.

14.2   RECOMMENDATION #1: INCLUDE REAL-TIME CLINICIAN-TO-CLINICIAN COMMUNICATION FEATURES AS PART OF THE REFERRAL SYSTEM

Providers often prefer traditional face-to-face or synchronous communication, such as telephone conversations. While excessive reliance on the EHR and other health information technology may diminish the use of real-time communication, certain critical situations require the interactivity afforded by direct conversation. In fact, some estimates propose that up to 60% of providers' time in clinic is devoted to synchronous conversation [51]. In some cases, such as when a referral is urgent, real-time communication may be required to expedite the referral process [52,53]. Specialists may also want to speak directly to referring providers if there is any doubt about a referral's appropriateness or urgency, even when PCPs and specialists share access to the patient's record. EHRs can facilitate real-time phone conversations or internet-based audio-, video-, or text-based conferencing interactions by providing easily accessible and updated contact information for specialists and PCPs (or their clinics) on the referral interface [54-57]. This flexibility should be specified in any policies and procedures governing outpatient referrals [58].

TABLE 1: Recommendations Summary and their relation to Socio-Technical dimensions

Recommendation		Primary Socio-Technical Dimension*
1	Include real-time clinician-to-clinician communication features as part of the referral system.	Hardware & Software
2	Design and use electronic standardized referral templates that include both structured and free-text fields.	Human-Computer Interface
3	Enforce electronic capture of the reason for the referral.	Clinical Content
4	Bring PCPs and specialists together to collaboratively develop referral guidelines for inclusion into the electronic referral system	People
5	Integrate patient communication into the electronic referral process	People
6	Use automation to pre-populate electronic referral requests with patient-specific data	Workflow & Communication
7	Include the capability of electronic consultations (information-only referrals).	Workflow & Communication
8	Close the communication loop by providing referral status tracking and feedback capabilities and integrating these tools into providers' workflows	Workflow & Communication
9	Standardize and maintain up-to-date institutional policies and procedures for electronic referrals.	Organization Policies & Procedures
10	Monitor electronic referral communication performance.	Measurement & Monitoring

Although recommendation may be associated with more than one dimension of the socio-technical mode, this table identifies the dimension each recommendation most directly relates to.

14.3 RECOMMENDATION #2: DESIGN AND USE STANDARDIZED ELECTRONIC REFERRAL TEMPLATES THAT INCLUDE BOTH STRUCTURED AND FREE-TEXT FIELDS

The content, form, and style of referral letters influences the referral process [5,16,59-61]. Several studies have shown increased provider satisfaction and more consistent and timely feedback from specialists when referral templates are used to standardize referral communication [16,62,63]. Electronic systems provide an excellent opportunity to create, maintain, and disseminate the use of standardized templates [64,65]. However, the interface of electronic referral templates should be designed to avoid excessive constraints that can limit providers' ability to explain and document relevant findings [4]. Thus, when designing electronic referral templates, human-computer interface designers must maintain a delicate balance between structured fields to capture required essential information and free-text fields to allow providers to qualify and expand on their findings freely.

14.4   RECOMMENDATION #3: ENFORCE ELECTRONIC CAPTURE OF THE REASON FOR THE REFERRAL

More than fifty years ago, Williams et al. determined that providing a clear reason for a referral was an essential step in the outpatient referral process [13]. Since then, multiple studies have shown that providers' failure to clearly state the reason for referral (a problem identified in 20-88% of referrals [7,8,21,50]) remains a major barrier to effective referral communication [20,66]. The inclusion of a clear reason to justify a referral is not only regarded as good professional practice but it has also been shown to expedite the referral process [2,7,22,67]. Therefore, electronic systems should be designed to prevent referrals from being transmitted unless they have a clearly defined reason to justify them. In addition to a standard set of generic choices, such as those proposed by Forrest et al. (to seek advice, to request a technical procedure, and to request co-management of the patient), electronic systems should give providers the option to expand and elaborate on their selection when needed [68].

14.5   RECOMMENDATION #4: BRING PCPS AND SPECIALISTS TOGETHER TO COLLABORATIVELY DEVELOP REFERRAL GUIDELINES FOR INCLUSION INTO THE ELECTRONIC REFERRAL SYSTEM

EHRs offer a robust platform for integrating referral guidelines into providers' workflows at the point of care, and referral guidelines can improve the referral process in several ways. For instance, they can help providers determine the appropriateness of a referral prior to initiating the request [42,47] or allow a provider to anticipate the specialist's referral information and patient work-up needs, improving efficiency and quality. People comprise one of the key dimensions of the socio-technical model. While EHRs are valuable delivery vehicles for referral guidelines, effective outcomes will only be achieved by collaborative efforts between referring providers and specialists to facilitate communication, decrease referral denials, and clarify referral expectations. While collaboration across different practice settings and institutions will be challenging to operationalize, it must also be encouraged keeping in line with the national focus on reducing health care costs and overutilization [19,69]. For instance, solo practitioners and small independent practices lacking formal organizational structures can leverage their existing networks of specialists to develop mutually agreed-upon referral guidelines. Additionally, third parties involved in regulatory, reimbursement, or quality improvement activities (e.g., regional extension centers, payers, or medical societies) can facilitate the development and dissemination of a basic set of guidelines as a starting point. Service agreements between PCPs and specialists that include referral guidelines can facilitate provider access to specialists and reduce inappropriate referrals by suggesting evidence-based pathways or alternatives to referrals [70-73]. However, given the complexity of some referrals, systems should remain sufficiently flexible to allow providers to bypass guidelines and submit a referral request that may not appear to adhere to guideline criteria by appropriately justifying its urgency and clinical need.

14.6 RECOMMENDATION #5: INTEGRATE PATIENT COMMUNICATION INTO THE ELECTRONIC REFERRAL PROCESS

As early as 1971, researchers pointed out that the success of outpatient referrals was related in part to patient-related variables, [2] such as patient's illness and socioeconomic background. However, subsequent work has paid little attention to the patient's role in outpatient referral communication. In recent years, the growth of personal health records and other consumer electronic communication tools have modernized and fundamentally transformed patient-provider communication [74]. Nevertheless, patient-related communication remains vulnerable to breakdowns. For instance, these communication failures can account for a substantial number of incomplete referrals resulting in missed appointments and delays in care [53,75]. Attributes similar to those expected of provider-to-provider electronic communication (i.e., secure, timely, reliable, and actionable) [76] must also be used to inform tools to enhance patient-centered communication [77]. These attributes should be the hallmark of effective electronic communication within the patient-centered medical home model [78-80]. Hence, EHRs aimed at supporting referral communication should include functionality to allow the patient to provide additional information if and when needed, and to permit patients to become an active decision-maker during the referral process (i.e. allow them to schedule and cancel appointments, select providers, ask questions). Given the low adoption and use of existing patient communication tools [81,82], novel methods beyond traditional web-based portals are needed. System developers and administrators should explore how to leverage technologies such as smart phone apps, social media portals, and electronic outreach programs [83,84] as well as consider alternative forms of patient access or outreach in order to make patient communication more reliable. This will enable patients to have secure and timely access to relevant information such as referral status updates, reminders to increase patient compliance, and tools to facilitate communication with their physician.

14.7 RECOMMENDATION #6: USE AUTOMATION TO PRE-POPULATE ELECTRONIC REFERRAL REQUESTS WITH PATIENT-SPECIFIC DATA

If used appropriately, electronic referrals have the potential to enhance provider workflow by automating certain tedious or repetitive steps where manual effort is unnecessary. The cognitive load imposed by the use of structured templates, referral guidelines, and use of computerized interfaces increases the time commitment and complexity of initiating and managing referrals [85]. In a recent study, referring PCPs and specialists both suggested the use of automation to pre-populate electronic referral requests in order to decrease both workload and cognitive load [9]. In a separate study, auto-population was commended by providers as a mechanism to improve the efficiency of the consultation process [86]. Electronic referrals should harness the benefits of EHR data and use it to automatically pre-populate fields in the referral template whenever possible (e.g., demographic data, current medication list, recent relevant laboratory test results [18]). Ultimately, more advanced EHRs could even use rule-based pre-population to supply additional relevant information based on the patient's diagnosis or age group.

14.8 RECOMMENDATION #7: INCLUDE THE CAPABILITY OF ELECTRONIC CONSULTATIONS (INFORMATION-ONLY REFERRALS)

The conceptual definition of "referral" implies an actual transfer of responsibility for some aspect of the patient's care and an encounter with another provider. In contrast, a strict consultation involves seeking a colleague's opinion about a particular aspect of the care of the patient, but at no time is the patient under the direct care of the consultant [1,87]. For example, certain referral questions are addressed more efficiently through consultation or information exchanges between the referring PCP and the specialist, which does not necessarily require a physical encounter between the patient and the specialist [9]. Workflow efficiency might be improved if electronic consultations are effectively used. Electronic health records can facilitate these consultations through more flexible and efficient electronic consultation processes that minimize delays (i.e., "information-only" referrals that do not require a patient visit). A successful example of this practice is the established telemedicine modality known as "store-and-forward" in which the provider exchanges relevant patient information with the consultant asynchronously and requests his or her opinion electronically [88,89]. These strategies, if implemented appropriately, can also minimize delays and inefficiencies in care related to unnecessary referrals [48].

14.9 RECOMMENDATION #8: CLOSE THE COMMUNICATION LOOP BY PROVIDING AND INTEGRATING REFERRAL STATUS TRACKING AND FEEDBACK CAPABILITIES INTO PROVIDERS' WORKFLOWS

Coordination of care is more effective when all interested parties are aware of the status of the referral request. Referring providers should receive timely feedback from the specialists upon denial, approval, or completion of each referral [9]. However, studies suggest that specialists fail to provide feedback in 15-45% of referrals [4,7,22,61]. Similarly, specialists may need to discuss requests with the referring providers before or after approving them. In engineering, a closed-loop control system is one in which feedback is needed to control the states or outputs of a dynamic system [90]. Often used in decision support systems, [91,92] closed-loop control can improve electronic referrals by ensuring that communication is coupled with timely and appropriate feedback. Effectively closing the loop on all outpatient referral communication requires considerable resources and efforts from all stakeholders; however, EHRs can help to close the referral communication loop in multiple ways. For example allowing providers to document and access each other's notes about encounters, orders, and other relevant information, or by automatically notifying providers of changes in the status of the referral as it progresses through the referral stages. Additionally, the EHR can notify the referring provider when the specialist has reviewed, approved, or denied a referral request or has asked for additional information [86]. These tools must integrate into providers' workflow in order to leverage improvements in reliability and efficiency. Nevertheless, as with other types of electronic communication in healthcare, it is important not to overload providers with excessive notifications about status updates [93]. Thus, while electronic referral communication must be comprehensive, it should be implemented in a non-intrusive manner so that information remains available to providers and patients on demand.

14.10 RECOMMENDATION #9: STANDARDIZE AND MAINTAIN UP-TO-DATE INSTITUTIONAL POLICIES AND PROCEDURES FOR ELECTRONIC REFERRALS

Within institutions, lack of clear policies and procedures can result in unnecessary heterogeneity across referral processes causing inefficiencies in patient care, provider dissatisfaction, and potential for delays in diagnosis and treatment [9]. Even when organizations develop policies and procedures governing referrals, the adoption of health information technology often translates into profound changes in performance and culture [94,95]. Organizations must carefully review and continuously update policies and procedures related to referrals to ensure they reflect appropriate use of electronic tools [40]. Referral policies and procedures should provide detailed guidance with respect to every facet of the use of technology supporting the referral process. For example, to assure compliance and effective use of health information technology for referrals, organizations need to have clearly documented roles and responsibilities for PCPs, specialists, and supporting staff during key stages of the referral process. Additionally, referral policies and procedures should outline the minimum information PCPs should include in the electronic referral request, as well as expected turnaround times for specialists to respond to the referral. They should also incorporate details about the tools available to providers to monitor timeliness and effectiveness of electronic referral communication [19]. Finally, they should allow the flexibility to account for different levels of urgency and importance across clinical problems and specialties, permitting providers to expedite a particular referral when necessary [40,52,96,97]. A clear and common understanding of referral processes with documented policies and procedures of how the technology should be used by PCPs, specialists, and supporting staff is essential for success.

14.11 RECOMMENDATION #10: MONITOR ELECTRONIC REFERRAL COMMUNICATION PERFORMANCE

Recent literature has revealed several serious health information technology-related errors that arose from faulty system design, configuration, or implementation processes [98-101]. Organizations must continuously monitor and evaluate the usability, performance, benefits, and drawbacks of their electronic referral systems [40]. As with any health information technology-related process, referral communication should be monitored and revised, as needed, [43] to ensure that all stakeholders' needs are being met in a safe and efficient manner. For instance, in our previous work we found that about 7% of electronic referrals at our institution had no follow-up action by specialists at 30 days [29]. Continuous monitoring and frequent assessments of several process measurements (e.g., completed referrals, no-shows/missed appointments, and denied or cancelled referrals) should be part of the organization's ongoing efforts to ensure the effectiveness of their electronic referral communication practices.

14.12 CONCLUSION

EHR-based referrals offer the possibility of greatly improving existing outpatient referral processes. However, technology-facilitated referral processes have not yet reached their potential and will soon be put to the test given the rapid adoption of EHRs. Our proposed recommendations highlight the need to consider the socio-technical context in which information technology-based tools are implemented. Allowing for some flexibility in the referral process and monitoring communication outcomes are vital to effective implementation. As healthcare organizations continue to adopt and use EHRs, the success of technology-enabled referral processes will depend on their ability to remain patient-centered and responsive to providers' needs. The recommendations presented address key areas within seven of the eight socio-technical dimensions, all of which must be performed while adhering to external rules and regulations (e.g., HIPAA or HITECH act), as suggested by the model's eighth dimension. We envision that these recommendations will be useful for several types of stakeholders as they move forward in designing, implementing, and improving their electronic referral systems.

REFERENCES

1. McWhinney IR: A textbook of family medicine. USA: Oxford University Press; 1997.
2. Shortell SM, Anderson OW: The physician referral process: a theoretical perspective. Health Serv Res 1971, 6:39-48.
3. Byrd JC, Moskowitz MA: Outpatient consultation: interaction between the general internist and the specialist. J Gen Intern Med 1987, 2:93-98. P
4. Newton J, Eccles M, Hutchinson A: Communication between general practitioners and consultants: what should their letters contain?
5. BMJ 1992, 304:821-824.
6. Westerman RF, Hull FM, Bezemer PD, Gort G: A study of communication between general practitioners and specialists. Br J Gen Pract 1990, 40:445-449.
7. Chen AHM, Yee HF Jr: Improving the primary care-specialty care interface: getting from here to there. Arch Intern Med 2009, 169:1024-1026. P
8. McPhee SJ, Lo B, Saika GY, Meltzer R: How good is communication between primary care physicians and subspecialty consultants? Arch Intern Med 1984, 144:1265-1268.
9. Gandhi TK, Sittig DF, Franklin M, Sussman AJ, Fairchild DG, Bates DW: Communication breakdown in the outpatient referral process. J Gen Intern Med 2000, 15:626-631.
10. Hysong SJ, Esquivel A, Sittig DF, Paul LA, Espadas D, Singh S, Singh H: Towards successful coordination of electronic health record based-referrals: a qualitative analysis. Implement Sci 2011, 6:84.
11. O'Malley AS, Reschovsky JD: Referral and consultation communication between primary care and specialist physicians: Finding common ground. Arch Intern Med 2011, 171:56-65.
12. Forrest CB, Majeed A, Weiner JP, Carroll K, Bindman AB: Comparison of specialty referral rates in the United Kingdom and the United States: retrospective cohort analysis. BMJ 2002, 325:370-371.
13. Roland M: General practitioner referral rates. BMJ. 1988, 297:437-438.
14. Williams TF, White KL, Fleming WL, Greenberg BG: The referral process in medical care and the university clinic's role. J Med Educ 1961, 36:899-907.
15. Deckard GJ, Borkowski N, Diaz D, Sanchez C, Boisette SA: Improving timeliness and efficiency in the referral process for safety net providers: application of the Lean Six Sigma methodology. J Ambul Care Manage 2010, 33:124-130.
16. Javalgi R, Joseph WB, Gombeski WR Jr, Lester JA: How physicians make referrals. J Health Care Mark 1993, 13:6-17.
17. Jenkins S, Arroll B, Hawken S, Nicholson R: Referral letters: are form letters better? Br J Gen Pract 1997, 47:107-108.
18. Munro C: Referral of Patients-A Neglected Aspect of Medical Practice. Hong Kong Prac 1989, 11:523-6.
19. Sittig DF, Gandhi TK, Franklin M, Turetsky M, Sussman AJ, Fairchild DG, Bates DW, Komaroff AL, Teich JM: A computer-based outpatient clinical referral system. Int J Med Inform 1999, 55:149-158.

20. Kim Y, Chen AH, Keith E, Yee HF Jr, Kushel MB: Not perfect, but better: primary care providers' experiences with electronic referrals in a safety net health system. J Gen Intern Med 2009, 24:614-619.

21. Lee T, Pappius EM, Goldman L: Impact of inter-physician communication on the effectiveness of medical consultations. Am J Med 1983, 74:106-112.

22. Conley J, Jordan M, Ghali WA: Audit of the consultation process on general internal medicine services. Qual Saf Health Care 2009, 18:59-62.

23. Cummins RO, Smith RW, Inui TS: Communication failure in primary care. Failure of consultants to provide follow-up information. JAMA 1980, 243:1650-1652.

24. Barnett ML, Song Z, Landon BE: Trends in Physician Referrals in the United States, 1999–2009. Arch Intern Med 2012, 172:163-170.

25. Public Inspection: Medicare and Medicaid Programs: Electronic Health Record Incentive Program -Stage 2 [https:/ / www.federalregister.gov/ articles/ 2012/ 03/ 07/ 2012-04443/ electronic-health-record-incentive- program--stage-2-medicare-and-medic aid-programs

26. Kalogriopoulos NA, Baran J, Nimunkar AJ, Webster JG: Electronic medical record systems for developing countries: review. Conf Proc IEEE Eng Med Biol Soc 2009, 2009:1730-1733.

27. McCullough JS, Casey M, Moscovice I, Prasad S: The effect of health information technology on quality in U.S. hospitals. Health Aff (Millwood) 2010, 29:647-654.

28. Roberts J: Personal electronic health records: from biomedical research to people's health. Inform Prim Care 2009, 17:255-260.

29. Blumenthal D: Launching HITECH. N Engl J Med 2010, 362:382-385.

30. Singh H, Esquivel A, Sittig DF, Murphy D, Kadiyala H, Schiesser R, Espadas D, Petersen LA: Follow-up actions on electronic referral communication in a multispecialty outpatient setting. J Gen Intern Med 2011, 26:64-69.

31. Novak LL: Improving health IT through understanding the cultural production of safety in clinical settings. Stud Health Technol Inform 2010, 157:175-180.

32. Callahan D: Medical progress: unintended consequences. Hastings Cent Rep 2009, Suppl:13-14.

33. Bernstam EV, Hersh WR, Sim I, Eichmann D, Silverstein JC, Smith JW, Becich MJ: Unintended consequences of health information technology: a need for biomedical informatics. J Biomed Inform 2010, 43:828-830.

34. Weiner M, El Hoyek G, Wang L, Dexter PR, Zerr AD, Perkins AJ, James F, Juneja R: A web-based generalist-specialist system to improve scheduling of outpatient specialty consultations in an academic center. J Gen Intern Med 2009, 24:710-715.

35. Shaw LJ, de Berker DAR: Strengths and weaknesses of electronic referral: comparison of data content and clinical value of electronic and paper referrals in dermatology. Br J Gen Pract 2007, 57:223-224.

36. Campbell EM, Sittig DF, Guappone KP, Dykstra RH, Ash JS: Overdependence on technology: an unintended adverse consequence of computerized provider order entry. AMIA Annu Symp Proc 2007, 94-98.

37. U.S. Congress: Patient Protection and Affordable Care Act. 2010.

38. Fisher ES, Shortell SM: Accountable Care Organizations. JAMA 2010, 304:1715-1716.

39. Mountford J, Davie C: Toward an Outcomes-Based Health Care System. JAMA 2010, 304:2407-2408.

40. Chen AH, Kushel MB, Grumbach K, Yee HF Jr: Practice profile. A safety-net system gains efficiencies through "eReferrals" to specialists. Health Aff (Millwood) 2010, 29:969-971.

41. Sittig DF, Singh H: Eight rights of safe electronic health record use. JAMA 2009, 302:1111-1113.

42. Berg M, Aarts J, van der Lei J: ICT in health care: sociotechnical approaches. Methods Inf Med 2003, 42:297-301.

43. Grimshaw JM, Winkens RAG, Shirran L, Cunningham C, Mayhew A, Thomas R, Fraser C: Interventions to improve outpatient referrals from primary care to secondary care. Cochrane Database Syst Rev 2005. CD005471

44. Sittig DF, Singh H: A new sociotechnical model for studying health information technology in complex adaptive healthcare systems. Qual Saf Health Care 2010, 19(Suppl 3):i68-74.

45. Armijo D, McDonnell C, Werner K: Electronic Health Record Usability: Interface Design Considerations. Rockville, MD: Agency for Healthcare Research and Quality; 2009. AHRQ Publication No. 09(10)-0091-2-EF

46. Schumacher RM, Lowry SZ: NIST Guide to the Processes Approach for Improving the Usability of Electronic Health Records. Gaithersburg, MD: National Institute of Standards and Technology; 2010:5-10.

47. Chen AH, Yee HF Jr: Improving primary care-specialty care communication: lessons from San Francisco's safety net: comment on "Referral and consultation communication between primary care and specialist physicians. Arch Intern Med 2011, 171:65-67.

48. Kim-Hwang JE, Chen AH, Bell DS, Guzman D, Yee HF Jr, Kushel MB: Evaluating electronic referrals for specialty care at a public hospital. J Gen Intern Med 2010, 25:1123-1128.

49. Katz MH: How can we know so little about physician referrals? Arch. Intern. Med. 2012, 172:100.

50. Augestad KM, Revhaug A, Vonen B, Johnsen R, Lindsetmo R-O: The one-stop trial: does electronic referral and booking by the general practitioner (GPs) to outpatient day case surgery reduce waiting time and costs? A randomized controlled trial protocol. BMC Surg 2008, 8:14.

51. Gandhi TK, Keating NL, Ditmore M, Kiernan D, Johnson R, Burdick E, Hamann C: Improving referral communication using a referral tool within an electronic medical record. In Advances in Patient Safety: New Directions and Alternative Approaches Edited by Henriksen K, Battles JB, Keyes MA, Grady ML Rockville MD. 2008, 4. [Agency for Healthcare Research and Quality]

52. Tang PC, Jaworski MA, Fellencer CA, Kreider N, LaRosa MP, Marquardt WC: Clinician information activities in diverse ambulatory care practices. Proc AMIA Annu Fall Symp 1996, 12-16.

53. Coiera E: Communication systems in healthcare. Clin Biochem Rev 2006, 27:89-98.

54. Singh H, Petersen LA, Daci K, Collins C, Khan M, El-Serag HB: Reducing referral delays in colorectal cancer diagnosis: is it about how you ask? Qual Saf Health Care 2010, 19:e27.
55. Robertson KJ: Diabetes and the Internet. Horm Res 2002, 57:110-112.
56. Saxena S, Kumar V, Giri V: Telecardiology for effective healthcare services. J Med Eng Technol 2003, 27:149.
57. Forti S, Galvagni M, Galligioni E, Eccher C: A real time teleconsultation system for sharing an oncologic web-based electronic medical record. AMIA Annu Symp Proc 2005, 2005:959.
58. Gwozdek AE, Klausner CP, Kerschbaum WE: The utilization of Computer Mediated Communication for case study collaboration. J Dent Hyg 2008, 82:8.
59. Coiera E: When conversation is better than computation. J Am Med Inform Assoc 2000, 7:277-286.
60. Esquivel A, Dunn K, McLane S, Te'eni D, Zhang J, Turley JP: When your words count: a discriminative model to predict approval of referrals. Inform Prim Care 2009, 17:201-207.
61. Graham PH: Improving communication with specialists. The case of an oncology clinic. Med J Aust 1994, 160:625-627.
62. Epstein RM: Communication between primary care physicians and consultants. Arch Fam Med 1995, 4:403-409.
63. Tan GB, Cohen H, Taylor FC, Gabbay J: Referral of patients to an anticoagulant clinic: implications for better management. Qual Health Care 1993, 2:96-99.
64. Elcuaz Viscarret R, Beorlegui Aznárez J, Cortés Ugalde F, Goñi Murillo C, Espelosín Betelu G, Sagredo Arce T: Analysis of emergency referrals to dermatology. Aten Primaria 1998, 21:131-136.
65. Cameron JR, Ahmed S, Curry P, Forrest G, Sanders R: Impact of direct electronic optometric referral with ocular imaging to a hospital eye service. Eye (Lond) 2009, 23:1134-1140.
66. Scott K: The Swansea electronic referrals project. J Telemed Telecare 2009, 15:156-158.
67. Piterman L, Koritsas S: Part II. General practitioner-specialist referral process. Intern Med J 2005, 35:491-496.
68. Goldman L, Lee T, Rudd P: Ten commandments for effective consultations. Arch Intern Med 1983, 143:1753-1755.
69. Forrest CB: A typology of specialists' clinical roles. Arch Intern Med 2009, 169:1062-1068.
70. Salerno SM, Hurst FP, Halvorson S, Mercado DL: Principles of effective consultation: an update for the 21st-century consultant. Arch Intern Med 2007, 167:271-275.
71. Mitus AJ: The birth of InterQual: evidence-based decision support criteria that helped change healthcare. Prof Case Manag 2008, 13:228-233.
72. CM protocol results in decreased denials Healthcare Benchmarks Qual Improv 2009, 16:20-22.
73. Lucassen A, Watson E, Harcourt J, Rose P, O'Grady J: Guidelines for referral to a regional genetics service: GPs respond by referring more appropriate cases. Fam Pract 2001, 18:135-140.

74. Fertig A, Roland M, King H, Moore T: Understanding variation in rates of referral among general practitioners: are inappropriate referrals important and would guidelines help to reduce rates? BMJ 1993, 307:1467-1470.

75. Reti SR, Feldman HJ, Ross SE, Safran C: Improving personal health records for patient-centered care. J Am Med Inform Assoc 2010, 17:192-195.

76. Singh H, Hirani K, Kadiyala H, Rudomiotov O, Davis T, Khan MM, Wahls TL: Characteristics and Predictors of Missed Opportunities in Lung Cancer Diagnosis: An Electronic Health Record–Based Study. J Clin Oncol 2010, 28:3307-3315.

77. de Meyer F, Lundgren PA, de Moor G, Fiers T: Determination of user requirements for the secure communication of electronic medical record information. Int J Med Inform 1998, 49:125-130.

78. Tang PC, Ash JS, Bates DW, Overhage JM, Sands DZ: Personal health records: definitions, benefits, and strategies for overcoming barriers to adoption. J Am Med Inform Assoc 2006, 13:121-126.

79. Davis K, Schoenbaum SC, Audet A-M: A 2020 vision of patient-centered primary care. J Gen Intern Med 2005, 20:953-957.

80. Nutting PA, Miller WL, Crabtree BF, Jaen CR, Stewart EE, Stange KC: Initial lessons from the first national demonstration project on practice transformation to a patient-centered medical home. Ann Fam Med 2009, 7:254-260.

81. Reid RJ, Fishman PA, Yu O, Ross TR, Tufano JT, Soman MP, Larson EB: Patient-centered medical home demonstration: a prospective, quasi-experimental, before and after evaluation. Am J Manag Care 2009, 15:e71-87.

82. Carrell D, Ralston JD: Variation in Adoption Rates of a Patient Web Portal with a Shared Medical Record by Age, Gender, and Morbidity Level. AMIA Annual Symposium Proceedings 2006, 2006:871.

83. Kaelber DC, Jha AK, Johnston D, Middleton B, Bates DW: A Research Agenda for Personal Health Records (PHRs). Journal of the American Medical Informatics Association 2008, 15:729-736.

84. Eysenbach G: Medicine 2.0: Social Networking, Collaboration, Participation, Apomediation, and Openness. Journal of Medical Internet Research 2008, 10(3):e22.

85. Gibbons MC: Use of Health Information Technology among Racial and Ethnic Underserved Communities. Perspectives in Health Information Management / AHIMA, American Health Information Management Association; 2011:8.

86. Patel VL, Kushniruk AW: Interface design for health care environments: the role of cognitive science. Proc AMIA Symp 1998, 29-37.

87. Warren J, White S, Day KJ, Gu Y, Pollock M: Introduction of Electronic Referral from Community Associated with More Timely Review by Secondary Services. Applied Clinical Informatics 2011, 2:546-564.

88. Palen TE, Price D, Shetterly S, Wallace KB: Comparing virtual consults to traditional consults using an electronic health record: an observational case¿control study. BMC Medical Informatics and Decision Making 2012, 12:65.

89. Hersh W, Helfand M, Wallace J, Kraemer D, Patterson P, Shapiro S, Greenlick M: A systematic review of the efficacy of telemedicine for making diagnostic and management decisions. J Telemed Telecare 2002, 8:197-209.

90. Callahan CW, Malone F, Estroff D, Person DA: Effectiveness of an Internet-based store-and-forward telemedicine system for pediatric subspecialty consultation. Arch Pediatr Adolesc Med 2005, 159:389-393.

91. The control handbook. New York\: CRC Press; 1996.

92. Gardner RM: Clinical decision support systems: the fascination with closed-loop control. Yearb Med Inform 2009, 17-21.

93. Gaudinat A: Closing the loops in biomedical informatics from theory to daily practice. Yearb Med Inform 2009, 37-39.

94. Murphy DR, Reis B, Sittig DF, Singh H: Notifications received by primary care practitioners in electronic health records: a taxonomy and time analysis. Am J Med 2012, 125(209):e1-7.

95. Brynjolfsson E, Hitt LM: Beyond computation: Information technology, organizational transformation and business performance. J Econ Perspect 2000, 14:23-48.

96. Southon FC, Sauer C, Grant CN: Information technology in complex health services: organizational impediments to successful technology transfer and diffusion. J Am Med Inform Assoc 1997, 4:112-124.

97. Toussaint PJ, Coiera E: Supporting communication in health care. Int J Med Inform 2005, 74:779.

98. Ash JS, Berg M, Coiera E: Some Unintended Consequences of Information Technology in Health Care: The Nature of Patient Care Information System-related Errors. J Am Med Inform Assoc 2004, 11:104-112.

99. Magrabi F, Ong M-S, Runciman W, Coiera E: An analysis of computer-related patient safety incidents to inform the development of a classification. J Am Med Inform Assoc 2010, 17:663-670.

100. Magrabi F, Ong M-S, Runciman W, Coiera E: Using FDA reports to inform a classification for health information technology safety problems. J Am Med Inform Assoc 2012, 19:45-53.

101. Sittig DF, Singh H: Defining health information technology-related errors: new developments since to err is human. Arch Intern Med 2011, 171:1281-1284.

102. Sittig DF, Ash JS, Zhang J, Osheroff JA, Shabot MM: Lessons from "Unexpected increased mortality after implementation of a commercially sold computerized physician order entry system.". Pediatrics 2006, 118:797-801.

Esquivel, A., Sittig, D. F., Murphy. D. R., Singh, H. Improving the Effectiveness of Electronic Health Record-Based Referral Processes. BMC Medical Informatics and Decision Making 2012, 12:107 doi:10.1186/1472-6947-12-10.7. Re-used as per the Creative Commons Attribution License.

PART VI

LABORATORY TEST RESULT MANAGEMENT

CHAPTER 15

EIGHT RECOMMENDATIONS FOR POLICIES FOR COMMUNICATING ABNORMAL TEST RESULTS

HARDEEP SINGH and MEENA S. VIJ

Failures of communication and follow-up of abnormal diagnostic test results can lead to errors, adverse events, and liability claims.[1–5] Therefore, The Joint Commission has prioritized safe and timely communication of critical test results as a National Patient Safety Goal (NPSG.02.03.01), "Report critical results of tests and diagnostic procedures on a timely basis." [6] Although communication breakdowns are deemed largely preventable, this goal remains one of the most commonly cited areas of noncompliance in routine surveys. [7] The evolving definition of "critical" results adds further complexity to the problem. In laboratory medicine, a critical (or panic) laboratory value represents a "pathophysiologic state at such variance with normal as to be life threatening if an action is not taken quickly and for which an effective action is possible." [8[(p. 709) It is now thought that this definition should include equally important but less time-sensitive "vital" values. [9–12]

Emerging evidence highlights vulnerabilities in test-result communication practices along the entire spectrum of testresult abnormality and severity. [5,13–17] The risks of communication breakdowns apply not only to critical values but also to abnormal but non–life-threatening test results. The latter are especially pertinent in the outpatient setting. For example, many test results (for example, chest x-ray with a suspicious shadow), although neither immediately life threatening nor requiring immediate attention, require a response by the provider in a relatively short (1–2 week) period of time. These results may not warrant direct verbal communication to providers; other means of indirect communication such as secure fax, e-mail, or the electronic medical record (EMR) are appropriate for this intermediate level of urgency. In March 2009, the Veterans Health Administration (VHA) released a directive recommending that test results be communicated to providers "within a timeframe allowing prompt attention and appropriate action to be taken" and to patients so that "they may participate in health care decisions." [13] Although apparently reliable electronic systems are used to communicate abnormal test results, breakdowns in test result follow-up persist. [15,18] For example, our recent work on automated EMR–based notifications of diagnostic test results within the Department of Veterans Affairs (VA) outpatient setting showed that 7% of abnormal laboratory results and 8% of abnormal imaging results lacked timely follow-up despite evidence of transmission to providers. [19,20] This is consistent with work in non–VA settings, where approximately 7% of abnormal diagnostic test results were either never communicated to the patient or the disclosure was undocumented. [14]

TABLE 1: Types of Definitions Useful in the Introductory Section of a Policy

Term	Description
Critical test result	Any result or finding that may be considered life threatening or that could result in severe morbidity and require urgent or emergent clinical attention
Significantly abnormal test result	Nonemergent, non–life-threatening results that need attention and follow-up action as soon as possible, but for which timing is not as crucial as critical results. They generate a mandatory notification in the electronic health record but are not required to be reported verbally.
Critical tests	Tests that require rapid communication of results, whether normal, abnormal, or critical
Read-back	The process of an individual receiving the results of a critical or significantly abnormal result or a critical test by writing down and reading back the information to the individual providing this information
Diagnostic area	Pathology and laboratory medicine, imaging, cardiology, and other diagnostic areas as defined by the organization

Therefore, evidence-based and practical institutional policies must uphold effective processes to guide communication of abnormal test results. [21] In 2004, we implemented a policy at our institution (Michael E. DeBakey VA Medical Center, Houston) in response to two separate incidents of small lung nodules detected on chest x-rays that went on to develop into unresectable lung carcinomas in the absence of any follow-up. We recently revised this policy in light of new guidance from the VA Central Office, updated Joint Commission National Patient Safety Goal requirements, and evidence from both within and outside our institution. This article describes the rationale of our institutional policy and provides general recommendations, on the basis of our previous work, other literature, and sound clinical practice, for creating or updating similar policies at other institutions.

15.1 RECOMMENDATION 1. POLICIES SHOULD BE INTRODUCED WITH CLEAR DEFINITIONS OF KEY TERMS

Test-result policies should provide key definitions up front. This not only lends credibility to the policy but also standardizes understanding across many users. Although the Joint Commission, the College of American Pathologists, and the Clinical Laboratory Improvement Act all require that laboratories and hospitals have procedures in place for immediately conveying critical results to the responsible provider, [22–24] what constitutes "critical" should be defined explicitly.

For example, in our new policy a section of key terms appears immediately after the statement of purpose (Table 1), and specific critical values for laboratory and pathology tests are listed in a set of appendices. Our policy also distinguishes critical results from "significantly abnormal" test results, such as positive cancer screens, that may require timely action but that are essentially nonemergent. It is important that policies address both degrees of abnormality to ensure that appropriate clinical responses occur within a reasonable time line. Our work has shown that many imaging results lacking timely follow-up were "suspicious for a new cancer diagnosis," and providers may perceive a lack of urgency for these types of test results because they may have less immediate implications. [20,25]

15.2 RECOMMENDATION 2. POLICIES SHOULD CLEARLY OUTLINE PROVIDER RESPONSIBILITIES

Ambiguous responsibility for test result follow-up can threaten patient safety. [20] For example, we found cases in which an ordering provider other than the primary care physician (PCP)—that is, a specialist or covering provider—believed that follow-up was the PCP's responsibility; meanwhile, the PCP, who did not order the test, believed otherwise, and no followup action was taken. Clarifying providers' responsibilities for follow-up is crucial in this scenario and in other situations when test results are communicated to more than one provider. We found that our institution's well-intentioned "dual notification" feature actually increased the odds that abnormal imaging results would not receive timely follow-up. [20]

Our policy has since been clarified to identify the ordering provider—regardless of specialty or routine relationship to the patient—as the person with whom responsibility rests for initiating follow-up of abnormal results.

15.3 RECOMMENDATION 3. POLICIES SHOULD SPECIFY PROCEDURES FOR FAIL-SAFE COMMUNICATION OF ABNORMAL TEST RESULTS

Ensuring delivery of test results can be challenging. It is sometimes difficult to identify the correct ordering provider or his or her contact information or to ensure he or she received the message. [25,26] Institutions must ensure that personnel involved in reporting test results have access to regularly updated contact information for ordering providers and their surrogates. In addition, transmission of information must be accompanied by backup procedures to ensure delivery. Computerized order entry and the use of an EMR may overcome some of these challenges. [26] For in-stance, critical and significantly abnormal results generate a "mandatory" alert, that is, the alert cannot be customized to be turned off by the receiv-ing provider.

Processes at our institution allow providers to assign surrogates for both electronic and verbal notifications. Within the EMR, patients are as-signed to a permanent staff PCP, and every mandatory test result is also sent to the PCP if he or she is not the ordering provider (with clear respon-sibilities for follow-up, as described). Similarly, trainees are assigned a supervising permanent staff physician so that every mandatory test-result alert is automatically transmitted to the staff physician in the trainee's ab-sence; this practice is well accepted and works well given the duty hour requirement for trainees.

Clear identification and read-back procedures for verbal notification ensure accurate transmission. For example, our policy for reporting criti-cal laboratory values states that clinical laboratory personnel must iden-tify themselves, state the emergency nature of the call, verify the name of the person receiving the report (either the ordering provider or his or her designee or surrogate), and give the name of the laboratory test and the test results. The person receiving the report must then read back the patient's name and the critical result. This interaction must be documented with the date and time of the call and the full names of both parties. Per our institutional policy, failed attempts to verbally communicate critical results to the responsible provider are documented on the Critical Values Documentation Form. In general, we have found laboratory result read-back procedures somewhat easier to implement because of their almost invariably numerical critical results.

For after-hours situations, structured algorithms with "escalation to su-pervisory level" provide guidance for sustaining communication attempts and avoiding loss of follow-up after repeated failures to reach the ordering or surrogate provider. These algorithms may include the use of licensed caregivers, such as nurses and mid-level providers, to receive results. [27] Such algorithms are especially useful for tests from outpatient settings, which traditionally take twice as long to report, [27] or when test results return after the patient has been discharged from the hospital, a particular area of vulnerability. [28]

15.4   RECOMMENDATION 4. POLICIES MUST DEFINE VERBAL AND/OR ELECTRONIC REPORTING PROCEDURES FOR BOTH CRITICAL AND SIGNIFICANTLY ABNORMAL LABORATORY, IMAGING, AND OTHER TEST VALUES

For any potentially life-threatening result, verbal notification of abnormal values is far more likely than electronic notification to initiate a response and is therefore a necessity. [20] For significantly abnormal results, at minimum some form of mandatory electronic notification is necessary [9,29]—such as alerting the provider through the EMR, an alphanumeric pager, or a secure fax. EMR systems can be configured to generate an alert automatically on entry of test results that meet or exceed certain preset values (for example, prostate-specific antigen [PSA] > 15ng/mL). Automated notification ensures that significantly abnormal findings are communicated consistently, but it does not eliminate certain gray areas, such as abnormal findings that do not really meet the threshold for a mandatory alert.[19] Furthermore, notifications of repeat critical or abnormal values may not be necessary. [12] Certain details of the procedures that we find useful for reporting diagnostic tests are now outlined.

15.4.1   LABORATORY AND PATHOLOGY RESULTS.

Our institutional policy establishes the clinical executive board's responsibility for creating and maintaining a list of tests and their defined high and/ or low critical values for both verbal and mandatory electronic notification. This list is subject to review at least annually. Many laboratories already use a critical value list, and several references are available in the literature, [12,30,31] although institutions may need to customize their own laboratory and pathology lists. [9,10,32,33] Our policy requires that critical results be transmitted to the ordering provider both verbally (that is, by telephone or face to face) and through the EMR. Any new pathologically confirmed malignancy in a patient with no existing definitive diagnosis of malignancy is communicated to the ordering provider through the EMR and, for some malignancies, verbally as well. Selected nonemergent but significantly abnormal laboratory results trigger a mandatory alert in the EMR (Table 2)

TABLE 2: Significantly Abnormal Laboratory Values That Trigger Mandatory Electronic Notification*

Test	Reportable High
Occult Blood	Positive
PSA, total	> 15 ng/mL
TSH	> 15 ulU/mL
Hemoglobin A1C	> 15%
HCV AB	Positive
HCV-PCR	Positive
Western Blot	Positive
RPR	Reactive
BUN	≥ 40 mg/dL
Creatinine	≥ 2 mg/dL
CPK	≥ 1,000 U/L

* *PSA, prostate-specific antigen; TSH, thyroid-stimulating hormone; Hemoglobin A1C, glycosolated hemoglobin; HCV AB, hepatitis C virus antibody; PCR, polymerase chain reaction; RPR, rapid plasma reagin; BUN, blood urea nitrogen; CPK, creatine phosphokinase.*

15.4.2 DIAGNOSTIC IMAGING RESULTS

Radiologists are now strongly advised to expedite reports that indicate significant or unexpected findings to ordering providers "in a manner that reasonably ensures timely receipt of the findings." [34(p. 3)] Radiologists and nuclear medicine physicians at our institution use a voicerecognition dictation system when reporting their interpretations in the EMR. Reporting priority is given to tests requested as "stat" and "urgent." An official interpretation (final report) is generated and archived as soon as possible following any examination, procedure, or officially requested consultation, regardless of where the exam was performed.

Pertinent diagnostic reporting codes (Table 3) are applied to the majority of imaging studies, with negative studies left uncoded. These codes, in turn, generate automated notifications to the provider in the EMR and have been adopted by other VA facilities in our south-central network. Verbal notification is required in cases of critical abnormalities and new reportable infectious abnormalities, and the details of the notification (date, time, and provider name) are documented in the final imaging report. In response to the VHA directive, [13] all VA facilities are developing abnormal diagnostic imaging codes.

Imaging reports are sometimes amended by a radiologist, especially when the test was initially read by a resident after hours. Any amendment to a report generates a mandatory notification to the ordering provider per our policy. Our policy also addresses standards for communicating results of studies performed outside our institution. Specifically, patients at our institution who require mammography are referred to providers in the community who have agreed to communicate their findings according to our policy. A separate set of diagnostic codes are used to trigger electronic and/or verbal notification of abnormal results from these studies (Table 3). The mammography codes are now standardized across the VA.

15.4.3   OTHER ABNORMAL TEST RESULTS

Policies should be tailored to address the needs of the institution and need not be limited to imaging and laboratory results. Because our patients tend to be older and at higher risk for cardiac problems, we have implemented procedures to streamline reporting of certain electrocardiogram and echocardiogram findings when the interpreting cardiologist finds a critical abnormality.

15.5   RECOMMENDATION 5. POLICIES SHOULD SPECIFY "CRITICAL TESTS" AND ACCEPTABLE LENGTH OF TIME BETWEEN THEIR ORDERING AND REPORTING

"Critical tests" are those that require communication of results regardless of finding (for example, normal, abnormal, or critical). The term was introduced in a Joint Commission National Patient Safety Goal in 2008 for implementation in 2009.

At our institution, a critical imaging test is defined as any imaging study requested as a STAT order, called in to the radiologist by telephone as a STAT exam and reading. These orders must clearly provide the complete contact information for the ordering provider. To determine whether these studies are being completed and reported within acceptable time limits, our policy identifies three such critical tests for routine monitoring of timeliness, as follows:

1. Radiograph in the operating room for retained foreign body (completed within 30 minutes of order and reported within time lines defined in other policies)
2. Ultrasound examination to rule out ectopic pregnancy (completed within 60 minutes of order and reported within 60 minutes of completion)
3. Post-trauma cross-table radiograph of the cervical spine in the emergency department (completed within 60 minutes of order and reported within 60 minutes of completion)

All pathology frozen sections are also considered critical tests and are monitored for timeliness of completion and reporting.

15.6   RECOMMENDATION 6. POLICIES SHOULD DEFINE TIME LINES BETWEEN THE AVAILABILITY OF TEST RESULTS AND PATIENT NOTIFICATION, AND INSTITUTIONS SHOULD SPECIFY PREFERRED MECHANISMS FOR PATIENT NOTIFICATION

Recommended timeliness standards for patient notification are available for certain types of critical results (ranging from 15 minutes to 60 minutes), but these may need to be customized to some extent by institutions. [21,27] For other significantly abnormal results, time frames are less well defined. One exception is VHA Directive 2009-019, which requires communication of non–life-threatening outpatient test results to patients no later than 14 calendar days from the date when results are available to the ordering provider. [13]

Policies should provide specific guidance on preferred means of communicating with patients or their designated representatives (for example, in-person, telephone, written, or secure portal). Although communication of test results through secure e-mail or Web-based portals has several advantages, previous research has shown that physicians tend to favor direct reporting to patients only when test results are normal, have less diagnostic severity, or have less potential for emotional impact. [35] Nevertheless, best practices in patient notification are evolving and are significantly likely to influence practice in future.

TABLE 3: Diagnostic Reporting Codes for Imaging Studies*

Code	Diagnostic Reporting Code Definition	Mandatory Verbal Notification	Mandatory Electronic Notification
	Critical Abnormality		
201	Any new finding that may be considered life threatening or could result in severe morbidity and require urgent or emergent clinical attention (e.g., cerebral hemorrhage, pneumothorax, pulmonary embolism, significant misplacement of tubes or catheters)	Y	Y
	New Reportable Infectious Abnormality		
202	Active tuberculosis or other reportable infectious disease that requires urgent follow-up	Y	Y
	Findings Suspicious for New Malignancy		
203	An unexpected abnormality that is suspicious or highly suggestive of malignancy	N	Y
	Abnormality		
204	An abnormality or unexpected finding that is not considered to be an urgent and immediate life-threatening finding but needs attention and follow-up action as soon as possible (e.g., acute fracture, new pneumonia, aortic aneurysm)	N	Y
Mammography Diagnostic Reporting Codes			
	BI-RADS 4 Mammogram		
1104	Suspicious abnormality; biopsy should be considered	Y	Y
	BI-RADS 5 Mammogram		
1105	Highly suggestive of malignancy; appropriate action should be taken	Y	Y
	BI-RADS 6 Mammogram		
1106	Known biopsy-proven malignancy; appropriate action should be taken	Y	Y

* Y, yes; N, no; BI-RADS, Breast Imaging–Reporting and Data System.

15.7 RECOMMENDATION 7. POLICIES MUST BE OF "REAL WORLD" VALUE AND WRITTEN WITH FEEDBACK FROM KEY STAKEHOLDERS

Policies are often geared toward regulatory compliance rather than operational value. Implementation of a sustainable and effective policy hinges on education and reinforcement of its users, which necessitates a concise, user-friendly, and easily referenced document. Policies should reflect feedback from representatives of key stakeholders including providers (both primary care and subspecialists), laboratory personnel, radiologists, quality improvement personnel, and residency training program personnel (in teaching institutions).

At our institution, the diagnostic committee [including H.S., M.S.V.] represents many of the aforementioned clinical and administrative stakeholders involved with management of diagnostic tests and is responsible for the content of the policy. This committee met every month during a six-month period in 2009 to reach consensus on certain new changes. Members sought current literature for guidance and solicited feedback from other stakeholders when necessary. We also obtained buyin from personnel who were being given responsibility for afterhours notification. For example, we learned that when the ordering or surrogate provider is not available after hours, reporting emergent results to the on-call senior resident may not be the best option, because it might add to his or her work load and thereby jeopardize compliance with Accreditation Council for Graduate Medical Education regulations. [36] Our critical value list was made current and finalized after consultation with relevant services and subspecialists. Recommendations were forwarded to leadership for feedback and approval, after which they were officially implemented.

15.8 RECOMMENDATION 8. POLICIES SHOULD ESTABLISH RESPONSIBILITIES FOR MONITORING AND EVALUATING COMMUNICATION PROCEDURES

Although electronic notification provides a means of ensuring that test results are transmitted, it provides no guarantee of follow-up. Thus, communication processes must be audited to ensure not only compliance with reporting procedures but also the timeliness of follow-up actions on abnormal test results, including patient notification. Monitoring and evaluation procedures must take into account work flow and practical management issues at the receiving end of the communication. In studies of both laboratory and imaging abnormal results, we found that electronically "acknowledged" and nonacknowledged test-result alerts were equally associated with a lack of timely follow-up. [19,20] When we discussed this with providers, they expressed the need for better systems to track follow-up actions and patient notification. We plan to address these needs in future work.

Finally, institutions must continuously learn from the intended and unintended consequences of their policies over time and identify failure modes and actual performance. Particularly when data suggest a potential system failure, the enlistment of end users to provide feedback on system performance is key for continuous quality improvement. For instance, in another study we found that system interventions including mandatory notification to improve follow-up of positive fecal occult blood test results did not dramatically reduce the high proportion of positive tests with no documented follow-up after two weeks. [17] Through consultation with end users and representatives from administration and information technology, we discovered and fixed a glitch in our software that had prevented the transmission of a certain subset of abnormal test results. [26]

15.9   CONCLUSIONS

We offer eight recommendations for health care institutions to design effective policies for ensuring safe and timely test-result communication. These recommendations are based on our recent work, experiences with a previous policy, and current literature, and they address the Joint Commission's National Patient Safety Goal (NPSG.02.03.01) of ensuring safe communication of critical diagnostic test results. We caution that many lessons learned are from experiences at a single VA facility and may not fully generalize to other VA or non–VA facilities. Although policy content may overlap between VA facilities because they respond to the VHA

Directive, details of policy implementation are not standardized across the VA system, and facilities may design policies and procedures to best address local needs. However, certain best practices could potentially be standardized and applied across VA facilities in the future without eliminating important areas of flexibility. There is already a move toward standardizing the use of certain computerized codes used by radiologists across our region and nationally. Moreover, the principles that underlie these recommendations can be useful for a wide variety of institutions and health care practices and apply to inpatient and outpatient care, EMR and non–EMR users, and private and public settings. Thus, despite the limitations of our work, some of these practical suggestions and best practices may be a useful guide for institutions to design or amend their policies for safe test-result communication

REFERENCES

1. 1. Gandhi T.K., et al.: Missed and delayed diagnoses in the ambulatory setting: A study of closed malpractice claims. Ann Intern Med 145:488–496, Oct. 2006.
2. Singh H., et al.: Reducing diagnostic errors through effective communication: Harnessing the power of information technology. J Gen Intern Med 23:489–494, Apr. 2008.
3. Singh H., et al.: Missed opportunities to initiate endoscopic evaluation for colorectal cancer diagnosis. Am J Gastroenterol 104:2543–2554, Oct. 2009. Epub Jun. 23, 2009.
4. Singh H., et al.: Errors in cancer diagnosis: Current understanding and future directions. J Clin Oncol 25:5009–5018, Nov. 2007.
5. Hickner J., et al.: Testing process errors and their harms and consequences reported from family medicine practices: A study of the American Academy of Family Physicians National Research Network. Qual Saf Health Care 17:194–200, Jun. 2008.
6. The Joint Commission: 2010 National Patient Safety Goals (NPSSGs). http://www.jointcommission.org/PatientSafety/NationalPatientSafetyGoals/ (last accessed Mar. 19, 2010).
7. The Joint Commission: Approved: 2010 National Patient Safety Goals. Jt Comm Perspect 29:1, 20–31, Oct. 2009.
8. Lundberg G.D.: Critical (panic) value notification: An established laboratory practice policy (parameter). JAMA 263:709, Feb. 2, 1990.
9. Piva E., et al.: Evaluation of effectiveness of a computerized notification system for reporting critical values. Am J Clin Pathol 131:432–441, Mar. 2009.
10. Visscher D.W.: What values are critical? Am J Clin Pathol 130:681–682, Nov. 2008.
11. Lundberg G.D.: It is time to extend the laboratory critical (panic) value system to include vital values. MedGenMed 9:20, Jan. 2007.

12. Howanitz P.J., Steindel S.J., Heard N.V.: Laboratory critical values policies and procedures: A College of American Pathologists Q-Probes study in 623 institutions. Arch Pathol Lab Med 126:663–669, Jun. 2002.

13. Department of Veterans Affairs, Veterans Health Administration: VHA Directive 2009-019: Ordering and Reporting Test Results. Mar. 24, 2009. http://www1.va.gov/vhapublications/ViewPublication.asp?pub_ID=1864 (last accessed Mar. 19, 2010).

14. Casalino L.P., et al.: Frequency of failure to inform patients of clinically significant outpatient test results. Arch Intern Med 169:1123–1129, Jun. 2009.

15. Gordon J.R., et al.: Failure to recognize newly identified aortic dilations in a health care system with an advanced electronic medical record. Ann Intern Med 151:21–27, W5, Jul. 2009.

16. Moore C., et al.: Timely follow-up of abnormal outpatient test results: Perceived barriers and impact on patient safety. J Patient Saf 4:241–244, Dec. 2008.

17. Singh H., et al.: Using a multifaceted approach to improve the follow-up of positive fecal occult blood test results. Am J Gastroenterol 104:942–952, Apr. 2009. Epub Mar. 17, 2009.

18. Kuperman G.J., et al.: How promptly are inpatients treated for critical laboratory results? J Am Med Inform Assoc 5:112–119, Jan.–Feb. 1998.

19. Singh H., Thomas E., Petersen L.A.: Notification of laboratory test results in an electronic health record: Do any safety concerns remain? Am J Med 123:238–244, Mar. 2010.

20. Singh H., et al.: Timely follow-up of abnormal diagnostic imaging test results in an outpatient setting: Are electronic medical records achieving their potential? Arch Intern Med 169:1578–1586, Sep. 28, 2009.

21. Hanna D., et al.: Communicating critical test results: Safe practice recommendations. Jt Comm J Qual Patient Saf 31:68–80, Feb. 2005.

22. The Joint Commission. NPSG.02.03.01: Critical Tests, Results and Values. Dec. 2009. http://www.jointcommission.org/AccreditationPrograms/ LaboratoryServices/Standards/09_FAQs/NPSG/Communication/ NPSG.02.03.01/Critical_tests_results_values.htm. (last accessed Mar. 19, 2010).

23. Clinical Laboratory Improvement Amendments of 1988 Final Rule (42 CFR Part 405). Fed Reg 57:7001–7186, Feb. 1992.

24. Commission on Laboratory Accreditation, College of American Pathologists: Laboratory General Checklist—Questions Related to Reporting of Results Only, Mar. 2005. http://www.cap.org/apps/docs/pathology_reporting/LabGeneralChecklist_Reporting.pdf (last accessed Mar. 19, 2010).

25. Singh H., et al.: Communication outcomes of critical imaging results in a computerized notification system. J Am Med Inform Assoc 14:459–466, Jul.–Aug. 2007. Epub Apr. 25, 2007.

26. Singh H., et al.: Improving follow-up of abnormal cancer screens using electronic health records: Trust but verify test result communication. BMC Med Inform Decis Mak 9:29, Dec. 2009.

27. Valenstein P.N.: Notification of critical results: A College of American Pathologists Q-Probes study of 121 institutions. Arch Pathol Lab Med 132:1862–1867, Dec. 2008.

28. Roy C.L., et al.: Patient safety concerns arising from test results that return after hospital discharge. Ann Intern Med 143:121–128, Jul. 19, 2005.
29. Kuperman G.J., et al.: Improving response to critical laboratory results with automation: Results of a randomized controlled trial. J Am Med Inform Assoc 6:512–522, Nov.–Dec. 1999.
30. Kost G.J.: Critical limits for urgent clinician notification at US medical centers. JAMA 263:704–707, Feb. 2, 1990.
31. Emancipator K.: Critical values: ASCP practice parameter. American Society of Clinical Pathologists. Am J Clin Pathol 108:247–253, Sep. 1997.
32. Huang E.C.: Critical diagnoses in surgical pathology: A retrospective single- institution study to monitor guidelines for communication of urgent results. Am J Surg Pathol 33:1098–1102, Jul. 2009.
33. Association of Directors of Anatomic and Surgical Pathology: Critical diagnoses (critical values) in anatomic pathology. Hum Pathol 37:982–984, Aug. 2006. Epub Jun. 2, 2006.
34. American College of Radiology: ACR Practice Guideline for Communication of Diagnostic Imaging Findings. 2005 (Res. 11). http://www.acr.org/SecondaryMainMenuCategories/quality_safety/guidelines/dx/comm_diag_rad.aspx (last accessed Mar. 19, 2010).
35. Sung S., et al.: Direct reporting of laboratory test results to patients by mail to enhance patient safety. J Gen Intern Med 21:1075–1078, Oct. 2006.
36. Acccreditation Council for Graduate Medical Education (ACGME): Resident Services Menu: Resident Duty Hours Documents. http://www.acgme.org/acWebsite/navPages/nav_residents.asp (last accessed Mar. 24, 2010).

Singh, H., and Vij, M. S. Eight Recommendations for Policies for Communicating Abnormal Test Results. Joint Commission Journal on Quality and Patient Safety. 2010 May;36(5):226-32. Reprinted with permission.

CHAPTER 16

IMPROVING FOLLOW-UP OF ABNORMAL CANCER SCREENS USING ELECTRONIC HEALTH RECORDS: TRUST BUT VERIFY TEST RESULT COMMUNICATION

HARDEEP SINGH, LINDSEY WILSON, LAURA A. PETERSEN, MONA K. SAWHNEY, BRIAN REIS, DONNA ESPADAS, and DEAN F. SITTIG

16.1 BACKGROUND

Fewer than 75% of patients with abnormal cancer screening examinations receive follow-up diagnostic care subsequent to the initial screening [1-5]. This inadequate follow-up of abnormal cancer screens compromises the benefits of population-based screening programs [6-9]. For instance, the rate of follow-up for positive fecal occult blood test (FOBT) results in the Veterans Affairs health care system is low; more than 40% of veterans with positive FOBTs may not be receiving timely diagnostic colonoscopies [10,11]. Lack of timely follow-up has also been documented outside the VA system [12,13].

An important, largely preventable but relatively unexplored reason for lack of follow-up is a problem in communication of the positive test result from the laboratory to the clinician who ordered it [14,15]. The use of electronic health records, especially those that utilize such features as automated communication of abnormal results from laboratories to clinicians, can potentially improve follow-up of abnormal cancer screens [16-19]. Electronically "alerting" the ordering provider about an abnormal test result such as positive FOBT can improve the availability of vital information at the point of care [18]. As one of several multifaceted interventions to improve follow-up of positive FOBTs, our institution previously implemented standard operating procedures for the electronic health record's test result communication system [19], including the transmission of a mandatory alert to the patient's clinician for every positive FOBT result. This procedure was expected to reduce breakdowns in communication between the laboratory and clinicians.

A significant increase in timely responses to positive FOBT notifications (defined as a documented response within two weeks of the test) followed implementation of this and several related interventions. However, we found that 40% of automated notifications of FOBT results had no documented response by a treating clinician at two weeks even though all of the patients with these positive FOBT tests were eligible to receive a diagnostic colonoscopy. Our research question was to determine why a large number of FOBT alerts were not followed by clinician response at 2-weeks and to investigate if technical and workflow-related aspects of automated communication in the electronic health record were responsible. We also sought to implement and evaluate a potential solution to the issue(s) we identified.

16.2   METHODS

The study was conducted at the Michael E. DeBakey Veterans Affairs Medical Center and its satellite clinics and was approved by the local institutional review board. We used a mixed methods approach analogous to root cause analysis [20] to uncover potential workflow or technical reasons for lack of clinician response to positive FOBT results. We conducted eleven semi-structured interviews with key informants from the laboratory, primary care, and information technology sections to gather details related to FOBT alert generation, transmission, and receipt. Concurrently, we obtained quantitative data to track the alert receipt and follow-up actions by providers.

Clinicians in the VA health care system receive notifications of high-priority information such as abnormal test results in a "View Alert" window of the electronic health record. To understand the technical issues surrounding electronic communication, we analyzed and mapped the associated system-level processes involved. We discovered that the FOBT alert communication system is driven by an underlying component of the electronic health record that continually monitors test order and result entry. Alerts are automatically generated and recipients selected based on a set of predefined rules and parameters. For instance, entry of a test result such as positive FOBT (which was pre-determined to be a high-priority test result) will generate an automated notification to one or more clinicians. The proper recipients for this notification are chosen based on the setting of certain system parameters. After delivery to recipients, alerts stay active in the clinician's inbox up to two weeks, or until acknowledged.

Using the alert tracking system of the electronic health record, we identified all positive FOBT alerts transmitted daily during our study period. Approximately three weeks after alert generation, a trained physician reviewed the electronic health record for evidence of timely FOBT follow-up using a standardized data collection form that had been pilot tested in previous work [19]. Any documented response to the FOBT, such as colonoscopy referral, patient notification, or mention of exclusion criteria for colonoscopy, was considered timely follow-up. If no follow-up action was documented, an additional investigator confirmed the findings and called the ordering clinician (usually the primary care practitioner-PCP). If the clinician gave convincing information to support any undocumented actions, we considered this response as evidence of timely follow-up as well. We also recorded clinicians' comments and actions.

Following a trail of positive FOBTs that were found to have lack of timely follow-up, we used purposeful sampling and snowball techniques to identify our study subjects [21]. We initially purposefully sampled three PCPs whose FOBT results were found on chart review to have not received follow-up. Information from these PCPs led to further interviews with 1 additional provider (a subspecialist) and representatives that were involved with FOBT performance (laboratory personnel) and FOBT reporting (laboratory and Information Technology personnel). Additionally, 3 institutional representatives from leadership and administration that oversee workflow related to FOBT results were also interviewed.

We gathered data from interviews, clinicians' comments and FOBT tracking to uncover reasons for lack of timely follow-up (Figure 1). Using themes generated from this data, we found that five steps contributed to the problem, one of which was a software configuration error in the alert communication system. The latter step was the most significant one in the final common pathway and most amenable to a systems based intervention

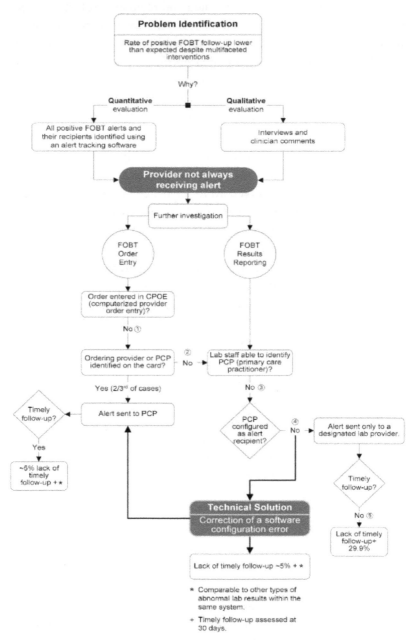

FIGURE 1: Workflow and technical analysis to investigate root cause of high rates of non- response to positive FOBT (fecal occult blood test). Contributing steps 1-5 identified.

to improve communication and follow-up of positive FOBTs. To assess effect of the intervention we implemented, we compared rates of follow-up of positive FOBTs pre- and post-intervention using a Z test of two proportions.

16.3   RESULTS

16.3.1   PROBLEM IDENTIFICATION

Data from PCP interviews and reported comments suggested that PCPs were not receiving positive FOBT alerts consistently, leading us to further investigate the processes associated with FOBT alert generation. Workflow analysis revealed that a large number of patients who are given FOBT cards never return them to the lab for processing, and therefore an order for the test (through a computerized order-entry system) is only placed upon receipt of the card by the lab. However, in the absence of a provider-generated computerized order, the ordering provider is not easily identifiable unless written on the card. Because lab technicians use a different order-entry system, it is difficult for them to identify the ordering provider (and hence the primary recipient of the alert).

Further analysis of alert generation revealed that, regardless of an identifiable ordering provider in the system, the alert management software is designed to communicate all high priority alerts to the PCP as long as a primary alert recipient is identified. We discovered that in positive FOBTs where the ordering provider was not identified, a laboratory staff member served as the designated "ordering" provider, i.e. the primary recipient for the alert. This workaround (nonstandard procedures typically used because of deficiencies in system or workflow design) [22] was intended to enable the completion of the order and subsequent transmission of any alert generated to the patient's PCP; a fail-safe or safety-net mechanism designed to prevent loss of FOBT follow-up.

However, additional technical analysis of the alert tracking data revealed that in all cases where the designated lab provider was alerted as the "ordering" provider, there was no concomitant alert transmission to the PCP. Thus, only the lab provider was receiving the positive FOBT results and had no knowledge of this technical problem. We categorized such alerts as designated lab provider alerts and found that lack of timely follow-up was much more prevalent in this subgroup of alerts (29.9% vs. 4.5% in non-designated lab provider alerts).

16.3.2   INTERVENTION

We surmised that a lack of PCP awareness (in over a third of cases with positive FOBTs) contributed substantially to the prevalence of FOBT results with no documented follow-up, and that a software configuration error was the root of the problem. Once the electronic health record determines the need to generate an alert, proper recipients are selected based on their relationship to the patient (i.e., ordering provider, PCP, etc.). We found an improper configuration of the parameter that defines these default recipients, such that the PCP was not selected as a recipient for designated lab provider alerts (i.e. when PCPs were not listed as ordering providers). However, we could not determine when and how this error occurred in the system. Nevertheless, we posited that a problem-specific fix of this incorrect software configuration would reduce the risk of loss of follow-up for these alerts. The solution to this problem, an addition of a code to link patients to their PCP for tests ordered by others, was implemented on November 28, 2008 (date of intervention).

16.3.3   EVALUATION

We reviewed 360 alerts (117 designated lab provider alerts) pre-intervention and 130 alerts (55 designated lab provider alerts) post-intervention. Figure 2 shows the monthly prevalence of designated lab provider and non- designated lab provider alerts without timely follow-up pre- and post-intervention. Pre-intervention, lack of timely follow-up was observed for 29.9% of the designated lab provider alerts and 4.5% of non- designated lab provider alerts group. However, in the time period following the intervention, the percentage of designated lab provider alerts without timely

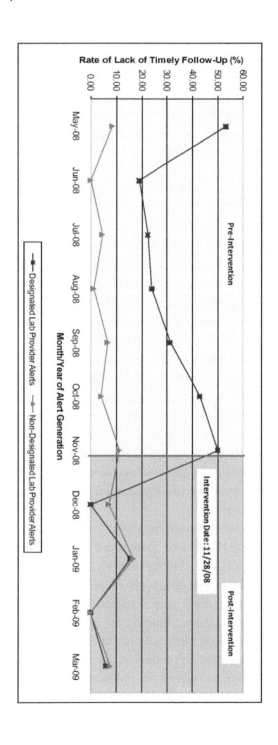

FIGURE 2: Follow Up of Positive Fecal Occult Blood Tests Pre- and Post-Intervention to Correct Software Configuration Error.

follow-up decreased to 5.4% (p < 0.01) and was not statistically significantly different from that of non- designated lab provider alerts (6.6%; p = 0.9). This rate decrease occurred immediately following the intervention and remained stable (i.e. lower than pre-intervention levels) in the subsequent four months (Figure 2). Post-intervention tracking data confirmed that alerts assigned to the designated lab provider were now also being transmitted to the patient's PCP.

16.4　DISCUSSION

We investigated reasons why follow-up actions on a large proportion of positive FOBT results that needed a diagnostic colonoscopy were not documented by clinicians despite the use of a system to electronically communicate positive results. In addition to order-entry workarounds in the electronic health record, we discovered that the communication system intended to alert PCPs of positive FOBT results was not configured correctly, leading to certain situations in which PCPs never received the test result. Upon correction of the software configuration error, the percentage of positive FOBT results lacking follow-up were dramatically reduced. Although the rate did not drop to zero, it was comparable to the rate of lack of timely follow-up we found for other types of non-life threatening, high-priority lab notifications in the same system [23]. Our findings suggest that communication of cancer-related test results in the electronic health record must be monitored to avoid compromising the promise of cancer screening programs.

Of the over 800 patients each year who have positive FOBTs at our institution, about 10-15% of them are eventually diagnosed with some form of colon disease (including cancer). None of the patients in our study had any delay in cancer diagnosis or related harm. Although it is possible that follow-up may have occurred beyond our 30 day "timely response" window had we not intervened, previous work suggests that many of these findings would ultimately never be followed-up [10,11,19]. Thus, our seemingly small intervention could potentially have a large impact on decreasing time to referral for colonoscopy, thereby reducing the risk of a missed or delayed diagnosis of colorectal cancer, a common reason for ambulatory malpractice claims [24-26]. Previous literature has high-lighted the need for system-based interventions to improve follow-up of positive cancer screens and our study is one of few that contributes to this body of knowledge [6].

Our findings also highlight how electronic health record use can have dramatic effects on follow-up care of patients. Electronic health records have potential to address the fragmented and discontinuous care that usually characterizes care in the outpatient setting. Critical information flow between different practitioners, settings and systems of care is essential to high quality care. Through good decision support systems, transmission of information to the right provider at the right time is within the reach of integrated electronic health records. However, as we find, electronic health record use must take into account the effect electronic communication will have on workflow and vice versa. Not doing this correctly would lead to circumstances that reduce the situational awareness of providers and perhaps other unintended adverse effects.

A limitation of our study was a lack of comparable data from other VA or non-VA facilities. However, our work illustrates how electronic test result communication systems are susceptible to errors that may limit their intended outcomes. Furthermore, it should be noted that other VA investigators [10,11] have demonstrated high rates of lack of positive FOBT follow-up, so it is possible that this problem exists at other VA sites. We are currently investigating whether this problem exists in other VA facilities or if this was an isolated event. Additionally, in this study we did not address many other systems issues that should be considered to address follow-up of abnormal test results in addition to provider, technology and work-flow. In our work, we are now using a socio-technical model that accounts for many other systems issues beyond the responsible provider, including the role of organizations and policies and procedures to address monitoring of abnormal test results [27]. For instance, an institutional policy that all FOBTs are ordered through computerized order entry would be another intervention to address this area. In our future work, we will propose multifaceted solutions to address the many complex issues related to abnormal test result follow-up.

Although electronic health records likely offer many benefits over paper-based systems for improving communication of abnormal cancer screening results [17], our findings highlight the need to account for inherent complexities of clinical practice. This complexity may introduce circumstances requiring special attention to EHR workflow to prevent loss of follow-up of important clinical information. In our setting, several workarounds of the FOBT ordering and reporting process resulted in disruption of the normal electronic health record workflow, creating a reliance on a secondary PCP notification system, which was not functioning as intended. The challenge of recognizing these complexities and their effects underscores the need for continuous monitoring of key electronic health record features that may impact safety. The work described here was a direct result of quality assurance work that is highly regarded in the VA health care system. Other institutions could use our methods to track the effectiveness of electronic communication. However, quality monitoring procedures such as used by the VA to ensure system safety must also be used to identify red flags that would lead to similar future investigations. Without the safeguards used by the VA, the problems related to test result communication may go undetected.

Health care systems should aim to achieve a high reliability for tracking delivery of abnormal cancer screening results. An example viewed as an ideal model for tracking systems is that of FedEx, which is considered to have 99.6% tracking reliability for its packages [28]. To achieve such high tracking reliability would not only require implementation of comprehensive technology-based systems for communication, but also formal policies and procedures regarding their use [28]. The test result communication system evaluated in our study addressed several criteria [28] for effective critical results reporting systems, such as computerized tracking and backup procedures. However, to achieve tracking comparable to other industries, cancer screening programs should continuously monitor and oversee the timely delivery of positive cancer screening results to the right clinicians. For example, we recommend that cancer screening programs using electronic health record systems should develop and monitor multiple metrics of performance of automated communication processes. Failure to implement such monitoring systems could lead to sub-optimal screening success, which may otherwise be difficult if not impossible to trace.

16.5 CONCLUSION

In conclusion, we believe that electronic health records are beneficial in communicating abnormal cancer screening results to clinicians and will improve their follow-up care; however, we cannot assume that electronic communication is always working exactly as expected especially when workarounds are used. To achieve the most benefits of cancer screening programs, robust monitoring systems are necessary in electronic health record systems to ensure that abnormal cancer screening results are being delivered to the correct providers in a timely manner.

REFERENCES

1. Yabroff K, Washington KS, Leader A, Neilson E, Mandelblatt J: Is the Promise of Cancer-Screening Programs Being Compromised? Quality of Follow-Up Care after Abnormal Screening Results. Med Care Res Rev 2003, 60:294-331.
2. Baig N, Myers RE, Turner BJ, et al.: Physician-reported reasons for limited follow-up of patients with a positive fecal occult blood test screening result. The American Journal of Gastroenterology 2003, 98:2078-2081.
3. Levin B, Hess K, Johnson C: Screening for colorectal cancer. A comparison of 3 fecal occult blood tests. Arch Intern Med 1997, 157:970-976.
4. Morris JB, Stellato TA, Guy BB, Gordon NH, Berger NA: A critical analysis of the largest reported mass fecal occult blood screening program in the United States. Am J Surg 1991, 161:101-105.
5. Burack RC, Simon MS, Stano M, George J, Coombs J: Follow-up among women with an abnormal mammogram in an HMO: is it complete, timely, and efficient? Am J Manag Care 2000, 6:1102-1113.
6. Bastani R, Yabroff KR, Myers RE, Glenn B: Interventions to improve follow-up of abnormal findings in cancer screening. Cancer 2004, 101:1188-1200.
7. Mandel JS, Church TR, Bond JH, et al.: The effect of fecal occult-blood screening on the incidence of colorectal cancer. N Engl J Med 2000, 343:1603-1607.
8. Mandel JS, Bond JH, Church TR, et al.: Reducing mortality from colorectal cancer by screening for fecal occult blood. Minnesota Colon Cancer Control Study. N Engl J Med 1993, 328:1365-1371.
9. Kronborg O, Jorgensen OD, Fenger C, Rasmussen M: Randomized study of biennial screening with a faecal occult blood test: results after nine screening rounds. Scand J Gastroenterol 2004, 39:846-851.
10. Etzioni D, Yano E, Rubenstein L, et al.: Measuring the Quality of Colorectal Cancer Screening: The Importance of Follow-Up. Diseases of the Colon & Rectum 2006, 49:1002-1010.

11. Fisher DA, Jeffreys A, Coffman CJ, Fasanella K: Barriers to full colon evaluation for a positive fecal occult blood test. Cancer Epidemiol Biomarkers Prev 2006, 15:1232-1235.

12. Myers RE, Hyslop T, Gerrity M, et al.: Physician Intention to Recommend Complete Diagnostic Evaluation in Colorectal Cancer Screening. Cancer Epidemiol Biomarkers Prev 1999, 8:587-593.

13. Myers RE, Turner B, Weinberg D, et al.: Impact of a physician-oriented intervention on follow-up in colorectal cancer screening. Prev Med 2004, 38:375-381.

14. Jimbo M, Myers RE, Meyer B, et al.: Reasons Patients With a Positive Fecal Occult Blood Test Result Do Not Undergo Complete Diagnostic Evaluation. Ann Fam Med 2009, 7:11-16.

15. Wahls T: Diagnostic errors and abnormal diagnostic tests lost to follow-up: a source of needless waste and delay to treatment. J Ambul Care Manage 2007, 30:338-343.

16. Poon EG, Wang SJ, Gandhi TK, Bates DW, Kuperman GJ: Design and implementation of a comprehensive outpatient Results Manager. J Biomed Inform 2003, 36:80-91.

17. Singh H, Arora HS, Vij MS, Rao R, Khan M, Petersen LA: Communication outcomes of critical imaging results in a computerized notification system. J Am Med Inform Assoc 2007, 14:459-466.

18. Singh H, Naik A, Rao R, Petersen L: Reducing Diagnostic Errors Through Effective Communication: Harnessing the Power of Information Technology. Journal of General Internal Medicine 2008, 23:489-494.

19. Singh H, Kadiyala H, Bhagwath G, et al.: Using a multifaceted approach to improve the follow-up of positive fecal occult blood test results. Am J Gastroenterol 2009, 104:942-952.

20. Bagian JP, Gosbee J, Lee CZ, Williams L, McKnight SD, Mannos DM: The Veterans Affairs root cause analysis system in action. Jt Comm J Qual Improv 2002, 28:531-545.

21. Ash JS, Smith AC, Stavri PZ: Performing subjectivist studies in the qualitative traditions responsive to users. In Evaluation Methods in Biomedical Informatics. 2nd edition. Edited by Friedman CP, Wyatt JC. Springer New York; 2006:267-300.

22. Koppel R, Wetterneck T, Telles JL, Karsh BT: Workarounds to Barcode Medication Administration Systems: Their Occurrences, Causes, and Threats to Patient Safety. J Am Med Inform Assoc 2008, 15:408-423.

23. Singh H, Thomas E, Petersen LA: Automated Notification of Laboratory Test Results in an Electronic Health Record: Do Any Safety Concerns Remain? American Journal of Medicine, in press.

24. Gandhi TK, Kachalia A, Thomas EJ, et al.: Missed and delayed diagnoses in the ambulatory setting: A study of closed malpractice claims. Ann Intern Med 2006, 145:488-496.

25. Phillips RL Jr, Bartholomew LA, Dovey SM, Fryer GE Jr, Miyoshi TJ, Green LA: Learning from malpractice claims about negligent, adverse events in primary care in the United States. Qual Saf Health Care 2004, 13:121-126.

26. Singh H, Sethi S, Raber M, Petersen LA: Errors in cancer diagnosis: current understanding and future directions. J Clin Oncol 2007, 25:5009-5018.

27. Sittig DF, Singh H: Eight Rights of Safe Electronic Health Record Use. JAMA 2009, 302:1111-1113.

28. Bates DW, Leape LL: Doing better with critical test results. Jt Comm J Qual Patient Saf 2005, 31:66-67.

Singh, H., Wilson, L., Petersen, L. A., Sawhney, M. K., Reis, B., Espadas, D., and Sittig, D. F. Improving Follow-Up of Abnormal Cancer Screens Using Electronic Health Records: Trust But Verify Test Result Communication. BMC Medical Informatics and Decision Making 2009 Dec 9;9:49. doi: 10.1186/1472-6947-9-49. Re-used as per the Creative Commons Attribution License.

PART VII

BAR CODED MEDICATION ADMINISTRATION

CHAPTER 17

FIFTEEN BEST PRACTICE RECOMMENDATIONS FOR BAR-CODE MEDICATION ADMINISTRATION IN THE VETERANS HEALTH ADMINISTRATION

EMILY S. PATTERSON, MICHELLE L. ROGERS, and MARTA L. RENDER.

Estimates of rates of adverse events in hospital settings range from 3.7% based on chart review [1] to 17.7% based on direct observation, [2] with medication errors the most commonly documented cause of adverse events in hospitals. [3] In an analysis of 334 medication errors from 11 acute care wards, 38% of the problems occurred at the time of administration by nursing personnel. [4] Although some believe that bar-code technology reduces medication errors and tracks near misses, supporting empirical evidence is limited. [5,6]

Bar-code scanning is the oldest machine-readable identification system and has been widely used in industrial manufacturing, shipping, and inventory control. [7,8] Compared with typing, which produces about one error every 300 keystrokes, bar-code scanning error rates range from one character in 15,000 to one in 36 trillion. [9] The use of bar-code medication administration (BCMA) systems to improve patient safety has been recommended by many organizations, including the Institute of Medicine, the National Patient Safety Foundation, the American Society of Health-System Pharmacists, and the National Alliance for Health Information Technology. On February 25, 2004, the U.S. Food and Drug Administration finalized a rule for bar-code labeling medications and blood components to prevent adverse events. [10] The rule requires placement of a linear bar-code label containing the National Drug Code number on most prescription drugs and certain over-the-counter drugs within two years. In addition, the Joint Commission on Accreditation of Healthcare Organizations is considering requiring that bar-code technology for patient identification and for matching patients to their medications and other treatments be operational in all health care accreditation programs by January 1, 2007. [11]

VHA has used its relatively mature BCMA system since 2000, and BCMA is deployed in all VHA facilities across the United States. Nurses access BCMA software by using a laptop computer attached to a wheeled medication cart and linked by a wireless network to electronic databases. If the scanned medication bar-code data do not match what is ordered for a patient identified by scanning a bar-coded wristband, the nurse is alerted to the discrepancy by the software (Figure 1, page 357).

As with any new technology, system effectiveness is dependent on myriad design, implementation, and maintenance choices. In addition, the introduction of any new technology, regardless of how effective the technology, generates negative, unanticipated side effects because of the complex, interconnected nature of the medication administration process. Recent research has identified five unintended side effects from the introduction of BCMA in VHA: [12]

- Missed doses when nurses were unaware of the automated removal of medications after a period of time
- Reduced access to medication administration data for physicians
- Nurses employing workaround strategies to increase efficiency during busy periods
- Nurses prioritizing activities that can be monitored with BCMA data over activities that are not able to be easily monitored
- Reduced efficiency for nonroutine activities
- Nursing "workaround" strategies reduce the effectiveness of various BCMA systems in acute care and long term care settings. [13,14] To address challenges identified from these studies and the collective VHA BCMA experience, a set of best practice recommendations is offered for VHA and other organizations considering the implementation and use of BCMAs.

17.1   IDENTIFYING BARRIERS TO BCMA'S EFFECTIVENESS

Between 1999 and 2003, data were collected on potential barriers to BCMA's effectiveness in VHA by direct observation of medication administration, simulations of BCMA use in a laboratory, a survey of nursing informatics specialists on policies and procedures, and unstructured interviews (Table 1). To address the challenges identified from these data, in March 2004 a set of best practice recommendations was proposed to the VHA's Office of Information and then disseminated by the Director of the National BCMA Joint Program Office to points of contact at every VHA facility.

17.2 RECOMMENDATIONS

Fifteen practices to maximize the effectiveness of the use of BCMA and reduce the risk of iatrogenic injury to patients are proposed (Table 2). The practices are grouped into the following categories: implementation and continuous improvement, training, troubleshooting, contingency planning, equipment maintenance, medication administration, and maintenance of paper patient wristbands. The rationale and supporting data are summarized in each recommendation to help non–VHA hospitals considering or using other systems to gauge their potential applicability.

17.2.1 *PUT IN PLACE A STANDING INTERDISCIPLINARY COMMITTEE*

17.2.1.1 RECOMMENDATION

A standing interdisciplinary committee composed of nursing, pharmacy, computer support, and, when possible, biomedical representatives should implement and proactively conduct continuous improvement on implementation and use. One method for obtaining feedback from front-line staff should include rounds on the floors on a frequent and continuous basis (for example, weekly or biweekly). Actions taken to address problems should be reported back to end users (for example, through e-mail and handouts).

17.2.1.2   RATIONALE

Integrating BCMA into medication administration is extremely complex and requires changes to how work is conducted by nurses and other personnel. Proactive attempts to solicit feedback and improve systems will reduce workaround strategies that circumvent system use.

17.2.1.3   SUPPORTING DATA

The supporting data are as follows:

- 11 of the 16 VHA hospitals have a standing interdisciplinary committee to troubleshoot when problems arise and to discuss opportunities for continuous improvement.
- 7 of the 16 VHA hospitals have instituted rounds on a routine basis.
- 10 of the 16 VHA hospitals use a mail group to identify problems and to alert users to problems and, less frequently, to communicate what has been done in response to the problems.

17.2.2   TRAIN ALL USERS. CROSS-TRAIN PHARMACISTS AND CERTAIN PHYSICIANS

17.2.2.1   RECOMMENDATION

All personnel administering medications, medicated ointments, or respiratory treatments need to receive significant training on BCMA software. Develop a process for informing personnel about software updates, particularly for "super-users" (nurses who serve as resources to other nurses) and temporary (agency) nurses. Cross-train all pharmacists on the nursing features in BCMA. Recruit certain physicians to serve as super-users and informal trainers on how to write orders in the provider order entry software programs that are compatible with BCMA.

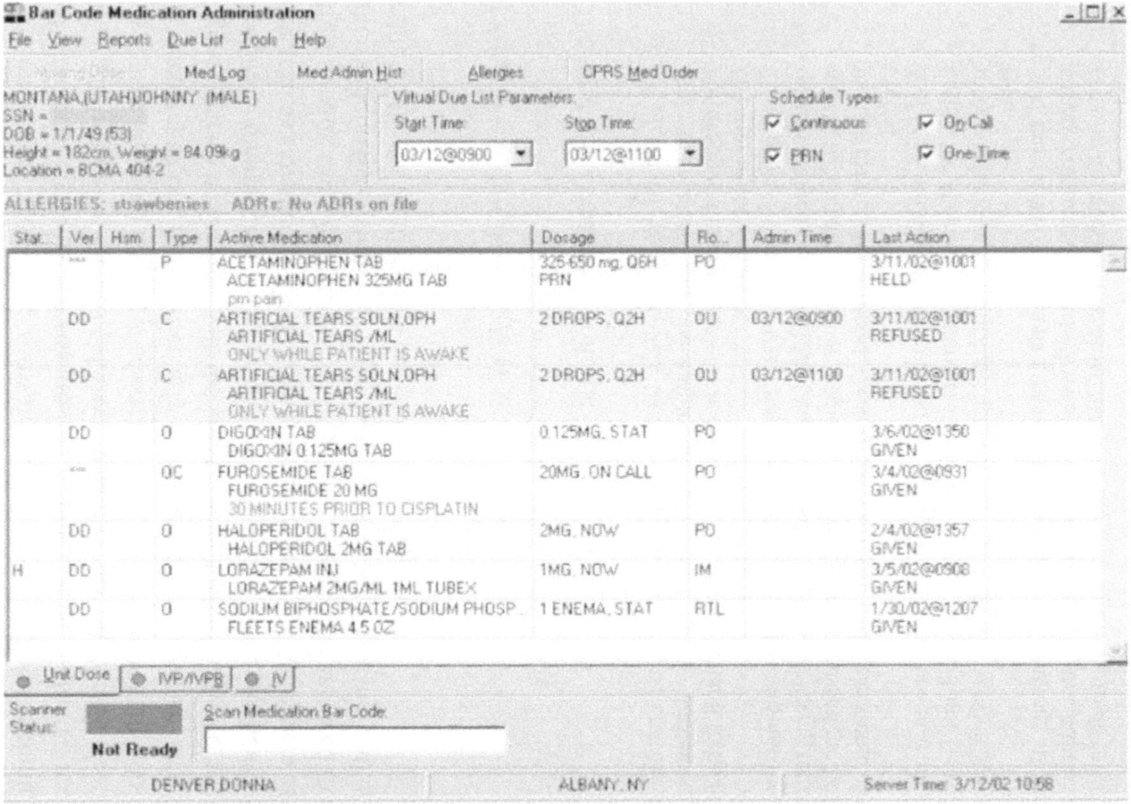

FIGURE 1: This sample screen shot displays the physician-ordered and pharmacist-verified 9–11 A.M. medications for a patient identified by scanning a bar-coded wristband.

17.2.2.2   RATIONALE

The BCMA software is sufficiently complex that new paths to medica-tion errors can result from software use without adequate training. Use of alternative systems that require less training, such as printed medica-tion administration records (MARs), to administer medications can lead to missed dose and double-dose errors and confusing gaps in the electron-ic documentation. It is particularly important that super-user nurses and agency nurses be familiar with the latest changes to the software. In many hospitals, pharmacists help nurses to troubleshoot when medications do not scan as expected, and it is helpful for them to know the system as seen by a nursing user. The use of BCMA affects how physicians need to enter their orders (for example, 20 mg needs to be written as "20 mg" rather than "20mg" for the medication's bar code to scan correctly).

17.2.2.3   SUPPORTING DATA

The supporting data are as follows:

- 11 of the 16 VHA hospitals formally employ superusers, one has infor-mal super-users, and one employed super-users during implementation but dropped the program later because of the complexity and frequency of changes to the software.
- Two agency nurses at a VHA hospital reported that they did not feel ade-quately trained to use BCMA. One of the nurses had the covering registered nurse (R.N.) administer her medications, and the other passed medications using a printed MAR report, thereby leaving a gap in the electronic medical record.
- 5 of the 5 nursing participants did not administer at least one ordered medi-cation for at least one simulated patient because they did not look on all three medication tabs during a usability test of a BCMA version 2.0 proto-type.
- 3 of the 16 VHA hospitals cross-train pharmacists. A nursing informatics survey respondent noted, "I would recommend that all sites train pharma-cists on the nursing side of BCMA. We are just beginning to do this."

TABLE 1: Summary of Methods*

Method	Description
Direct observation of medication administration by 3 trained observers with Ph.D.'s in human factors engineering	Prior to implementation, observation of the following: • 21 hours, 7 nurses on acute care wards at a 155-bed hospital with 9,000 admissions per year • 25 hours, 5 nurses in the medical ICU and surgical ICU of a 327-bed hospital with more than 12,000 admissions per year After implementation, observation of the following: • 24 hours, 5 nurses on acute care wards with 99 beds and 5 nurses on long term care wards with 460 beds at a hospital with 3,000 admissions per year • 48 hours, 19 nurses on acute care wards with 155 beds with 9,000 admissions per year • 33 hours, 5 nurses on acute care wards at a 327-bed hospital with more than 12,000 admissions per year and 3 nurses on long term care wards at a 180-bed nursing home
Simulations of BCMA use in a laboratory	After implementation, observing simulated use of the following: • The initial version of BCMA software; 5 nursing participants Prior to implementation, observing simulated use of the following: • BCMA Version 2.0 early prototype with additional IV medication features and a multitabbed interface; 5 nursing participants • BCMA Version 2.0 revised prototype with an additional pop-up warning dialog box when there were active medications on background tabs; 4 nursing participants • BCMA Version 2.0 advanced prototype with a feature that allowed ICU nurses to scan bar-coded medications prior to physician order entry and pharmacy verification; 2 nursing participants • Wireless medication administration for a handheld device designed by an external vendor to simulate BCMA functionality; 5 nursing participants
Open-ended survey of hospital policies and procedures for BCMA on challenging issues	• 16 e-mail responses to survey posting to 578 nursing informatics listserv recipients from most VHA medical centers • 1 phone, 1 e-mail response to survey posting to National Patient Safety Foundation listserv with nearly 2,000 recipients
Interviews on perceived barriers to intended system use and reactions to draft recommendations	• 30 unstructured interviews with nurses, nurse managers, pharmacists, computer support personnel, administrators, patient safety experts, and physicians from public and private hospitals

* *ICU, Intensive care unit; BCMA, bar-code medication administration.*

TABLE 2: Summary of Recommendations

Topic	Recommendation
Implementation/continuous improvement	1. Standing interdisciplinary committee
Training	2. Train all nurses; cross-train others
Troubleshooting	3. Communicate known problems
	4. Contact information for types of problems
Contingency planning	5. No double documentation as a backup
	6. Schedule downtimes to minimize disruptions
Equipment maintenance	7. Replace malfunctioning equipment during its servicing
	8. Procedures to clean equipment
Medication administration	9. Scan wristbands and medications prior to administration
	10. Caregiver documents at time of administration
	11. Verify displayed allergy information
	12. Use printed worksheet as overview
	13. Print missed medications report once a shift
	14. Alert nurses to new stat orders
Wristband maintenance	15. Periodic replacement of wristbands

17.2.3   COMMUNICATE KNOWN PROBLEMS

17.2.3.1   RECOMMENDATION

Develop a process (for example, Web site, help line) for interested people to view examples of national problems at any time (24 hours a day, seven days a week).

17.2.3.2   RATIONALE

Although there already is a VHA national help desk that is continuously staffed, technology can be used to build a "community of knowledge" that enables easy viewing of known problems, the status of resolution of those problems, other frequently asked questions (FAQs), and locally developed solutions. This approach would reduce calls to the help desk and make it more efficient to see whether problems are national or local. Knowing national problems reduces time wasted trying to troubleshoot locally, while knowing that problems are not national makes it easier to troubleshoot and resolve local problems.

17.2.3.3   SUPPORTING DATA

The supporting data are as follows:

- VHA Hospital 9: "Other problems are usually in line with nationally reported issues, and we wait for solutions. We recommend actions locally until national solutions are programmed."
- VHA Hospital 11: "Core group of staff communicate findings and responds to questions. This group includes the nursing education coordinator, two nurses in nursing informatics, pharmacy (computer specialist), inpatient pharmacy supervisor, and a computer equipment specialist. Nurses are encouraged to contact this core group and staff pharmacist and nurse supervisor. Problems are handled in real time by any of these personnel. If the problem cannot be resolved, the national help desk is contacted for resolution. Patient safety alerts to all clinical users are sent if system problem is presently uncorrectable."

17.2.4   DISPLAY CONTACT INFORMATION FOR RESOURCES TO RESOLVE DIFFERENT TYPES OF PROBLEMS

17.2.4.1   RECOMMENDATION

Prominently display contact information for resources to resolve recurring types of problems. Update list as necessary.

17.2.4.2   RATIONALE

Time spent locating appropriate resources to aid in troubleshooting reduces the available time to provide patient care. This process can be facilitated, particularly for nurses new to an organization or when systems are first implemented, by making it easier to identify appropriate resources to contact (for example, computer personnel for hardware problems, clerks for problems in scanning wristbands, pharmacy for problems in scanning medication bar codes, specialized personnel for software problems, engineering or computer personnel for problems with the wireless network).

17.2.4.3   SUPPORTING DATA

The supporting data are as follows:

- VHA hospital: "We believe that we have a best practice for this issue. We staff a help desk for everything related to the electronic medical record. . . Three nurses, a dietitian, a social worker, and a radiology technician comprise the clinical informatics staff, which responds to help desk calls continuously 6:30 A.M.-5:30 P.M. Monday through Friday. Rather than a system of "page me if you need help" and then wait for them to get back to you, you dial 'H-E-L-P' and someone immediately answers the line. We can resolve the problem in 5 rather than 45 minutes this way. If not, we can forward the problem to the technical or hardware staff. Nursing supervisors perform this function on off-tours. We have information resource management (IRM) on-call during off tours and weekends. We think of IRM as the hardware people and clinical informatics as the software people. People who answer the help desk also do the teaching for the software and know the ins and outs of the software packages they support. This allows them to better assist the users and to troubleshoot problems in the software."
- One cluster of VHA hospitals made mouse pads with troubleshooting hints on them.
- One VHA hospital instituted a hot-line number in pharmacy and an e-mail address for scanning problems and provided a sheet on each medication cart with names and numbers to contact for specific issues.

17.2.5   DO NOT EMPLOY A DOUBLE-DOCUMENTATION SYSTEM

17.2.5.1 RECOMMENDATION

Do not employ a paper-based medication administration system in parallel with a BCMA for more than a few weeks.

17.2.5.2   RATIONALE

A double-documentation system reduces nursing productivity. Different nurses will use different systems as the primary system, leading to the possibility of missed medications, double-dose medications, and confusing documentation gaps.

17.2.5.3   SUPPORTING DATA

The supporting data are as follows:

- At one hospital with a double documentation system that had been in place for approximately one year, documentation was done only on the paper MAR and not BCMA for the following reasons:
  - BCMA was unavailable because of maintenance.
  - Nurse was unable to log in.
  - Staff members administering medications were not trained on BCMA.
  - Patient record was unavailable because it was in use by another user.
  - Nurse had problems scanning a medication.
  - Medication was ordered but not in BCMA, in some cases because the orders were automatically dropped from BCMA several hours after the scheduled administered time.
  - Administration time was not changed in BCMA.
  - Covering nurse administered a medication for another nurse.
  - "Batch documentation" was done on the paper record in the absence of the realization that one medication was not administered using BCMA.
  - A nurse forgot to scan a medication and so the administration was only documented in the paper record.
- During the same observations, documentation was done only in BCMA and not on the paper MAR because of the following:
  - A nurse forgot to document a medication on the MAR.
  - A nurse documented in BCMA that a nursing assistant in a long term care facility administered a topical cream, a standard practice in some VHA long term care facilities, that was not actually administered.
  - A set of medications was scanned for a patient who was not available, and so the medications were documented as administered but not administered at that time.
  - A patient refused a scanned medication, and so the medication was documented as administered although it was not.
  - A medication was held due to vital sign data after it was scanned, so it was documented as administered although it was not.

17.2.6 SCHEDULE PLANNED DOWNTIMES TO MINIMIZE DISRUPTIONS

17.2.6.1 RECOMMENDATION

Planned downtimes should be scheduled to minimize disruptions to the hospital, with the possible exception of testing back-up plans. The specific plan for downtime should take into account facilityspecific factors such as availability of troubleshooting support and medication administration schedules.

17.2.6.2 RATIONALE

Planned downtimes are less disruptive than unplanned downtimes. Unexpected downtimes may result in missed doses or double doses due to confusing gaps in documentation.

17.2.6.3 SUPPORTING DATA

The supporting data are as follows:

- 13 of the 16 VHA hospitals schedule downtimes during low-volume medication administration times.

17.2.7 REPLACE MALFUNCTIONING EQUIPMENT DURING ITS SERVICING

17.2.7.1 RECOMMENDATION

Each hospital should have a minimum of two complete replacement units (laptop, mouse or stylus, battery, scanner, cables, power pack) available in a location that is accessible at any time (24 hours a day, seven days a week) so that malfunctioning equipment can be serviced without reducing nursing productivity.

17.2.7.2   RATIONALE

Productivity is reduced if users must wait for equipment to be serviced. Equipment taken out of circulation can undergo spot checks of the entire setup, with reduced time pressure to put the equipment back in circulation, including verifying that equipment is reliably functional and that all software upgrades have been properly installed. Ideally, equipment can also be cleaned by biomedical personnel, which may reduce the risk of nosocomial infections. Some facilities might need substantially more than two backup units, depending on their size and structure.

17.2.7.3   SUPPORTING DATA

The supporting data are as follows:

- VHA Hospital 6: "Since there are no backups, we can't take any to biomed to clean it, so unless it's being fixed it's never cleaned."
- VHA Hospital 9: "We [nursing informatics personnel] keep extra supplies, mouse hardware, laptops, batteries, scanners, cables, power packs, etc. in our office, and as each nurse has a problem we go to the ward and fix or replace. We save the user time by just taking a new setup and bringing the old one back to our office, where either we identify and fix the problem, or we enter a [service request]. . . . Our nursing supervisors have access to our backup equipment and help the staff on evenings, nights, weekends, and holidays."
- VHA Hospital 10: "Upon patch install [software upgrade] the technical support person inspects every laptop and scanner."

17.2.8   DEVELOP A PROCEDURE FOR CLEANING BCMA-RELATED EQUIPMENT

17.2.8.1   RECOMMENDATION

A procedure should be developed, ideally in collaboration with experts in infection control, to routinely clean BCMA-related equipment to reduce the risk of nosocomial infections. This procedure should include a process for monitoring that the tasks are carried out as planned.

17.2.8.2   RATIONALE

Maintenance of equipment cleanliness will be variable and difficult to monitor without explicit standards of practice and clear communication and monitoring of expectations. Risks of nosocomial infections can be reduced by improving cleanliness.

17.2.8.3   SUPPORTING DATA

The supporting data are as follows:

- 3 of the 16 VHA hospitals had policies that nurses were responsible for maintaining a clean work area in general, which implicitly includes BCMA equipment.
- 8 of the 16 VHA hospitals reported that their hospitals' policies and procedures regarding cleaning BCMArelated equipment were inadequate.

17.2.9   SCAN WRISTBANDS AND MEDICATIONS PRIOR TO MEDICATION ADMINISTRATION

17.2.9.1   RECOMMENDATION

Nurses should scan a bar-coded wristband on the patient to verify patient identity prior to medication administration. Nurses should scan barcoded medication immediately prior to medication administration to verify that it is the same name, dose, route, and time as the ordered medication. If not, the nurse should identify the discrepancy and apply professional judgment as to how to proceed. If the nurse cannot identify the discrepancy personally, other personnel (e.g., nurse manager, pharmacy) should be recruited to help troubleshoot before medication administration when the delay to administration will not adversely affect the patient. Exceptions to this practice include the following:

- Patients in isolation. In this case, a wireless device (scanner or handheld) can be used that is protected by a clear thin plastic bag that is thrown away after a single use. Alternatively, there can be a dedicated device in the patient's room if the patient is not in contact isolation.
- Patients who physically cannot wear a wristband, patients who have a disruptive behavioral response to scanning, when a scanner is tethered to a medication cart that does not fit into a patient's room, or when a backup system is in use that does not enable scanning of wristbands.
- Incorrect or missing bar code on medication. In this case, pharmacy should be alerted to the problem, in order to better detect if incorrect bar codes have been applied to multiple medications, to improve bar coding of medications, and to help identify cases where the nurse has erroneously assumed that the bar code is incorrect.
- Pharmacy unavailable to resolve discrepancies (for example, no pharmacy personnel on "off-tours"). In this case, problems should be communicated to pharmacy personnel when available and an alternative plan designed by the facility should be used.

17.2.9.2   RATIONALE

BCMA is designed to reduce medication errors by having the machine verify the identity of the patient and of the ordered medications immediately prior to administration. In exceptional circumstances, the system cannot be used as designed, in which case alternative plans are required.

17.2.9.4   SUPPORTING DATA

The supporting data are as follows:

- 6 of the 16 VHA hospitals have nurses type the social security number for patients that are in isolation.
- 5 of the 16 VHA hospitals have a clear thin plastic bag placed over a wireless scanner for patients that are in isolation.
- 2 of the 16 VHA hospitals have nurses scan patients that are in isolation without touching patients.

17.2.10   *CAREGIVERS SHOULD PERSONALLY DOCUMENT AT THE TIME OF MEDICATION ADMINISTRATION*

17.2.10.1   RECOMMENDATION

Caregivers (for example, R.N.'s, licensed practical nurses, respiratory therapists, nursing assistants who administer ointments in long term care facilities) who administer medications, medicated ointments, or respiratory treatments should personally document administration at the time of administration.

17.2.10.2   RATIONALE

Relying on communication to know when a medication was administered is less reliable because of memory and communication limitations than having the person who administered it document it at the time of administration.

17.2.10.3   SUPPORTING DATA

The supporting data are as follows:

- 6 of the 16 VHA hospitals have nursing assistants selfdocument their administration of creams and ointments in long-term care facilities: two in BCMA and four on paper treatment sheets.
- 4 of the 16 VHA hospitals have licensed nursing personnel document administration of creams and ointments by nursing assistants in long term

care facilities, often with the requirement of adding a comment that it was administered by the nursing assistant.

17.2.11   VERIFY ALLERGY INFORMATION DISPLAYED IN BCMA PRIOR TO ADMINISTRATION

17.2.11.1   RECOMMENDATION

Nurses should verify the allergy information displayed in BCMA before administration with information from another source (for example, allergy bracelet, asking patients to recite allergies before medication administration).

17.2.11.2   RATIONALE

The prominent display of allergy information in red on the primary BCMA interface is not sufficient to deter nurses from administering medications that are ordered to which a patient is known to be allergic. In addition, allergy information displayed in BCMA is not always accurate.

17.2.11.3   SUPPORTING DATA

The supporting data are as follows:

- All 15 nursing participants administered a medication to which a (simulated) patient was allergic during usability tests. All reported that they were unaware of the displayed information.
- 3 of the 16 VHA hospitals include allergy information on a wristband—either the BCMA wristband or an additional wristband.

17.2.12 SUPPORT STAFF PERSONNEL SHOULD PRINT A REPORT AT THE BEGINNING OF A SHIFT FOR NURSES TO USE AS AN OVERVIEW WORKSHEET

17.2.12.1 RECOMMENDATION

The long-term recommendation is for two-page overview reports to be designed that are tailored to the acute care, intensive care unit, and nursing home settings. In the short term, one of the currently available reports should be printed by support personnel for use by a nurse at the beginning of a shift to serve as an overview worksheet. This report should serve only as a supplementary tool because the information can be outdated within minutes and so should not be used for administration or documentation purposes. In addition, it is important for nurses to periodically refresh the information displayed in BCMA so that they are administering medications from the most current information.

17.2.12.2 RATIONALE

Nurses can better plan medication administrations if they can see at a glance an overview of the recent medication history and what medications are ordered for administration during their shift. They will also make fewer errors of omission if they quickly jot down notes in a temporary location because their notes will remind them to do activities, including pass along information during the handoff to the next shift.

17.2.12.3 SUPPORTING DATA

The supporting data are as follows:

- 8 of the 16 VHA hospitals had policies for nurses to use printed reports as overviews, and several hospitals had support staff print them for the nurses.
- 7 of the 16 VHA hospitals had no policy but observed that nurses frequently print paper reports to use as an overview sheet.

17.2.13   NURSES SHOULD PRINT MISSED MEDICATION REPORTS ONCE A SHIFT.

17.2.13.1   RECOMMENDATION

Like other systems, BCMA has a Missed Medication Report, which lists ordered medications that were not documented as administered. We recommend that organizations develop a process for tracking that this report is reviewed by nursing personnel. The process should not involve extensive documentation or time commitments by nursing personnel or add to the duties of the charge nurse without reducing patient load. In addition, nurse managers should not rely on missed medication reports to file medication error reports. To avoid reducing productivity, the tracking process should avoid extensive time or documentation commitments for nurses and charge nurses. In addition, to continually improve the safety culture, the reports must not be used for punitive purposes and so ideally would not contain practitioner identifiers.

17.2.13.2   RATIONALE

Missed medications, particularly onetime order and on-call medications that are removed one hour after the ordered time because of provider or pharmacist mis-entry and one-time orders that are needed to remain active for more than 12 hours can be reduced by nurses reviewing the medications that were ordered but not yet administered. Without a process for tracking (for example, nursing personnel might place printed reports in the nursing manager's mailbox, so that the reports are reviewed and thrown away once a week), report use will be variable and difficult to monitor.

17.2.13.3   SUPPORTING DATA

The supporting data are as follows:
- 7 of the 16 VHA hospitals require nurses to print and review missed medication reports.
- 9 of the 16 VHA hospitals monitor that nurses are printing and reviewing missed medication reports.

17.2.14   ALERT NURSES TO NEW STAT (URGENT) ORDERS

17.2.14.1   RECOMMENDATION

Particularly for urgent orders and orders in the intensive care unit, it is important for nurses to know when new medication orders have been written. In many hospitals with the paper-based MAR, this is accomplished by having printouts of new orders arrive on labels in a central location. Nurses are alerted to new orders by the sound of a new printout. With BCMA, it is no longer necessary to have labels printed, and seeing an updated view of orders sometimes requires a manual refresh command. Methods to alert nurses to new stat orders, such as by having an overview display on a dedicated monitor in a central location with information about new orders, should be developed. In addition, physicians should inform the nurse verbally when a new stat order has been written.

17.2.14.2   RATIONALE

Relying on nurses to continuously access the electronic medical record to detect new orders is inefficient and contributes to delayed or missed medication orders, some of which may be critical to patient safety.

17.2.14.3   SUPPORTING DATA

The supporting data are as follows:

- VHA Hospital 4: "During med[ication] pass, the nurse does a refresh . . . to see if new orders had been processed that did not appear on the due list."
- VHA Hospital 9: "We require that each nurse administering med[ication]s run a DUE List for their tour of duty and even rerun the list after morning physician rounds."
- VHA Hospital 15: "Routinely, nurses print at the start of their shift the "Due List," which lists all current meds both prn (as needed) and scheduled. This is very popular with all units. They are continually reminded that this is for planning purposes only as the due list is only current at the time printed."
- At two VHA hospitals, a dedicated monitor in a central location in the intensive care unit was observed to display new orders for patients (for example, "Mr. Smith has four new orders").

17.2.15   REPLACE WRISTBANDS AS NEEDED AND PERIODICALLY IN LONG TERM CARE

17.2.15.1   RECOMMENDATION

Wristbands in the VHA are printed on inexpensive paper with no folds. We recommend replacing worn, missing, or inaccurate wristbands as soon as discovered by any personnel. In long term care settings, support staff personnel should replace wristbands periodically (for example, weekly). Install wristband printers on every ward and allow nurses, nursing assistants, and ward clerks access privileges to print new wristbands. If wristbands cannot be applied (for example, when patients who physically cannot or refuse to wear a wristband), they may be applied to items unique to the patient (for example, stapled into the patient's paper charts) but not to items that are not unique to the patient (for example, on a bedside table, outside the room, in a patient's medication drawer, on top of a medication cart or computer console).

17.2.15.2   RATIONALE

Scanning wristbands to verify patient identity is more likely to occur when wristbands reliably scan on the first attempt. Wristbands become worn between several days and two weeks after application. Acute care patients rarely stay long enough to warrant periodic replacement, but long term care patients have longer lengths of stay. Application of wristbands is a potentially errorprone step. Facilities should consider how to increase the reliability of wristband replacement, such as by requiring verification of patient identity during application.

17.2.15.3   SUPPORTING DATA

The supporting data are as follows:
- 16 of the 16 VHA hospitals replace wristbands on asneeded basis in acute care.
- 11 of the 16 VHA hospitals replace on an as-needed basis in long term care, 4/16 VHA hospitals replace once a week in long term care (3 printed by clerk, one by morning shift).
- 16 of the 16 VHA hospitals have installed wristband printers on every ward.

17.3   DISCUSSION

Deployment of technology in the clinical setting requires a thoughtful and comprehensive approach. In addition to the need to tailor technologies to particular contexts, it is important to identify opportunities to continuously improve the use of a technology over time. We believe that the lessons learned from the VHA, the recognized leader—both in time and scope of implementation—in the use of bar-code technology to identify patients and medications, about challenges and best practices to address challenges should be valuable to others considering procurement and implementation of bar-code technology.

There are several limitations to these recommendations. First, although the introduction of BCMA affects all hospital personnel, minimal research was conducted with non-nursing personnel. Second, these recommendations are solely based on experience with the BCMA system used in VHA hospitals. Because of context- specific variables, it is not expected that all recommendations will apply to all hospitals with BCMA in every situation. Third, none of these recommendations has been evaluated for its efficacy in improving quality of care or reducing iatrogenic injury and may even create unintended consequences that generate new paths to failure. Fourth, recommendations are based on Version 2.0 of Bar Code Medication Administration; future changes might necessitate changes to the recommendations. Fifth, in all the studies that informed these recommendations, the hospitals and participants were convenience samples and represented a small percentage of the overall hospitals and employees in the VHA and so might not be representative or might otherwise be biased. Finally, although we believe that these recommendations might be of interest to hospitals using software packages other than the BCMA software developed for VHA, generalization needs to be done with care because of diversity of organizational structures and infrastructure in hospitals and the myriad choices in design and implementation of a software package. For example, with respect to Recommendation 12, systems might already have overview worksheets available for printing or might have chosen not to remove nonadministered medications after a specified time window.

REFERENCES

1. Brennan T.A., et al.: Incidence of adverse events and negligence in hospitalized patients: Results of the Harvard Medical Practice Study I. N Engl J Med 324:370–376, Feb. 7, 1991.
2. Andrews L., et al.: An alternative strategy for studying adverse events in medical care. Lancet 349:309–313, Feb. 1, 1997.
3. Leape L.L., et al.: The nature of adverse events in hospitalized patients: Results of the Harvard Medical Practice Study II. N Engl J Med 324:377–384, Feb. 7, 1991.
4. Leape L., et al.: Systems analysis of adverse drug events. ADE Prevention Study Group. JAMA 274:35–43, Jul. 5, 1995.
5. Bates D.W., et al.: Reducing the frequency of errors in medicine using information technology. J Am Med Inform Assoc 8:299–308, Aug. 2001.

6. Johnson C.L., et al.: Using BCMA software to improve patient safety in Veterans Administration Medical Centers. J Healthcare Info Mgt 16:46–51, Winter 2002.
7. Rappoport A.: A hospital patient and laboratory machine-readable identification system (MRIS) revisited. J Med Syst 8:133–156, Apr. 1984.
8. Weilert M., Tilzer L.L.: Putting bar codes to work for improved patient care. Clin Lab Med 11:227–238, Mar. 1991.
9. Maffetone M.A., Watt S.W., Whisler K.E.: Automated sample handling in a clinical laboratory. Comput Healthc 9:48–50, Sep. 1988.
10. Bar code label requirement for human drug products and blood: Proposed rule. The Federal Register 68:12500–12534, Mar. 14, 2003.
11. Joint Commission on Accreditation of Healthcare Organizations: Potential 2005 National Patient Safety Goals Field Review. http://www.jcaho.org/accredited+organizations/05_npsg_fr.htm. (last accessed Apr. 21, 2004).
12. Patterson E.S., Cook R.I., Render M.L.: Improving patient safety by identifying side effects from introducing bar coding in medication administration. J Am Med Inform Assoc 9:540–553, Sep.–Oct. 2002.
13. Puckett F: Medication-management component of a point-of-care information system. Am J Health-Syst Pharm 52:1305–1309, Jun. 15, 1995.
14. Patterson E.S., Rogers M.L., Render M.L.: Simulation-based embedded probe technique for human-computer interaction evaluation. Cognition, Technology, and Work, in press.

Patterson, E. S., Rogers, M. L, Render, M. L. Fifteen Best Practice Recommendations for Bar-Code Medication Administration in the Veterans Health Administration. Joint Commission Journal on Quality and Patient Safety. 2004 Jul;30(7):355-65. Reprinted with permission.

PART VIII

COMPUTER-BASED PROVIDER ORDER ENTRY

CHAPTER 18

COMPUTERIZED PROVIDER ORDER ENTRY ADOPTION: IMPLICATIONS FOR CLINICAL WORKFLOW

EMILY M. CAMPBELL, KENNETH P. GUAPPONE, DEAN F. SITTIG, RICHARD H. DYKSTRA, and JOAN S. ASH

18.1 INTRODUCTION

Health care providers use computerized provider order entry (CPOE) systems to place orders for medications, laboratory tests and other ancillary services. [1] CPOE has been shown to decrease medication ordering errors and redundant test ordering, promote practice standardization, and reduce overall healthcare costs. [2–4] Despite these benefits, CPOE systems have yet to be widely adopted for several reasons, including the high cost of implementation, clinician resistance to technology, worry regarding practice disruption and loss of productivity, fear of technology failure, and the inability of some CPOE implementations to integrate with existing healthcare systems. [5–7] Furthermore, there is evidence that unintended adverse consequences can surround the implementation and ongoing maintenance of these systems. [8–10] Recent, conflicting reports about the role of CPOE in the reduction of medication errors and associated costs have cast some doubt on the actual scale of improvements to be gained as CPOE systems have generated new kinds of medical errors, negatively affected patient outcomes, and resulted in higher overall medical costs for those institutions implementing them. [9,11–13] Thus, there remains a need for ongoing analysis of CPOE to understand the causes of these issues and help find solutions.

A growing body of research explores the impact of integrating clinical information systems, including CPOE, within healthcare. [1,14–17] Regardless of the study focus, one theme consistently emerges: embedding CPOE in healthcare fundamentally changes the way clinicians coordinate their work activities and collaborate to deliver care. [18–21] Indeed, in our prior work we identified nine broad categories of unintended adverse consequences related to CPOE, negative impact on workflow emerged as the most frequently occurring theme. [18,22] The purpose of this current study was to explore these workflow issues in greater detail.

18.2   BACKGROUND

We broadly define workflow as the activities, tools, and processes needed to produce or modify work, products, or services.23 More specifically, clinical workflow encompasses all of the 1) activities, 2) technologies, 3) environments, 4) people, and 5) organizations engaged in providing and promoting health care.

A sociotechnical evaluation framework [18,23–25] views these five components of clinical work as a single work system; that is, the components cannot be effectively analyzed in isolation. To understand the effects of embedding CPOE into existing care delivery systems, we must focus on how the systems as a whole responds to the change. When using this approach, one should not separate the information technology system from its implementation. Even exquisitely designed and coded software can be implemented poorly. Conversely, poorly engineered software can promote process improvements if it is well implemented. Thus any evaluation of a CPOE system must study the system as configured, implemented and used [26].

TABLE 1: Description of sites studied

Hospital	Size (beds)	Type of Institution	CPOE system	Up since	Percent orders entered
Wishard Memorial, Indianapolis, IN	340	Acute care county teaching hospital associated with Indiana University School of Medicine	Homegrown: Regenstrief Medical Records System (RMRS)	1973	100%
Massachusetts General Hospital, Boston, MA	893	Large, academic, general hospital; part of Partners HealthCare System; associated with Harvard Medical School	Homegrown: Clinical Application Suite	1994	100%
The Faulkner, Boston, MA	150	Community teaching hospital with a private medical staff, affiliated with Harvard Medical School	Meditech	2003	95%
Brigham $ Women's Hospital, Boston, MA	725	Large, academic, general hospital; part of Partners HealthCare System; associated with Harvard Medical School	Homegrown: BICS	1991	90%
Alamance Regional Medical Center, Burlington, NC	238	Community hospital	Eclipsys	1998	95%

18.3 METHODS

18.3.1 SITE SELECTION

Over the past three years, we visited five hospitals in three different healthcare delivery organizations using CPOE. The sites were selected based on their reputations for excellence in the use of CPOE; all sites have fully operational and functional systems that capture a minimum of 90% of all medical orders, and have been operating at this level for several years. In addition, we wanted to evaluate different types of CPOE systems (e.g., commercially built as well as "home-grown") in different types of hospitals. The research sites included Wishard Memorial Hospital in Indianapolis, IN, using the locally developed Regenstrief system, Brigham and Women's and Massachusetts' General hospitals in Boston, both using in-house developed systems, The Faulkner Hospital in Boston, MA, using MediTech (Westwood, MA), and Alamance Regional Medical System in Burlington, NC, using Eclipsys (Boca Raton, FL). Complete site details are presented in Table 1.

18.3.2   DATA COLLECTION

The Institutional Review Boards of Oregon Health & Science University as well as each of our study sites approved this study. The research team consisted of two physicians, a nurse, a pharmacist, a librarian, a public health researcher, and a technically-oriented informaticist.

Our fieldwork used two approaches to data collection. The first consisted of hour-long, semi-structured oral history interviews with hospital administrators, physicians, nurses, pharmacists, and others suggested to us by local principal investigators. Our team leader (JA) conducted these interviews to elicit historical and current perspectives on the unintended consequences, whether positive or negative, related to CPOE implementation at each of the institutions. Table 2 includes a list of questions that served as a starting point for these interviews. Interviewee responses generated additional probing questions which differed during each interview. Interviews were recorded and later transcribed. All interviewees were formally consented.

Our second approach to data collection involved shadowing clinicians and other personnel interacting with CPOE systems during their work. The clinicians shadowed were selected by prior arrangement with study collaborators so that skeptics as well as accepting users were included. Subjects who agreed to be shadowed were formally consented. Researchers then unobtrusively observed the subjects for periods from 2–6 hours at various times during the day and night. When clinicians offered comments about the systems, we noted them. In addition, when we were unclear about specific activities, we asked questions for clarification. In addition to shadowing individuals, we also observed general work activities in ambulatory care centers, hospital wards, emergency rooms, surgical recovery areas, and other critical care units.

TABLE 2: General interview guide for semi-structured interviews

Interview subject	Question topic	Introductory question
All interviewees	Personal background	Could you please briefly describe your background and professional experience?
End-users	System changes	Could you please describe what it's like for a user when changes are made in the CPOE system?
Various personnel*	System history	Could you please give us a brief history of your experience with the system?
Various personnel*	System implementation	Can you describe lessons learned in the implementation process?
Various personnel*	Surprises	Could you tell us about your memories of any surprises?
Various personnel*	End-user perceptions	What are your perceptions of how people felt about the consequences of CPOE?
Various personnel*	Problem resolution	Can you tell us how problems identified by critics were solved?
Various personnel*	Future issues	How do you describe the future of CPOE here?

Various personnel: End-users, information and technology leaders and implementers

Data were collected from August 2004 through April 2005. During this time we conducted 32 semi-structured oral history interviews totaling 43 hours. We performed over 400 hours of observation that included shadowing 95 clinical providers (40% medical residents and staff physicians, 30% nurses, 10% pharmacists, and 20% other clinical personnel or IT staff) using CPOE systems in diverse settings. All transcripts and field notes were analyzed using N6 software (N6, QSR International Pty. Ltd., Melbourne, Australia, 2002).

18.3.3 DATA ANALYSIS

Each project team member independently reviewed an assigned selection of transcribed field notes or interviews to identify unintended consequences. The entire project team then met 36 times to collectively determine which data represented unintended consequences, and how the data could be meaningfully categorized. We specifically focused on unintended adverse consequences because these need to be carefully managed. We ultimately identified 324 instances of these related to CPOE. We used a card sort method [22] to develop provisional categories for those consequences that appeared to relate to the same content. Once initial groupings were assigned, the team iteratively reviewed each item in each category using a grounded theory approach, to confirm commonality among elements and to allow themes to emerge from the data. [22] Nine categories emerged and have been described in detail elsewhere. [18] Following this initial categorization we performed in-depth analysis of the nine categories using axial coding techniques [25] to better understand the properties and dimensions of each. As noted, the largest unintended consequence category was workflow, which is our focus here. Axial coding resulted in five themes within that category.

18.4 RESULTS

We discuss each of the five themes below and provide representative examples of each. Although we note that general themes existed in all settings we studied, the representative examples we use to elaborate the themes are site-specific.

18.4.1 CPOE INTRODUCTION EXPOSES HUMAN–COMPUTER INTERACTION PROBLEMS

We found that ergonomic issues can disrupt workflow. For example, some disruptions arise when environments designed prior to the computer era cannot adequately accommodate new hardware. Mobile computers have little flat space to accommodate paper charts. One physician noted: "A computer that doesn't have a place to put the chart down is no computer I am willing to use." In addition, when workstations are in short supply, contention for computers can be high in busy work areas, especially after morning rounds.

We noticed many issues related to poor CPOE usability. These included overly cluttered screen design, poor use of available screen space, and inconsistencies in screen design. More specifically, we saw lists that could not be easily sorted, screens that were hard to read or annotate, minimum availability of system defaults, and lack of appropriate safeguards to prevent selecting the wrong patient or entering incorrect data, to name just a few. Not all of these problems occurred at all sites, though all sites reported software design issues that made some work processes awkward. For example, a researcher observed this example of suboptimal design: "I notice that the resident has to perform four mouse clicks to access an element on a list: 1) click on the pick list, 2) open the list with the down arrow, 3) select an item from the list, and 4) hit the return key to exit the pick list. Normally, this wouldn't be much of a problem, but the list only contains one element!"

18.4.2 CPOE CHANGES WORK PACE, SEQUENCE, AND DYNAMICS

With some CPOE systems, providers find it difficult to access patient information housed in clinical systems that are not integrated with CPOE, require separate system logins, or cannot be accessed simultaneously. A physician explained: "For me to get lab values I would have to exit out of the discharge summary, [look up the lab values] then bring [the discharge summary] up again. It is just easier for me to look up values on a separate computer."

In addition, CPOE can force the provider to accommodate the system. For example, many systems provide minimal space for free-text entry or limit the use of timesaving shorthand (such as abbreviations or acronyms) and instead require data entry using nested menus, order sets, and preconfigured pick lists. A resident noted "...the order sets are organized in a linear fashion, for one problem at a time...most of [my patient's] problems are multidimensional...I have to fill out several different order sets...one for each problem."

The CPOE systems we studied often do not smoothly handle transitions in level or location of care. For example, it is quite common for an admitting clinician to begin to write orders for an emergency department patient prior to transfer to an inpatient bed. Because some CPOE implementations associate orders with a patient's physical location, the system may prevent the admitting clinician from entering these orders. "There is a major problem with confusion over whether it is the floor accepting the patient or the ER transferring. The difference is who is responsible."

CPOE systems can force rigid scheduling of tests and medications. Some systems assign medication start times when the order becomes active (as opposed to when the medication is given) making it difficult for staff to alter the timing to match reality. This may cause delays in medication administration. "One problem was that the start time in our system doesn't mean the time the medication is first administered—it means the time the order becomes active and then the administration times are automatically calculated based on that. [A physician ordered] a Q 12 medication. The first scheduled administration time was about 11 hours later so the patient's post-transplant medication was delayed 11 hours." In addition some CPOE systems make it difficult for clinical staff to alter the timing of doses when they cannot be given on schedule, such as when patients are absent from the nursing unit when medications are due. Even in systems where medication dosage times can be changed, often the system cannot automatically reschedule subsequent doses after this modification, requiring staff to alter each of the remaining dosage times manually to match the new, corrected administration schedule.

18.4.3   CPOE PROVIDES ONLY PARTIAL SUPPORT FOR THE WORK ACTIVITIES OF INVOLVED CLINICAL STAFF

These systems do not fully support the activities of all clinical staff who must process orders entered in the system. Nurses were the most vocal of the non-physician groups: "This is not a nursing system… the nurses are just saying 'Give me a template nurses can use. Give me standard order sets I can sign off with a single review. Get the standard nursing orders into the doctor's order templates, so we don't have to remind them to write an order for something like drawing arterial blood gases every 8 hours unless the patient condition changes.'"

Non-physician staff found it bothersome to receive alerts not applicable to them or their clinical setting. For example, some drug–drug interaction alerts may be highly desirable in one context and not another. One intensive care nurse observed: "… the [alerts] warning against prescribing heparin and aspirin—these are CCU patients, the system should know we are going to give these two meds together on this floor and quit warning us about them." In addition, because nurses do not prescribe medications, this alert is targeted at the wrong clinician.

18.4.4   CPOE REDUCES SITUATION AWARENESS

Dourish and Bellotti define situation awareness as "the understanding of the activities of others which provides a context for your own activity." [27] Collaboration understandably improves when people develop and maintain awareness of what is going on around them. [28] We found that CPOE systems, because they allow orders to be entered at any time by providers located outside of the hospital, can contribute to loss of situation awareness. For example: "It was not at all unusual in the paper world to have two or three people generate orders very close to each other but the common thing they had was a paper or a sheet. In the emergency department [there] was literally a different workstation about every two inches down there. We had a lot more instances of within thirty seconds of each other, two, sometimes three providers would enter the same order at approximately the same time and so it really forced us to go back and do more education on being careful to look and see what [orders are] active before you enter a new order."

Finally, interesting situation awareness issues emerge when providers from different clinical services use CPOE to enter orders simultaneously on the same patient. The orders might appear to conflict, when in fact they do not. "I was sitting there in the ICU looking at my patient and …boom, an order for dopamine shows up. I didn't write that…and I look at it…and turned out that it was written by the anesthesiologist getting ready for the case tomorrow. So I was seeing all of the pre-op medicines…a good thing, right? Except it surprised me. I'd never seen those orders before, and [the patient] looked like he didn't need dopamine to me, so I just cancelled the order."

18.4.5 CPOE CAN HIGHLIGHT INEFFECTIVE IMPLEMENTATION OF POLICY AND PROCEDURES

CPOE systems help to formalize organizational policies and procedures. [29] In many cases, actual practice does not match this rigid "letter of the law," so the CPOE system may introduce a significant amount of extra work (perceived or real): "We found that [obstetrics] was one of the most complex places in the hospital because patients were going from the screening room to the pod room to a labor room to the delivery room to postpartum and each of those are a different level of care and so orders need to be rewritten. Although nurses are very good about blending the orders as need be from one [level] to the other, the computer isn't nearly as flexible."

Difficulties arise when standards are hard to interpret or implement, as when one clinician initiates patient care that must be monitored by other specialists: "Some orders [are] written by certain specialists like anesthesiologists [for] epidurals. No one wants to rewrite those orders. So how should those [orders] traverse the levels of care when the epidural catheter moves with the patient?" In such cases, CPOE can complicate already difficult issues.

18.5 DISCUSSION

By observing and interviewing clinicians, we found that embedding CPOE systems in clinical practice can disrupt work processes in several general ways, regardless of the site studied. Specifically: 1) CPOE systems can expose new human–computer interaction problems and exacerbate space constraints, 2) CPOE can alter the pacing, sequencing, and dynamics of work patterns,3) Despite the fact that these systems are ostensibly provider systems, they remain, at least in the sites we studied, predominantly physician systems, such that the workflow needs of non-physician personnel are not yet being addressed, 4) CPOE can impact situation awareness for providers, so that clinicians cannot guarantee that they are acting on complete information at all times, and 5) CPOE can be leveraged to poorly implement organizational policies and procedures, creating extra work or slowing down current work processes for providers. We observed these types of workflow disruptions at all institutions we visited, regardless of the CPOE system in use. As a result, these general themes provide the following focus points for improvements in CPOE system design, implementation, and evaluation.

18.5.1   CPOE INTRODUCTION EXPOSES HUMAN–COMPUTER INTERACTION PROBLEMS

End-users struggle with many human–computer interface issues when moving from a pen and paper environment that is flexible and highly portable to an electronic system that is much more rigid and fixed. Poor system interface design (e.g., overly complex screens, inconsistencies in the interface, poor grouping of like terms, etc.) can exacerbate this transition. It is imperative that system engineers use proven usability design standards to avoid implementing systems that violate basic principles. We look forward to the development of explicit interface design and usability criteria that must be met in order to certify CPOE systems through such organizations as the Certification Commission for Healthcare Information Technology (http://www.cchit.org).

18.5.2   CPOE CHANGES WORK PACE, SEQUENCE, AND DYNAMICS

Alterations in work pace, sequence, and dynamics represent changes that emerge primarily from the difficulties inherent in attempting to customize the non-linear, iterative, ad hoc, interruption and exception driven activities of clinical care. [18,23] Computerization of ordering can dramatically affect the care delivery process, as patterns of communication, cooperation, and collaborative work must shift to accommodate the technology. It is not surprising that the National Health Policy forum reported that clinician productivity can drop approximately 20% within the first three months of CPOE implementation, [6] though other studies [29,30] have indicated that productivity often improves over time as users gain proficiency with the system. CPOE can be improved through development of interoperability with and access to other clinical information systems and research about how users circumvent the system to get their work done. We acknowledge that these systems are relatively new, and that as they mature, they should be able to handle more complex care scenarios. We encourage careful design that incorporates non-standard scenarios into the workflow mix.

18.5.3   CPOE DESIGN AFFECTS ALL CLINICAL PERSONNEL

Healthcare delivery is a complex activity system requiring the expertise of various professionals whose respective skills are interrelated and inseparable. Indeed, this distribution of work adds to the robustness of the health care system. However, current CPOE systems do not always accommodate the work needs of all levels of clinical personnel. In fact, many CPOE systems seem to provide support for only the physician's work activities. Although physicians bear the legal responsibility for ordering and have the expertise needed for the decision-making required, the entire ordering-to-completion process includes many different levels of healthcare personnel. For these reasons, it is paramount that the roles of nursing, clerical, pharmacy and other ancillary staff are considered when CPOE systems are designed, implemented, and modified if clinical workflow is to proceed with minimal disruption. This does not imply that all care activities for all personnel must be incorporated into CPOE; instead, those activities pertaining to order management must be considered.

18.5.4 CPOE CAN IMPACT SITUATION AWARENESS

CPOE systems can vastly improve situation awareness through functionality that integrates with other systems and subsequently displays information derived from these differing sources in a single location. In addition, clinical decision support tools can alert clinicians to potential problems that might otherwise go unnoticed (e.g., drug–drug or drug–allergy interactions). Because CPOE can standardize practice (e.g., through order sets, codification of procedures, etc.), it can provide a level of consistency in practice that can enhance situation awareness, as users can "expect" certain CPOE behavior, and adapt to CPOE processes. However, CPOE can also contribute to a general loss of situation awareness as it can change the pattern, style and timing of provider interactions. A certain degree of iterative and interactive communication among the various players is essential to promote and support situation awareness in medical work and decision making. Such awareness is vitally important for effective performance in any complex and dynamic environment. [31] Without careful design to facilitate multiple provider communication the computerization of the health record can serve to isolate users from each other, depriving each of the benefit of coworkers' understanding and insights regarding the clinical situation.

18.5.5 CPOE CAN HIGHLIGHT INEFFECTIVE OR INCOMPLETE IMPLEMENTATION OF POLICY AND PROCEDURES

While CPOE can be a highly effective and efficient tool for implementing organizational policy or procedure, using CPOE in this manner can bias workflow design towards an organizational perspective, one that emphasizes an explicit view of work: "those things that are documented, visible, and articulable [sic]," [20] such as procedures and methods. This view fails to acknowledge the more tacit aspects of work processes-those activities carried out in everyday practice, which rely on human ingenuity and depend on rules of thumb or individual judgment for synthesis and completion. [20] As a result, rote implementation of policy or procedure can highlight pronounced differences between organizational intention and provider practice, leading to the adoption of system workarounds by clinicians struggling to use a system that does not fully support their work. [26] Any implementation of organizational rules or directives should be undertaken only after careful assessment of the impact of such changes on actual clinical work, to determine whether or not these rules can be practically integrated into workflow. In addition, care must be taken to assure that work practices mandated in CPOE systems are actually formally required, as opposed to representing "the way things have always been done." CPOE can make it easy to implement organizational changes. It is thus imperative that organizational mandates implemented through CPOE are rigorously tested using real-time scenarios to assure that these requirements not only make practical sense, but do not negatively impact workflow. [18]

18.6   LIMITATIONS

In this study, we only observed users interacting with CPOE systems. It is possible we might find different unintended adverse consequences had we evaluated user interactions with other systems. As a qualitative study, this investigation produced rich, in depth knowledge about five carefully selected sites. It is possible that these sites are not truly representative of all sites using CPOE.

18.7   CONCLUSION

The introduction of CPOE into the healthcare environment has a dramatic effect on clinical workflow. CPOE systems are tools intended to support and improve the delivery of care, and are not solutions for all problems related to clinical practice. We must take care to continually improve these systems if they are to fit seamlessly into clinical workflow. As we identify how, when, and where workflow problems arise, we gain insight for better system design and implementation. As CPOE systems evolve, ongoing care must be taken to reduce or resolve the many unintended adverse effects these systems have on clinical workflow. The five kinds of unintended and unanticipated consequences related to workflow with CPOE can be mitigated by iteratively altering both clinical workflow and the CPOE system until a comfortable and optimized fit is achieved.

REFERENCES

1. Poon E, Blumenthal D, Jaggi T, Honour M, Bates D, Kaushal R. Overcoming barriers to adopting and implementing computerized physician order entry systems in U.S. hospitals. Health Aff. 2004;23(4): 184–90.
2. Committee on Quality Health Care in America. To Err is Human: Building a Safer Health System. Washington, DC: Institute of Medicine; 1999.
3. Committee on Quality Health Care in America. Crossing the Quality Chasm: A New Health System for the 21st Century. Washington, DC: Institute of Medicine; 2001.
4. The Leapfrog Group. Factsheet: Computer physician order entry. 2004 [accessed August 29, 2008]; Available from: http://www.leapfroggroup.org/media/file/Leapfrog-Computer_Physician_Order_Entry_Fact_Sheet.pdf
5. Oren E, Shaffer E, Guglielmo B. Impact of emerging technologies on medication errors and adverse drug events. Am J Health Syst Pharm. 2003;6014:1447–58.
6. Sprague L. Electronic health records: How close? How far to go. NHPF Issue Brief. 2004;800:1–17.
7. Wears R, Berg M. Computer technology and clinical work: still waiting for Godot. JAMA. 2005;293(10):1261–1263.
8. Ash J, Berg M, Coiera E. Some unintended consequences of information technology in health care: the nature of patient care information system-related errors. J Am Med Inform Assoc. 2004;11(2):104–112.
9. Koppel R, Metlay J, Cohen A, Abaluck B, Localio A, SE K. Role of computerized physician order entry systems in facilitating medication errors. JAMA. 2005;293:10:1197–1203.
10. Kremsdorf R. CPOE: not the first step toward patient safety. Health Manag Technol. 2005;26(1):66.
11. Berger R, Kichak J. Computerized physician order entry: helpful or harmful. J Am Med Inform Assoc. 2004;11(2):100–3.
12. Han Y, Carcillo J, Venkataraman S, Clark R, Watson R, Nguyen T, et al. Unexpected increased mortality after implementation of a commercially sold computerized physician order entry system. Pediatrics. 2005;116(6):1506–12.

13. Wang J, Lee H, Huang F, Chang P, Sheu J. Unexpected mortality in pediatric patients with postoperative Hirschsprung's disease. Pediatr Surg Int. 2004;20(7):525–8.

14. Aarts J, Berg M. A tale of two hospitals: a sociotechnical appraisal of the introduction of computerized physician order entry in two Dutch hospitals. 2004;11(Pt 2):. Stud Health Technol Inform. 2004;107(Pt 2):999–1002.

15. Ash J, Anderson J, Gorman P, Zielstorff R, Norcross N, Pettit J, et al. Managing change: analysis of a hypothetical case. J Am Med Inform Assoc. 2000;7(2)125–34.

16. Lorenzi N, Smith J, Conner S, Campion T. The success factor profile for clinical computer innovation. Stud Health Technol Inform. 2004;107(Pt 2)1077–80.

17. Poon E, Blumenthal D, Jaggi T, Honour M, Bates D, Kaushal R. Overcoming the barriers to the implementing computerized physician order entry systems in US hospitals: perspectives from senior management. AMIA Annu Symp Proc. 2003:975.

18. Campbell E, Sittig D, Ash J, Guappone K, Dykstra R. Types of unintended consequences related to computerized provider order entry. J Am Med Inform Assoc. 2006;13(5):547–56. Sep–Oct.

19. Rinkus S, Walji M, Johnson-Throop K, Malin J, Turley J, Smith J, et al. Human-centered design of a distributed knowledge management system. J Biomed Inform. 2005;38(1)4–17.

20. Sachs P. Transforming work: Collaboration, learning, and design. Commun ACM. 1995;38(9):36–44.

21. Pratt W, Reddy M, McDonald D, Tarczy-Hornoch P, Gennari J. Incorporating ideas from computer-supported cooperative work. J Biomed Inform. 2004;37(2):28–37.

22. Lincoln Y, Guba E. Natualistic Inquiry. Newbury Park, CA: Sage Publications, Inc.; 1985.

23. Berg M. Medical work and the computer-based patient record: a sociological perspective. Methods Inf Med. 1998;37(3)294–301.

24. Berg M. Patient care information systems and health care work: a sociotechnical approach. Int J Med Inform. 1999;55(2):87–101.

25. Crabtree B, Miller WL. Doing Qualitative Research. 2nd ed. Thousand Oaks, CA: Sage Publications, Inc; 1999.

26. Harrison M, Koppel R, Bar-Lev S. Unintended consequences of information technologies in health care—An Interactive sociotechnical analysis. J Am Med Inform Assoc. 2007;14(5):542–9.

27. Dourish P, Bellotti V. Awareness and coordination in shared work spaces. ACM Conference on Computer-Supported Cooperative Work (CWSW '92). 1992:107–14.

28. Endsley M. Toward a theory of situation awareness in dynamic systems. Hum Factors. 1995;37(1)32–64.

29. Kuperman G, Gibson R. Computer physician order entry: Benefits, costs, and issues. Ann Intern Med. 2003;139(1):31–9.

30. Overhage J, Perkins S, Tierney W, McDonald C. Controlled trial of direct physician order entry: effects on physicians' time utilization in ambulatory primary care internal medicine practices 2001;8(4):361–71.

31. Hazlehurst B, McMullen C, Gorman P. Distributed cognition in the heart room: How situation awareness arises from coordinated communications during cardiac surgery. J Biomed Inform. 2007;40(5):539–51.

CHAPTER 19

LESSONS FROM "UNEXPECTED INCREASED MORTALITY AFTER IMPLEMENTATION OF A COMMERCIALLY SOLD COMPUTERIZED PHYSICIAN ORDER ENTRY SYSTEM"

DEAN F. SITTIG, JOAN S. ASH, JIAJIE ZHANG,
JEROME A. OSHEROFF, and M. MICHAEL SHABOT,

We are writing in response to the article "Unexpected Increased Mortality After Implementation of a Commercially Sold Computerized Physician Order Entry System" by Han et al. [1] The authors are to be congratulated for their courage in bringing their compelling account of computerized physician order entry (CPOE) implementation problems to the medical literature as they tried to interpret their results concerning mortality. Their article is as much a search for answers as it is a recitation of the shortfalls in their implementation process and computer systems. It is critically important to understand that the types of problems described by Han et al are not limited to their institution. In fact, setbacks and failures in the implementation of clinical information systems (CISs) and CPOE systems are all too common (eg, see refs 2–4). Although it is tempting to focus solely on the role of new technology in the problems highlighted by this example, there are also important lessons to be learned about related organizational and workflow factors that affect the potential for danger associated with CPOE implementation.

There are many previous publications about troubled or failed implementations. The account by Han et al is unique in that an adverse change in mortality rate was associated in time with CIS and CPOE implementation. We may question the study's methodology and conclude that causality was not proven, yet the assignment of CPOE to a severity-adjusted odds ratio of 3.71 for patient death simply cannot be ignored. Regardless of what was or was not proven, if only one unnecessary death were caused by the implementation process or CIS and CPOE modules, that is one too many.

The question that must be asked is how can intelligent and well-intentioned leaders at all levels of an institution make the kind of implementation decisions that ultimately place excellent patient care in jeopardy? Clearly, that was not their intent, so how could it happen? What is it about CIS and CPOE that makes implementation so risky? Why are these implementations prone to causing emotional distress, [5] rework, [6] delay, [7] user protest, [7] temporary system withdrawal, and later repeat implementation, [8] often at a cost of millions of dollars to the hospital or health system involved? How can institutions avoid these risks and additional costs? These are the questions that demand answers.

We posit that the primary reason CISs and CPOE are prone to failure is that they have the ability to profoundly alter patient care workflow processes. Although the intent of computerization is to improve patient care by making it safer and more efficient, the adverse effects and unintended consequences of workflow disruption may make the situation far worse.9 It is important to remember that the manual processes of patient care and documentation in place within an institution have been finely tuned over long periods of time, usually years to decades. Although paper charting forms, medication ordering, delivery and administration, and processes for patient admission and transfer are appropriate subjects for computerization, the transition from manual to computerized methods is notoriously complex. This is a severely underappreciated fact of CIS and CPOE implementation. In an ordinary business, employees, clients, revenue, and profits may be adversely affected by computerization. In a hospital, patients and caregivers are at risk. In other words, the stakes are much higher. Santayana once wrote, "Those who cannot remember the past are condemned to repeat it." [10] So perhaps what we should do in retrospect is to learn from mistakes that occurred in this implementation and others to help ensure that organizations implementing CIS and CPOE in the future do not fall prey to Santayana's admonition.

We can learn many things from the Han et al study. Each of the following lessons begins with a direct quote from the article by Han et al.

1. "Hospital-wide implementation of CHP's [Children's Hospital of Pittsburgh's] CPOE system (along with its clinical applications platform) occurred over a 6-day period."—Although few organizations have the luxury of pioneering institutions that spent 10 years or more rolling out a CIS and CPOE, attempting such a project in a few days goes beyond challenging and borders on the temerarious. [11] Previous studies have shown that the workflow of clinicians changes significantly after implementation of these types of systems. [12] Given such a huge change, clinicians must be given time to adapt to their new routines and responsibilities in a setting that is carefully managed to ensure that patient care is not harmed in any way. Contrary to isolated claims of success by several Health Information Technology vendors, rapid implementation of any CIS, let alone one that changes the way that orders are written and conducted, should not be attempted unless planning has been thorough and resources are abundant. [13,14] Furthermore, time is needed during the implementation process to evaluate whether the changes in workflow are positive or negative, safe or unsafe, and more or less efficient. This cannot be done in a few days, even on a single ward. Experience with countless previous CIS and CPOE implementations has shown that not all changes in workflow represent improvements (eg, see refs 15 and 16).

2. "After CPOE implementation, order entry was not allowed until after the patient had physically arrived to the hospital and been fully registered into the system."—Although accurate patient registration is clearly important to patient safety, the care and treatment of a severely ill patient should never be made to wait for a computer system. Analysis by multidisciplinary teams regarding the workflows that were successful before system implementation should have led clinicians and system administrators to develop a means to allow clinicians to continue to treat patients in the best way possible. This might require using old-fashioned paper orders in emergency situations with subsequent entry into the CPOE system after the patient is stable. Under no circumstances can the care of a patient be subordinated to the idiosyncrasies of a computer system.

3. "As part of CPOE implementation, all medications, including vasoactive agents and antibiotics, became centrally located within the pharmacy department."—It is important to recognize that the relocation of all medications including ICU vasoactive drugs to a central pharmacy, even if this were done for administrative reasons without implementation of a CIS and CPOE, could account for many of the adverse effects noted in this study. Considering that the hospital was already undertaking a huge disruptive organizational change affecting every caregiver in the institution, it was unfortunate that they would also try to institute a significant policy change regarding pharmacy workflow to accommodate CPOE more effectively. The additive effects of the CIS implementation, CPOE implementation, and pharmacy centralization could have been predicted to dramatically slow the delivery of drugs to all patients. Han et al's selection of interfacility transport patients as the patient population probably magnified the ill effects, because these patients can be predicted to be more severely ill at admission than other patients. Piggybacking organizational changes with significant potential for adverse workflow effects onto a CIS/CPOE implementation should be avoided if at all possible. CIS and CPOE are disruptive in and of themselves; interrelated workflows should be enhanced before implementation, when possible, or at least remain stable through the implementation period to minimize this disruption. Many hospitals use small "tests of change" on a single hospital unit to evaluate a new care process for both efficacy and potential adverse effects or unintended consequences. If pharmacy centralization had been evaluated in a single ICU in advance of CIS and CPOE implementation, it is likely that the operational problems described by Han et al would have been appreciated so that appropriate solutions could have been put into place.
4. "Because pharmacy could not process medication orders until they had been activated, ICU nurses also spent significant amounts of time at a separate computer terminal and away from the bedside."—This was clearly an unintended consequence of computerization. Careful sociotechnical analysis is required before clinical

systems are implemented to ensure that caregivers can do their basic job at least as well and as safely as they could before computerization. Whenever an organization commits to moving from a well-honed manual care delivery system to a new computer-based model, the organization should carefully review and modify all applicable practices, procedures, policies, and bylaws. Mock use, full dress drills, and trial use on individual patients and wards should precede wider implementation. The role of the computer in health care is not to ensure that rules and regulations that had never been completely followed are now rigorously followed. Rather, computerization highlights the need for review, careful consideration of purpose, and clear definition of intended policies. Allowing a computer to enforce rules and regulations without first working through all implications and potential unintended consequences for patient care is a prescription for disaster.

5. "After CPOE implementation, because order entry and activation occurred through a computer interface, often separated by several bed spaces or separate ICU pods, the opportunities for such face-to-face physician-nurse communication were diminished."—Clear, 2-way, face-to-face communication is the hallmark of high-quality, collaborative patient care. Assuming that ambiguities in the treatment process are removed because all the orders are now legible and available in a central database is inappropriate and potentially dangerous. As the importance and complexity of the information to be communicated increases, the necessity of face-to-face communication increases dramatically. Careful sociotechnical evaluation, or even trial use on a single ward, probably would have brought to light the need for better system design. In addition, recent advances in the capability and utility of mobile terminals, tablet computers, and other devices such as hands-free, wireless communication systems [17] may allow caregivers to remain in personal contact while doing their computer work. In fact, careful attention to these details has been shown to bring care teams together and make them more, not less, effective. [18,19] Computer systems need to be designed and implemented in such a way as to foster appropriate levels of communication, not hinder it.

6. "This initial time burden seemed to change the organization of bedside care. Before CPOE implementation, physicians and nurses converged at the patient's bedside to stabilize the patient. After CPOE implementation, while 1 physician continued to direct medical management, a second physician was often needed solely to enter orders into the computer during the first 15 minutes to 1 hour if a patient arrived in extremis."—Again, it is apparent that the consequences of CPOE were not appreciated until after implementation. Doubling physician workload, while slowing the delivery of life-saving medications, treatments, and diagnostic studies could not have been the original intent. Careful pilot studies could have revealed these issues so that solutions could have been devised before hospital-wide implementation. Although several studies have shown a small, but significant, increase in the time required on the part of clinicians to enter orders using a computer system, no one has ever documented a "doubling" of physician workload (see ref 12 for a review of several studies).

7. "The physical process of entering stabilization orders often required an average of ten "clicks" on the computer mouse per order, which translated to 1 to 2 minutes per single order as compared with a few seconds previously needed to place the same order by written form. However, no ICU-specific order sets had been programmed at the time of CPOE implementation."—Methods of entering frequently occurring orders should be as easy and fast as on paper, especially for sets of orders, with the added benefits of 100% legibility, instantaneous transmission to the ancillary department, dose-range checking, and potential drug, laboratory, and condition interaction checking. [20] Organizations must take the time to implement validated standard order sets for routinely occurring critical conditions to speed the ordering and care process. [21] Simply training users to overcome a steep learning curve and time-consuming process of entering many individual orders in the midst of critical patient care is not an optimal, or even effective, solution. Therefore, organizations must work to ensure that the clinical content (eg, order sets), default settings, and anticipated screen flows are designed, implemented, and tested to optimize speed, usability, and patient

safety. Again, this may require trial use of the system on one or a few well-defined and well-staffed wards by a variety of users and over a prolonged period of time. This cannot be done in a few days. A more reasonable estimate of the amount of time to fully develop and vet clinical policies and order sets and to configure, test, and implement CPOE systems is 1 to 3 years.6

8. "Because the vast majority of computer terminals were linked to the hospital computer system via wireless signal, communication bandwidth was often exceeded during peak operational periods, which created additional delays between each click on the computer mouse."—Technical issues such as this can also be anticipated and tested in advance. On top of all the other process and workflow changes involved in CPOE implementation, inadequate or unreliable computing capacity can be particularly frustrating to clinicians and other end-users. Testing a new CIS under peak load conditions is an important task that can not be overlooked.

Although it is not clear whether the increase in mortality rate was a direct result of the CPOE implementation or other concomitant organizational and system changes, the CPOE implementation may well have been responsible, and we applaud the authors for reporting their findings and their problems with implementation. Although it is easy to criticize organizations for reporting implementation decisions that in retrospect seem flawed, we must respect, appreciate, and encourage other institutions to share their experiences so that everyone can learn from them. Likewise, regardless of whether the technology has a direct role in adverse effects from a specific deployment, we can take the opportunity from case studies such as this one to learn how to develop better systems.

The complexity of the decisions that must be made by CIS implementation and management teams demands iterative ongoing dialogue and feedback over time. There is no substitute for careful workflow and sociotechnical analysis, and beyond those there is no substitute for trial or pilot use of a system to uncover hidden flaws, unintended consequences, and adverse effects.

One must avoid the inclination or temptation to blame the adverse effects noted in this article solely on the particular CIS or CPOE system used. This would be the equivalent to stating that a particular brand of tool from a hardware store was unsafe because an injury occurred while someone was misusing it.

To return to the central question, how can well-intentioned organizations avoid these problems? Beyond the solutions noted above, several collective publications on CIS and CPOE implementation are available to guide institutions in designing a safe and effective process. [22–25] The advice in these guides, along with a careful evaluation of caregiver workflows and trial implementation in limited hospital areas, should allow safe implementation for everyone involved, especially patients.

A very important lesson in the Han et al article is the need to measure overall hospital mortality and adverse-event rates when implementing major new systems. Indeed, these mortality rates could go up even when rates of adverse drug events (ADEs) go down, as concomitantly reported from Han et al's institution. [26] However, these particular findings need to be interpreted cautiously, because they relied on "self-reported" ADEs, which may have little to do with the true underlying rate. [27] Traditionally, the efficacy of CPOE systems has been measured in terms of ADE rates; Han et al have reminded us that we must consider the larger scope of patient outcomes to accurately evaluate safety and efficacy.

We believe that the problems observed in Han et al's and others' CPOE deployments can be overcome by systematically developing and applying human-centered design, implementation, and evaluation methods adapted to point-of-care CISs. Such a systematic approach, as advocated by experienced practitioners in the field of medical informatics, has been achieved in aviation, the military, nuclear power, and the consumer software industry; it can, and must, be achieved in health care as well.

REFERENCES

1. Han YY, Carcillo JA, Venkataraman ST, et al. Unexpected increased mortality after implementation of a commercially sold computerized physician order entry system [published correction appears in Pediatrics. 2006;117:594]. Pediatrics.2005;116 :1506–1512

2. Southon G, Sauer C, Dampney K. Lessons from a failed information systems initiative: issues for complex organisations. Int J Med Inform.1999;55 :33–46 e

3. Goddard BL. Termination of a contract to implement an enterprise electronic medical record system. J Am Med Inform Assoc.2000;7 :564– 568

4. Wager KA, Lee FW, White AW. Life After a Disastrous Electronic Medical Record Implementation: One Clinic's Experience. Charleston, SC: Idea Group Publishing; 2002

5. Sittig DF, Krall M, Kaalaas-Sittig J, Ash JS. Emotional aspects of computer-based provider order entry: a qualitative study. J Am Med Inform Assoc. 200;12:561–567

6. Payne TH, Hoey PJ, Nichol P, Lovis C. Preparation and use of preconstructed orders, order sets, and order menus in a computerized provider order entry system. J Am Med Inform Assoc.2003;10 :322– 329

7. Massaro TA. Introducing physician order entry at a major academic medical center: I. Impact on organizational culture and behavior. Acad Med.1993;68 :20– 25

8. Scott JT, Rundall TG, Vogt TM, Hsu J. Kaiser Permanente's experience of implementing an electronic medical record: a qualitative study. BMJ.2005;331 :1313– 1316

9. Ash JS, Berg M, Coiera E. Some unintended consequences of information technology in health care: the nature of patient care information system-related errors. J Am Med Inform Assoc.2004;11 :104– 112

10. Santayana G. Life of Reason: Reason in Common Sense. New York, NY: Scribner's; 1905:284

11. McDonald CJ, Overhage JM, Tierney WM, et al. The Regenstrief medical record system: a quarter century experience. Int J Med Inform.1999;54 :225– 253 e

12. Poissant L, Pereira J, Tamblyn R, Kawasumi Y. The impact of electronic health records on time efficiency of physicians and nurses: a systematic review. J Am Med Inform Assoc.2005;12 :505– 516

13. CPOE improves patient safety at top-ranked pediatric hospital [press release]. December 2, 2005. Available at: www.cerner.com/public/NewsReleases_1a. asp?id=257&cid=4668. Accessed June 14, 2006

14. Baker ML. Management plays key role in success of electronic patient record system Ziff Davis Internet. May 26, 2004. Available at: www.eweek.com/article2/0,1895,1600999,00.asp. Accessed June 14, 2006

15. Weingart SN, Toth M, Sands DZ, Aronson MD, Davis RB, Phillips RS. Physicians' decisions to override computerized drug alerts in primary care. Arch Intern Med.2003;163 :2625– 2631

16. Nebeker JR, Hoffman JM, Weir CR, Bennett CL, Hurdle JF. High rates of adverse drug events in a highly computerized hospital. Arch Intern Med.2005;165 :1111– 1116

17. Breslin S, Greskovich W, Turisco F. Wireless technology improves nursing workflow and communications. Comput Inform Nurs.2004;22 :275– 281

18. Ash JS, Stavri PZ, Dykstra R, Fournier L. Implementing computerized physician order entry: the importance of special people. Int J Med Inform.2003;69 :235– 250 e

19. Reddy M, Pratt W, Dourish P, Shabot MM. Sociotechnical requirements analysis for clinical systems. Methods Inf Med.2003;42 :437– 444

20. Bates DW, Boyle DL, Teich JM. Impact of computerized physician order entry on physician time. Proc Annu Symp Comput Appl Med Care.1994:996

21. Ali NA, Mekhjian HS, Kuehn PL, et al. Specificity of computerized physician order entry has a significant effect on the efficiency of workflow for critically ill patients. Crit Care Med.2005;33 :110– 114e

22. Lee F, Teich JM, Spurr CD, Bates DW. Implementation of physician order entry: user satisfaction and self-reported usage patterns. J Am Med Inform Assoc.1996;3: 42– 55

23. Osheroff JA, Pifer EA, Teich JM, Sittig DF, Jenders RA. Improving Outcomes With Clinical Decision Support: An Implementer's Guide. Chicago, IL: Healthcare Information and Management Systems Society; 2005

24. Metzger J, Fortin J. Computerized Physician Order Entry in Community Hospitals: Lessons From the Field. Oakland, CA: California Healthcare Foundation; 2003

25. Drazen E, Kilbridge P, Turisco F. A Primer on Physician Order Entry. Oakland, CA: California Healthcare Foundation; 2000

26. Upperman JS, Staley P, Friend K, Neches W, Kazimer D, Benes J, Wiener ES. The impact of hospitalwide computerized physician order entry on medical errors in a pediatric hospital. J Pediatr Surg.2005;40 :57– 59e

27. Classen DC, Pestotnik SL, Evans RS, Burke JP. Computerized surveillance of adverse drug events in hospital patients [published correction appears in JAMA. 1992;267:1922]. JAMA.1991;266 :2847– 2851

Sittig, D. F., Ash, J. S., Zhang, J., Osheroff, J. A.,and Shabot, M. M. Lessons From "Unexpected Increased Mortality After Implementation of a Commercially Sold Computerized Physician Order Entry System". Reprinted with permission from Pediatrics 2006 Aug;118(2):797-801. Copyright 2009 by the American Academy of Pediatrics.

AUTHOR NOTES

CHAPTER 1

Financial Disclosures
None reported.

Funding/Support
Dr Sittig is supported in part by grant R01-LM006942 from the National Library of Medicine. Dr Singh is supported by career development award K23CA125585, the VA National Center of Patient Safety, Agency for Health Care Research and Quality, and in part by the Houston VA HSR&D Center of Excellence (HFP90-020).

Role of Sponsors
None of the supporting agencies had any role in the preparation, review, or approval of the manuscript.

Disclaimer
The views expressed in this article are those of the authors and do not necessarily represent the views of the Department of Veterans Affairs or the National Institutes of Health.

Additional Contributions
We thank Laura A. Petersen, MD, MPH, VA HSR&D Center of Excellence, Michael E. DeBakey Veterans Affairs Medical Center, and Baylor College of Medicine, Michael Shabot, MD, Memorial Hermann Health Care System, and Eric Thomas, MD, MPH, University of Texas, Houston-Memorial Hermann Center for Healthcare Quality and Safety and Department of Medicine, University of Texas Medical School, Houston, for their valuable comments on an earlier version of this manuscript and Annie Bradford, PhD, Baylor College of Medicine, for assistance with medical editing, for which they received no compensation.

CHAPTER 2

Acknowledgments

We are very grateful to all participants who kindly gave their time and to the extended project and program teams of work we have drawn upon. We are also grateful to two anonymous expert peer reviewers who commented on a previous version of this manuscript.

Footnotes

Contributors AS conceived this work. AS is currently leading a National Institute for Health Research-funded national evaluation of electronic prescribing and medicines administration systems. KMC is employed as a researcher on this grant and led on the write-up and drafting of the initial version of the paper, with DWB and AS commenting on various drafts.

Funding

This work has drawn on data funded by the NHS Connecting for Health Evaluation Programme (NHS CFHEP 001, NHS CFHEP 005, NHS CFHEP 009, NHS CFHEP 010) and the National Institute for Health Research (NIHR)-funded Programme Grants for Applied Research scheme (RP-PG-1209-10099). The views expressed are those of the author(s) and not necessarily those of the NHS, the NIHR, or the Department of Health.

Competing interest

None.

Provenance and peer review

Not commissioned; externally peer reviewed.

CHAPTER 3

Author Contributions

Study concept and design: Sittig and Singh. Acquisition of data: Sittig. Analysis and interpretation of data: Sittig. Drafting of the manuscript: Sittig. Critical revision of the manuscript for important intellectual content: Singh. Obtained funding: Sittig.

Financial Disclosure

None reported.

Funding/Support

Dr Sittig is supported in part by grant R01-LM006942 from the National Library of Medicine and by Strategic Health IT Advanced Research Projects (SHARP) contract ONC 10510592 from the Office of the National Coordinator for Health Information Technology. Dr Singh is supported by National Institutes of Health K23 career development award K23CA125585, VA National Center of Patient Safety, Agency for Health Care Research and Quality grant R18-HS17820, SHARP contract ONC 10510592 from the Office of the National Coordinator for Health Information Technology, and in part by grant HFP90-020 from the Houston VA Health Services Research and Development Center of Excellence.

Role of the Sponsors

The funding institutions had no role in the preparation, review, or approval of the manuscript.

Disclaimer

The views expressed in this article are those of the authors and do not necessarily represent the views of the Department of Veterans Affairs or any of the other funding agencies.

Previous Presentation

Portions of this article were presented to the US Institute of Medicine Committee on Patient Safety and Health Information Technology; December 14, 2010; Washington, DC.

Additional Contributions

We thank Laura A. Petersen, MD, MPH, and Eric J. Thomas, MD, MPH, for their guidance in this work. We also thank Annie Bradford, PhD, who edited the paper for language and brevity for which she received a small compensation.

CHAPTER 4

Acknowledgments

Dr. Sittig was supported in part by a grant from the American Society for Healthcare Risk Management to the American Health Lawyers Association. Dr. Singh is supported by the VA National Center of Patient Safety, Agency for Health Care Research and Quality, and in part by the Houston VA HSR&D Center of Excellence (HFP90-020). These sources had no role in the preparation, review, or approval of the manuscript. We thank Annie Bradford, Ph.D., for assistance with medical editing.

CHAPTER 5

The authors thank Laurence Berg for his contributions to the data collection and analysis. The authors were supported in part by NCATS grants UL1 TR000371 (ABM, EVB, DFS), RC1 RR028254 (EVB), and UL1 TR000154 (MGK); NLM grant R00 LM009556-06 (JS); NSF grant III 0964613 (EVB); and ONC SHARP contracts #10510592 (ABM, AW, EVB, DFS) and #10510924 (EVB).

Footnotes

Contributors Conception and design: ABM, AW and DFS. Analysis and interpretation of data: ABM, AW, MGK, JSS, EVB and DFS. Drafting the article or revising it critically for important intellection content: ABM, AW, MGK, JSS, EVB and DFS. Final approval of the version to be published: ABM, AW, MGK, JSS, EVB and DFS.

Competing interests

None.

Ethics approval

UTHealth, Partners, Denver Childrens, Mt Sinai.

Provenance and peer review

Not commissioned; internally peer reviewed.

CHAPTER 6

Acknowledgments

The authors thank Dr. Ben Shneiderman for encouraging us to explore this topic. The authors also thank Drs. Elmer V. Bernstam, Annie Bradford, Gilad J. Kuperman, Daniel G. Miller, Laura A. Petersen, Ryan P. Radecki, Heidi V. Russell, M. Michael Shabot, Ben Shneiderman, Geeta R. Singhal and Eric J. Thomas for their helpful comments on early drafts of this manuscript.

Footnotes

This article has been peer reviewed.

Competing interests

Dean Sittig's institution received a Strategic Health IT Advanced Research Projects (SHARP) contract from the Office of the National Coordinator for Health Information Technology (ONC no. 10510592) and the National Library of Medicine (R01-LM006942). Hardeep Singh's institution received funds from the Mentored Patient-Oriented Research Career Development Award (K23) program from the National Institutes of Health (grant no. K23CA125585), the VA National Center for Patient Safety, the Agency for Healthcare Research and Quality (R18 HS 017820) and a SHARP contract from the Office of the National Coordinator for Health Information Technology (ONC no. 10510592). Dr. Singh is also supported by the Houston VA Health Services Research and Development Center of Excellence (HFP90-020). These funding sources had no role in the preparation, review or approval of the manuscript. The views expressed in this article are those of the authors and do not represent the views of the Department of Veterans Affairs or other funders.

Contributors

Both authors drafted the article, revised it critically for important intellectual content and approved the final version submitted for publication.

CHAPTER 7

Acknowledgments

The authors gratefully acknowledge the intellectual contributionsfromthe following reviewers:
Anne Bobb, R.Ph., Children's Memorial Hospital, Chicago, IL
Joseph Cafazzo, Ph.D., P.Eng., Healthcare Human Factors, University-Health Network, Toronto
Willa Drummond, M.D., University of Florida College of Medicine
Daniel Essin, M.A., M.D., USC Keck School of Medicine
Scott Finley, M.D., M.P.H., Westat and VHA, Office of Health Information
Anne B. Francis, M.D., Elmwood Pediatric Group, Rochester, NY

Ayse Gurses, Ph.D., Johns Hopkins University
Marta Hernanz-Schulman, M.D., Vanderbilt Children's Hospital
Kevin Jones, M.S., Ohio State University
Dean Karavite, M.S., Children's Hospital of Philadelphia
Ben-Tzion Karsh, Ph.D., University of Wisconsin
Yiannis L. Katsogridakis, M.D., M.P.H., Children's Memorial Hospital, Chicago, IL
Rainu Kaushal, M.D., M.P.H., Weill Cornell Medical College
George Kim, M.D., Johns Hopkins University Children's Center
Nancy F. Krebs, M.D., M.S., University of Colorado School of Medicine
David Kreda, Social Research Corporation, PA
Andrew Kroger, M.D., M.P.H., National Center for Immunization and Respiratory Diseases
Herschel R. Lessin M.D., The Children's Medical Group, Poughkeepsie, NY
Eugenia Marcus, M.D., Pediatric Health Care at Newton Wellesley, Newton, MA
Colleen McLaughlin, M.P.H., Ph.D., Patient Safety Center, New York State Dept. of Health
Deepa Menon, M.D., Johns Hopkins University
Mary Patterson, M.D., Med, Akron Children's Hospital
Sean Petty, R.N., Jacobi Medical Center, Bronx, NY
Debora Simmons, Ph.D., R.N., CCNS, St. Luke's Episcopal Health System
Dean Sittig, Ph.D., University of Texas Houston
Arthur Smerling, M.D., Columbia fUniversity College of Physicians and Surgeons
S. Andrew Spooner, M.D., M.S., Cincinnati Children's Hospital Medical Center
Jennifer Stinson, R.N., Ph.D., Hospital for Sick Children, Toronto
Susan Torrey, M.D., NYU Langone Medical Center
Michael S. Victoroff, M.D., University of Colorado School of Medicine
Roberts Wears, M.D., Ph.D., University of Florida Health Cente rJacksonville

Disclaimer
Certain commercial entities, equipment, or material may be identified in this document in order to describe a concept adequately. Such identifi-

cation is not intended to imply recommendation or endorsement by the National Institute of Standards and Technology, nor is it intended to imply that these entities, materials, or equipment are necessarily the best available for the purpose.

CHAPTER 8

Acknowledgments
Project funded by Baylor College of Medicine Center for Globalization Demonstration Project Grant, and in part by the Houston VA HSR&D Center of Excellence (HFP90-020).

CHAPTER 9

Footnotes
Supported in part by RO1 HS07107 from the Agency for Health Care Policy and Research.

CHAPTER 10

Financial Disclosure
The authors have indicated they have no financial relationships relevant to this article to disclose.

Opinions expressed in these commentaries are those of the authors and not necessarily those of the American Academy of Pediatrics or its Committees.

CHAPTER 11

Competing interests
The authors declare that they have no competing interests.

Authors' contributions
JSA, DFS, AW, and CM designed and conducted the study, analyzed the data, and wrote the paper. KPG, RHD, JR, JC, AB and MS assisted in the design of the study, gathered and analyzed the data, and reviewed versions

of the manuscript. AB also organized the data and contributed significantly to writing the paper. BM, with JSA, obtained funding for the study and reviewed and revised drafts of the manuscript. All authors except RHD, now deceased, have read and approved the final manuscript.

Acknowledgments

We are grateful to the participants who allowed us to observe and interview them during our research, and to Drs. Marc Overhage, Eric Pifer, Greg Fraser, Frank Sonnenberg, and Jason Saleem for their assistance with site visits. We thank the 17 experts who took part in our fifth Menucha conference: John Dulcey, Tom Payne, Mike Shabot, Jim Carpenter, Victor Lee, Scott Evans, Brian Patty, Eric Poon, Chuck Tucinda, Julie McGowan, Paul Nichol, Brian Churchill, Ken Guappone, Joanie Kapusnik, Dick Gibson, Gil Kuperman, and Randy Miller.

This work was supported by AHRQ contract #HHSA290200810010, NLM Research Grant 563 R56-LM006942 and Training Grant 2-T15-LM007088. AHRQ and NLM had no role in the design or execution of this study, nor in the decision to publish.

Finally, we would like to dedicate this paper to POET team member Richard H Dykstra, MD, MS, who was instrumental in developing the new theoretical framework but who unfortunately passed away before the paper was accepted for publication.

CHAPTER 12

Acknowledgments

We are grateful to the participants who allowed us to observe and interview them during our research. We also acknowledge and appreciate the assistance of J Coury, of the Kaiser Permanente Center for Health Research, who provided editorial assistance as we prepared this manuscript.

Footnotes

A portion of these data was presented as part of a panel at AMIA 2009 by AW, DFS, WPN, BM, and DWB

Funding

This work was supported by AHRQ contract #HHSA290200810010 and NLM Research Grant 563 R56-LM006942.

Competing interests
None.

Ethics approval
Approval was provided by Partners HealthCare; approval was also obtained at some of the sites (where not waived to Partners).

Provenance and peer review
Not commissioned; externally peer reviewed.

CHAPTER 13

Author contributions
A.W., J.F. and D.F.S. participated in all parts of the study, including study design, data cleaning/analysis, and manuscript preparation. J.E.P. participated in data cleaning and manuscript preparation. J.D.C., M.A.K., and B.M. participated in data analysis and manuscript preparation.

Conflict of interest
The authors have no conflicts of interest to report.

Acknowledgments
We are grateful to the participating sites that provided us with data order sets and utilization patterns at their institutions and to Stanislav Henkin for providing assistance with the editing of the manuscript. This work was supported by United States Agency for Healthcare Research and Quality (AHRQ) contract #HHSA290200810010 and United States National Library of Medicine (NLM) Research Grant 563 R56-LM006942. Neither the NLM nor AHRQ had a role in the design or execution of this study, nor in the decision to publish.

CHAPTER 14

Competing interests
The author(s) declare that they have no competing interests.

Author's contributions
AE participated in conceptualization and drafting of the manuscript. DFS participated in conceptualization and revising of the manuscript. DRM

participated in conceptualization and drafting of the manuscript. HS participated in conceptualization and revising of the manuscript.

Acknowledgments

Dr. Singh is supported by an NIH K23 career development award (K23CA125585), the VA National Center of Patient Safety, and in part by the Houston VA HSR&D Center for Excellence (HFP90-020). Dr. Sittig is supported in part by a SHARP contract from the Office of the National Coordinator for Health Information Technology (ONC #10510592).

CHAPTER 15

Dr. Singh is supported by the Department of Veterans Affairs (VA) National Center for Patient Safety, and in part by the Houston VA Health Services Research and Development Service (HSR&D) Center of Excellence (HFP90-020). Dr. Vij is supported by the Michael E. DeBakey VA Medical Center. These sources had no role in the preparation, review, or approval of the manuscript. The content is solely the responsibility of the authors and does not necessarily represent the official views of the Department of Veterans Affairs. The authors thank members of the Diagnostic Committee and other stakeholders at the Michael E. DeBakey VA Medical Center who provided valuable feedback for the local policy and Annie Bradford, Ph.D., for editorial assistance.

CHAPTER 16:

Competing interests

The authors declare that they have no competing interests.

Authors' contributions

HS conceived of the study, participated in its design and coordination, and drafted the manuscript. LW participated in the statistical analysis and qualitative data collection. LP participated in drafting and editing the manuscript as well as the design of the study. MS was involved in the qualitative data collection and analysis. BR was involved in qualitative data collection with Information Technology personnel and drafting the results of the manuscript. DE participated in the coordination of the study as well as qualitative data collection. DS participated in data analysis and provided edits to the final manuscript. All authors read and approved the final manuscript.

Authors' information

The study was supported by an NIH K23 career development award (K23CA125585) to Dr. Singh, the VA National Center of Patient Safety, and in part by the Houston VA HSR&D Center of Excellence (HFP90-020). These sources had no role in the design and conduct of the study; collection, management, analysis, and interpretation of the data; and the preparation, review, or approval of the manuscript. The views expressed in this article are those of the authors and do not necessarily represent the views of the Department of Veterans Affairs.

Acknowledgments

We would like to thank Ms. Roxy Pierce, Section of Information Technology for support of this work.

Data

All authors had full access to all of the data in the study and take responsibility for the integrity of the data and the accuracy of the data analysis.

CHAPTER 17

This work was supported by the Department of Veterans Affairs, Veterans Health Administration (VHA), Health Services Research and Development Service (Project no. SAF 20 - 049) and VHA Office of Information. A VAHSR&D Merit Review Entry Program Award supported Emily Patterson.The views expressed in this report are those of the authors and do not necessarily represent the views of the Department of Veterans Affairs. They also do not represent the views of any commercial or hardware vendors. The authors thank persons who openly discussed challenges with us, which is critical to improving patient safety. They also thank Patricia Ebright, Geraldine Coyle, Mary Heinen, April Hamilton, Mary Burkhardt, Chris Tucker, Russ Carlson, Richard Cook, Nance Widdowson, Ginny Creasman, Kimberly Zipper and Donna Calliari for their careful readings of drafts of these recommendations and helpful suggestions for revision

CHAPTER 18

Acknowledgments

We would like to thank all the individuals who allowed us to observe or interview them, and the experts who participated in the Menucha Conference. Special thanks go to the site principal investigators J. Marc Overhage, M.D., Ph.D., Eric G. Poon, M.D., M.P.H., and Carol Hudson, R.N. This work was funded by research grant LM06942 and training grant ASMM10031 from the U.S. National Library of Medicine, National Institutes of Health.

Conflict of Interest

The authors state no conflicts of interest regarding the research or publication of this manuscript.

CHAPTER 19

Financial Disclosure

Dr Shabot is a consultant for Philips Medical Systems and the Cerner Corp and has performed research funded by Eli Lilly & Company. The other authors have indicated they have no financial relationships relevant to this article to disclose.

Opinions expressed in these commentaries are those of the authors and not necessarily those of the American Academy of Pediatrics or its Committees

INDEX

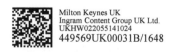